D1368126

TREATMENT
OF
MENTAL
DISORDERS

A REVIEW OF EFFECTIVENESS

TREATMENT OF MENTAL DISORDERS

A REVIEW OF EFFECTIVENESS

Edited by

Norman Sartorius, M.D., M.A., D.P.M., Ph.D., F.R.C.Psych.
Director, Division of Mental Health,
World Health Organization, Geneva, Switzerland

Giovanni de Girolamo, M.D.
Division of Mental Health,
World Health Organization, Geneva, Switzerland

Gavin Andrews, M.D., F.R.A.N.Z.C.P., F.R.C.Psych.
University of New South Wales, Sidney, Australia

G. Allen German, M.B.Ch.B.(Aber.Hons.),
F.R.C.P.(Edin.), F.R.C.Psych., F.R.A.N.Z.C.P.
University of Western Australia, Perth, Australia

Leon Eisenberg, M.D.
Harvard University, Boston, Massachusetts, United States

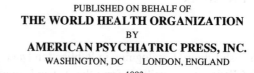

PUBLISHED ON BEHALF OF
THE WORLD HEALTH ORGANIZATION
BY
AMERICAN PSYCHIATRIC PRESS, INC.
WASHINGTON, DC   LONDON, ENGLAND
1993

Manufactured in the United States of America on acid-free paper
96   95   94   93   4   3   2   1
First Edition
American Psychiatric Press, Inc.
1400 K Street, N.W., Washington, DC   20005

Library of Congress Cataloging-in-Publication Data
Treatment of mental disorders : a review of effectiveness / edited by
   Norman Sartorius . . . [et al.].—1st ed.
        p.   cm.
   Includes bibliographical references and index.
   ISBN 0-88048-975-8 (alk. paper)
   1. Mental illness—Treatment.   I. Sartorius, N.   II. World Health
Organization.
   [DNLM: 1. Mental disorders—therapy.   WM 400 T78473 1993]
RC480.5.T747   1993
616.89′1—dc20
DNLM/DLC   93-2989
                                                                        CIP

British Library Cataloguing in Publication Data
A CIP record is available from the British Library.

Contents

Section I
Prevention

Section II
Biological Treatments

Section III
Psychological Treatments

Section IV
Psychosocial Treatments

Section V
Influence of Culture on Treatment

Section VI
Quality of Care and Care of Quality

Acknowledgments

The editors of the volume wish to acknowledge the valuable help and suggestions received by the following experts during the finalization of some chapters: William A. Anthony, Ph.D (Center for Psychiatric Rehabilitation, Boston University, Sargent College of Allied Health Professions, Boston, Massachusetts, United States); Alexander Boroffka, M.D. (Consultant Psychiatrist, Wishern Haus, Kiel, Germany); Marianne D. Farkas, Sc.D. (Center for Psychiatric Rehabilitation, Boston University, Sargent College of Allied Health Profession, Boston, Massachusetts, United States); Malcom H. Lader, M.D., Ph.D., D.Sc., F.R.C.Psych. (Institute of Psychiatry, University of London, London, England); Ian R.H. Falloon, M.D. (Buckingham Mental Health Service, Buckingham, United Kingdom); Paolo Migone, M.D. (Psychiatric Clinic, University of Bologna, Italy); Harold A. Sackheim, M.D. (College of Physicians and Surgeons, Columbia University and Department of Biological Psychiatry, New York State Psychiatric Institute, New York, New York, United States).

Contributors

Gavin Andrews, M.D., F.R.A.N.Z.C.P., F.R.C.Psych.
Clinical Research Unit for Anxiety Disorders,
University of New South Wales, Darlinghurst, Australia

José M. Bertolote, M.D., M.Sc., Ph.D.
Senior Medical Officer, Division of Mental Health,
World Health Organization, Geneva, Switzerland

Thomas G. Bolwig, M.D.
Rigshospitalet, University Hospital, Copenhagen, Denmark

Lorenzo Burti, M.D.
Istituto di Clinica Psichiatrica, Policlinico Borgo Roma,
Verona, Italy

Stephen F. Butler, Ph.D.
Northeast Psychiatric Associates at Brookside Hospital,
Nashua, New Hampshire, United States

Jean Cottraux, M.D., Ph.D.
Hôpital Neurologique, Laboratoire de Psychologie Médicale,
Lyon, France

Giovanni de Girolamo, M.D.
Division of Mental Health, World Health Organization,
Geneva, Switzerland

John P. Docherty, M.D.
Division of Psychiatry, National Medical Enterprises,
Santa Monica, California, United States

Leon Eisenberg, M.D.
Department of Social Medicine, Harvard Medical School,
Boston, Massachusetts, United States

Silvio Garattini, M.D.
Istituto "Mario Negri," Milan, Italy

**G. Allen German, M.B.Ch.B.(Aber.Hons.), F.R.C.P.(Edin.),
F.R.C.Psych., F.R.A.N.Z.C.P.**
Department of Psychiatry & Behavioural Science,
Queen Elizabeth II Medical Centre, Nedlands, Australia

Wilbur R. Grimson, M.D.
Vicente Lopez, Buenos Aires, Argentina

Jörgen Herlofson, M.D.
Department of Psychiatry, Danderyd General Hospital,
Umea, Sweden

Matthew Hodes, B.Sc., M.B.B.S., M.Sc., M.R.C.Psych.
Academic Unit for Child and Adolescent Psychiatry, St. Marys
Hospital Medical School, London, United Kingdom

Wolfgang G. Jilek, M.D.
Faculty of Medicine, University of British Columbia,
Vancouver, Canada

Donald G. Langsley, M.D.
American Board of Medical Specialties, Evanston, Illinois,
United States

Anthony J. Marsella, Ph.D.
Department of Psychology, University of Hawaii, Honolulu,
Hawaii, United States

Masahisa Nishizono, M.D.
Department of Psychiatry, Fukuoka University
School of Medicine, Fukuoka, Japan

Carlos Perris, M.D.
Department of Psychiatry, University of Umea, Umea, Sweden

Benedetto Saraceno, M.D.
Istituto "Mario Negri," Milan, Italy

Norman Sartorius, M.D., M.A., D.P.M., Ph.D., F.R.C.Psych.
Professor of Psychiatry and Director, Division of Mental Health,
World Health Organization, Geneva, Switzerland

Gianni Tognoni, M.D.
Istituto "Mario Negri," Milan, Italy

Joseph P. Westermeyer, M.D., M.P.H., Ph.D.
Department of Psychiatry, University of Oklahoma, Oklahoma
City, Oklahoma, United States

Narendra N. Wig, M.D., D.P.M., F.R.C.Psych., F.A.M.S.
formerly Regional Advisor for Mental Health, World Health
Organization Regional Office for the Eastern Mediterranean,
Alexandria, Egypt

Vasily S. Yastrebov, M.D.
Academy of Medical Sciences, Moscow, Russia

Introduction

Acceptance of psychiatry as a medical discipline rests on three premises: first, that its practitioners can reach a reliable diagnosis using tools that other branches in medicine use; second, that treatment of psychiatric disorders is possible and effective and that it can be evaluated, using criteria valid for the assessment of medical treatment; and third, that psychiatry can contribute to the improvement of public health by providing specific suggestions concerning the prevention (and the organization of treatment) of mental illness and the rehabilitation of those with it.

The past 20 years have brought major advances in the methods that are used to examine individuals with mental disorders. Valid and reliable techniques for the acquisition of data about mental illness suitable for use in a variety of cultures have been produced. A vast array of laboratory examinations, neuroimaging tests, and standardized procedures for the assessment of the mental state, personality traits, intellectual performance, social relations, and other characteristics important for reaching a diagnosis in psychiatry have become available. Diagnostic and classificatory systems have also changed; they are now accompanied by clear and unequivocal descriptions of psychiatric disorders and of the manner in which the syndromes can be recognized and classified.

The World Health Organization (WHO) has made a significant contribution to the development of a common technical language that makes it possible to convey findings of research and experience in the field of mental health in a universally understandable way. In the period between 1965 and 1972, WHO carried out a major international program directed at the standardization of psychiatric diagnosis, classification, and statistics, involving experts from some 30 countries (Kramer et al. 1979; Sartorius 1976). It has also initiated cross-cultural investigations of major mental disorders such as schizophrenia and depression (Sartorius 1989). It has, jointly with the U.S. Alcohol, Drug Abuse, and Mental Health Administration (ADAMHA), launched an international program (Jablensky et al. 1983) directed at the production of internationally applicable instruments for assessing psychiatric problems (Loranger et al. 1991;

Robins et al. 1988; Sartorius and Jablensky 1984; Wing et al. 1990).

WHO has also coordinated the work necessary to produce a set of definitions, clinical guidelines, and research criteria for the use in the *International Classification of Diseases* (Sartorius 1976; Sartorius et al. 1988; World Health Organization 1992). These guidelines were assessed in a field test involving more than 100 centers in some 40 countries (Sartorius et al. 1993) and proved to be easy to use, fitting clinical decisions and enabling clinicians to reach the same diagnoses in a remarkably high proportion of cases. Other WHO-coordinated studies have produced an array of useful information, including guidelines and materials for training to ensure that psychiatrists will be able to make their diagnoses reliably and in a manner that is explicit and demonstrable. The first requirement for the recognition of psychiatry as a medical discipline—creating a generally understandable, acceptable, and applicable system of diagnosis and classification—has thus been met; the challenge for the future is to make this system sufficiently well known so that practitioners and researchers the world over use it consistently, and through that endeavor, continue to improve it.

Satisfying the second prerequisite—developing methods for the treatment of mental illness that will eliminate the illness or reduce suffering—also seems to be more possible now than before. Unfortunately, as the true causes of mental illness, in many cases, remain unknown, treatments in psychiatry are still mainly symptomatic and often bring relief and comfort but not complete cure. The proportion of "cured" patients with psychiatric diseases depends on the theoretical position taken in relation to diseases that can reoccur in the same or similar form after a symptom-free period: if the disappearance of symptoms is seen as representing the end of a disease (which can then occur again), the proportion of "cures" will be higher; if the disappearance of symptoms is seen as a variation in the intensity of symptoms that are an integral part of a periodically florid disease, the proportion of "cures" will be lower. In view of the facts that most therapeutic interventions are not developed with knowledge of causes and that they do not lead to a complete disappearance of symptoms, it is necessary to assess their effectiveness in terms that allow comparisons with other treatment methods, that is, in terms of reduction of symptoms or of changes of functional capacity to perform well-defined tasks.

The methods necessary to undertake such assessments are now available. Their application is of particular importance at this point in time because of current revolutionary changes in the manner in which services to psychiatric patients are being provided. Earlier in this century psychiatric services were provided only for the most dramatic forms of mental disorder, usually in specialized institutions. Today, availability of appropriate care for all forms of mental disorders is seen as a human right that must be respected even if resources for health care are scarce (United Nations 1991). And this is not all; the fact that services should be made available to all who need them implies that they can no longer be provided exclusively, nor even mainly, through the psychiatric institutions. On the contrary, research in the past few decades has demonstrated that an overwhelming majority of people with mental disorders seek help from general health service providers (if at all). Research has also demonstrated that simply trained staff, if adequately supported and supervised, can effectively provide well-defined treatments for many of the mental disorders without referral to specialists.

The second requirement for the recognition of psychiatry—to define an array of effective treatment methods with clear indications and instructions about the manner of their application—has thus also been met. The same is true for the third requirement listed above; psychiatry can now provide clear indications about the way in which governments can develop programs of primary prevention of mental illness, treatment provision, and rehabilitation of those impaired by mental disorders. At the same time, the overall changes in health philosophy and organization of care, together with the growth of knowledge about the size of mental health problems and their links to other types of illness, have also begun to make it more likely than ever before that governments would be willing to invest in the application of well-proven methods of treatment of mental illness.

In the light of these developments, WHO convened a group of experts to define methods suitable for assessing methods of treatment in psychiatry (World Health Organization 1991). In preparation for this meeting the organization called on leading experts from different countries to review knowledge about treatments and scan literature, particularly in languages and journals that are less easy to access. The papers prepared by these experts reviewed the subject matter by disease group (e.g., treatment for schizophrenia), by level of care (e.g., treatment at primary care level), by discipline (e.g., pharmacotherapy), and by population group (e.g., treatment of mental disorders in the elderly). It was originally expected that it would be possible to publish all of the reviews in one place; a variety of reasons led to a change in this plan. Thus it was decided to use the material obtained in reviews of treatment by level of care in WHO's work on defining the essential treatments in psychiatry. The reviews of treatment methods and the results of their application to specific disorders have been published in a series of papers in scientific journals (de Girolamo 1992a, 1992b). Some of the materials concerning treatment of special population groups will be used in the development of manuals in these areas not published now. The reviews of treatment by discipline are less easy to find, and it has been felt that these could be usefully brought together in this volume.

The original papers have been reviewed by experts who were not involved in the project and revised where necessary. Some additional material was produced by the editors and invited experts. The list of contributors indicates this; in addition to those listed, however, other specialists and practitioners with whom the organization collaborates provided valuable comments and suggestions and deserve the editors' and readers' sincere thanks.

This book includes six sections, each containing several reviews. Section I deals with prevention: it is placed first because prevention is sadly neglected in mental health programs (Sartorius and Henderson 1992). The possibilities for preventive action identified in the chapter are only examples; there are a host of others.

Section II deals with biological treatment methods. These have been seen as the central (if not the only) method for treating mental disorders in many countries. The distinction between *biological* and *nonbiological* methods of treatment is not always easy to maintain. Also, no biological treatment can be given in isolation from social and situational influences and psychological factors (such as previous experience of the doctor and patient); these other factors are usually inextricably linked with the administration of biological treatment and the decision to apply it. The separation of this group of chapters from the chapters in Section III does not reflect the editors' view that biological and psychological treatments should be kept distinct; rather, it corresponds to the usual way of discussing these treatments and is meant to facilitate the use of the book.

Section III deals with psychological treatments. These have gained in importance over the years, not only in the treatment of mental disorders but also in general medicine, and now include a large number of techniques. This volume concentrates on those psychological treatments that have been examined in well-designed clinical trials.

The final three sections broaden the scope of the discussion. Section IV focuses on psychiatric rehabilitation and on psychosocial interventions, both of which have to involve several "actors" (family members, formal or informal patient groups, etc.) rather than only the doctor and the patient. Section V brings in the use of traditional medical procedures relevant for psychiatry and reviews the impact of the cultural variables on treatment delivery and treatment response. Section VI deals with the variation in treatment models and practices according to the level of care, and with the assessment of quality of care.

This book presents views of the authors of the different chapters who have reviewed the available literature. There are undoubtedly publications that have escaped the authors' attention because of limitations of language, difficulty of access, and other constraints. The anecdotal knowledge reflecting experience of doctors worldwide may also have been insufficiently reflected. This book therefore does not aim to present the "truth"; rather, it presents evidence—maybe not all of it—that should be examined and used in decisions about treatment, research on treatment, and training in treatment methods.

Norman Sartorius, M.D., M.A., D.P.M., Ph.D., F.R.C.Psych.

References

de Girolamo G (ed): Evaluation of treatment methods in Psychiatry: 1. International Journal of Mental Health 21:2, 1992a

de Girolamo G (ed): Evaluation of Treatment Methods in Psychiatry: 2. International Journal of Mental Health 21:3, 1992b

Jablensky A, Sartorius N, Hirschfeld R, et al: Diagnosis and classification of mental disorders and alcohol- and drug-related problems: a research agenda for the 1980s. Psychol Med 13:907–921, 1983

Kramer M, Sartorius N, Jablensky A, et al: The ICD-9 classification of mental disorders: a review of its development and contents. Acta Psychiatr Scand 59:241–262, 1979

Loranger A, Hirschfeld R, Sartorius N, et al: The WHO/ADAMHA International Pilot Study of Personality Disorders: background and purpose. Journal of Personality Disorders 5:296–306, 1991

Robins LN, Wing J, Wittchen HU, et al: The Composite International Diagnostic Interview. Arch Gen Psychiatry 45:1069–1077, 1988

Sartorius N: Classification: an international perspective. Psychiatric Annals 6:22–35, 1976

Sartorius N: Recent research activities in WHO's mental health program. Psychol Med 19:233–244, 1989

Sartorius N, Henderson AS: The neglect of prevention in psychiatry. Aust N Z J Psychiatry 26:550–553, 1992

Sartorius N, Jablensky A: Diagnostic et classification en psychiatrie: à propos notamment de certains problèmes qui ont surgi dans un projet conjoint OMS-ADAMHA. Confrontations Psychiatriques 24:131–139, 1984

Sartorius N, Jablensky A, Cooper JE, et al (eds): Psychiatric Classification in an International Perspective. Br J Psychiatry 152 (suppl 1), 1988

Sartorius N, Kaelber C, Regier D, et al: Progress towards achieving a common language in psychiatry: results from the ICD-10 clinical field trial of mental and behavioral disorders. Arch Gen Psychiatry 50:115–124, 1993

United Nations: The protection of persons with mental illness and the improvement of mental health care. United Nations Resolution UN/GA/46/119. New York, United Nations, 1991

Wing JE, Babor T, Brugha T, et al: SCAN: Schedule for Clinical Assessment in Neuropsychiatry. Arch Gen Psychiatry 47:589–593, 1990

World Health Organization: Evaluation of Methods for the Treatment of Mental Disorders: Report of a WHO Scientific Group (WHO Technical Report Series, No 812). Geneva, World Health Organization, 1991

World Health Organization: The ICD-10 Classification of Mental and Behavioral Disorders: Clinical Descriptions and Diagnostic Guidelines. Geneva, World Health Organization, 1992

Section I

Prevention

Introduction to Section I

Psychiatry has neglected prevention. It has been occupied with the treatment and rehabilitation of the mentally ill. Although there is a considerable body of literature on primary prevention of mental disorders, most of it consists of rhetoric or proposals for what is thought possible. But for what is demonstrably a major category of morbidity, the neglect of prevention is no longer defensible; the public health burden is too high. In this section, Eisenberg reviews the notion that prevention of mental disorders is possible, and proposes some specific interventions, many of which could be applied even in countries with few resources.

This section also includes the World Health Organization (WHO) Report "Prevention of Mental, Neurological, and Psychosocial Disorders." This important document was submitted by the Director-General of WHO to the Executive Board at its 77th session in January 1986. The Director-General then invited the Executive Board to make recommendations to the Health Assembly concerning actions to be taken at the national and international level in order to apply measures for preventing mental, neurological, and psychosocial disorders. The deliberations of the Executive Board were used in updating the report, which is now reproduced to show how vast are the possibilities of prevention in the mental health field.

CHAPTER 1

Prevention of Mental, Neurological, and Psychosocial Disorders[1]

Report by the Director-General of the World Health Organization to the World Health Assembly[2]

Mental, neurological, and psychosocial problems are of major public health importance. Methods for the prevention of a number of them have become available in recent years. The Director-General prepared a review of such problems, assessing their magnitude and specific measures of proven effectiveness that could be taken to prevent them. He submitted the report to the Executive Board at its 77th session in January 1986 and invited it to make recommendations to the Health Assembly concerning action to be taken at the national and international level and to apply those measures. The deliberations of the Board[3] were used in updating the report, which is reproduced here.

I. Introduction

Purpose and Scope

1.   This report has four purposes: a) to indicate the magnitude of the public health burden resulting from mental, neurological, and psychoso-

---

[1]See resolution WHA39.25.
[2]This report was originally prepared for the Thirty-Ninth World Health Assembly as document A39/9 and has been updated to include the Health Assembly's discussions on it.
[3]See document EB77/1986/REC/2, pp. 138–144.

5

cial disorders and problems; b) to demonstrate the extent to which this burden can be reduced by preventive methods; c) to recommend action on a set of prevention programs chosen because they address important problems, are cost-effective, and are not at present given the priority they merit; and d) to indicate research needs.

2.   The report focuses on methods that are effective in reducing the incidence, prevalence, or chronicity of mental and neurological disorders. Treatment is referred to only when it permits the prevention of secondary consequences which themselves are within the scope of the report (e.g., treating hypertension in order to prevent stroke). In such cases, the treatments themselves are listed rather than described. Because the emphasis is on disease prevention, the report does not examine issues concerning the promotion of mental health (e.g., methods to enhance normal function), an important topic in itself but beyond the present scope.

Definition of Prevention

3.   Primary prevention refers to methods designed to avoid the occurrence of disease or impairment (e.g., the provision of a balanced diet to avoid pellagra or of immunization against measles to avert mental retardation from measles encephalitis).

4.   Secondary prevention refers to early diagnosis and treatment to shorten illness episodes, to minimize the chance of transmission of disorder or disease, and to limit disease sequelae. Timely treatment of certain conditions may also have primary preventive effects on other conditions: control of hypertension can prevent the occurrence of cerebrovascular disease, and control of epileptic seizures can reduce work injuries, road accidents, and severe burns due to seizures.

5.   Tertiary prevention refers to measures to limit disability and handicap consequent upon impairment or disease which may not be fully treatable. For example, a rapid, relevant response in the community to sudden decompensations in personal and social functioning can prevent the development of a chronic social breakdown syndrome in people with schizophrenia and other serious mental disorders. In such cases it is not

so much the disease (e.g., schizophrenia or posttraumatic dementia) per se, but the way the patient care system responds, which determines the extent of the disability of the patient.

Feasibility and Urgency of Prevention of Many Mental, Neurological, and Psychosocial Problems

6. Proposals for prevention programs in the field of mental health often meet with negative attitudes and responses, partly because of unrealistic promises made several decades ago about the results to be expected from measures such as the introduction of child guidance clinics or from the application of intensive psychotherapy; also because it is still not possible to design effective programs for the primary prevention of certain severe mental disorders such as schizophrenia or the affective disorders. But this no more justifies overlooking measures that can prevent other neuropsychiatric disorders than the lack of an effective vaccine against certain parasitic diseases warrants abandoning immunization against measles or poliomyelitis.

7. Mental hospitals at the turn of the century were filled by many cases of general paresis and pellagra; both diseases have become rare in many countries, the first because of the effective treatment of syphilis, and the second because of improved diet. Many other important neuropsychiatric disorders such as cretinism can be sharply reduced by measures available today, if such measures were to be applied to all those who could profit from them. In the case of other mental disorders (e.g., the schizophrenias and the affective disorders), chronic loss of the ability for self-care and troublesome behavior can be minimized if the health team, community, and family provide prompt and constructive responses to the occurrence of the disorder. Education of the public to overcome entrenched prejudice against the mentally ill will also be necessary.

II. The Magnitude of the Problem

Mental and Neurological Disorders

8. The magnitude of problems linked to mental and neurological disorders is generally underestimated for at least three reasons:

1) Vital statistics traditionally measure mortality rather than morbidity—but many mental, neurological, and psychosocial disorders have a far greater effect on function and quality of life than on mortality per se;

2) Even where morbidity is recorded, health information systems usually do not appropriately monitor the extent of neuropsychiatric morbidity;

3) The tabulation of mortality or morbidity by disease often fails to indicate behavioral causes of physical disease: for example, acquired central nervous system lesions resulting from motor vehicle accidents which are secondary to unwise use of psychotropic drugs.

9.   This fact has to be borne in mind in trying to understand the discrepancy between common impressions about the size of the problem and the results of investigation and other evidence presented below.

Mental Retardation

10.   The prevalence of severe mental retardation below the age of 18 years (defined by an intelligence quotient [IQ] of less than 50 and major disabilities in intellectual and social function, usually associated with neurological abnormalities) is approximately 3 to 4 per thousand; the prevalence of mild and moderate mental retardation (defined by an IQ between 50 and 70 and by marginal performance at school in complex intellectual tasks) is approximately 20 to 30 per thousand. These figures are likely to be underestimates for many areas of the developing world because of the persistence of preventable mental retardation secondary to a) faulty delivery methods which lead to birth trauma and b) bacterial and parasitic infections of the central nervous system (1). Of greatest importance from the standpoint of prevalence is the mild mental retardation and behavioral maladaptation that results from the interrelated problems of malnutrition and cognitive understimulation in infants reared in severely disadvantaged families. The world population of retarded persons numbers between 90 and 130 million.

Acquired Lesions of the Central Nervous System

11. Damage to brain tissue—resulting from trauma, bacterial and parasitic infections, alcohol abuse, malnutrition, hypertensive encephalopathy, pollutants (e.g., carbon monoxide, heavy metals, chemical fertilizers, and insecticides), lack of essential nutrients and other conditions—constitutes a major source of mental and neurological impairment. It has been estimated that no less than 400 million people suffer from iodine deficiency, their children being at risk of mental and neurological disorders associated with fetal damage due to the deficiency (2). Debilitating effects of cerebrovascular accidents secondary to uncontrolled hypertension are a rapidly increasing problem in developing countries. Cerebrospinal meningitis, trypanosomiasis, and cysticercosis are major sources of brain disorders in a number of countries. Persistent infections, even when the brain is not directly invaded, impair cognitive efficiency.

Peripheral Nervous System Damage

12. Inadequate and/or unbalanced diet (e.g., cassava neuropathy), metabolic diseases (diabetes), infections (leprosy), trauma, and toxins can cause incapacitating peripheral neuropathies. Besides their direct effects on motor and sensory function, neuropathies can have numerous social and psychiatric consequences because of the impairments that may result (3).

The Psychoses

13. The prevalence of severe mental disorders such as schizophrenia, the affective disorders, and the chronic brain syndromes is estimated conservatively at not less than 1%; somewhat more than 45 million mentally ill people the world over suffer compromised social and occupational function because of these conditions. According to World Health Organization (WHO) data, the annual incidence of schizophrenia is approximately 0.1 per thousand in the population 15 to 54 years of age, and the prevalence, according to several surveys is 2 to 4 per thousand. There are no demonstrable differences in these figures between developing and developed countries (4). The rate for depressive disorders is severalfold higher. Moreover, the incidence of depressive disorders has shown a

striking increase in some countries. The amount and kind of treatment services, as well as the attitude of family and community towards patients suffering from these disorders, are important determinants of their outcome.

The Dementias

14. Dementia is not part of normal aging, but represents a disease, the cause of which should be sought and if possible treated; metabolic, toxic, infectious and circulatory diseases can all be the cause of impaired mental function (5). These disorders constitute an ever greater burden on health services as an increasing proportion of the population survives to older ages and becomes vulnerable to senile dementias of the Alzheimer type.

The prevalence of senile dementias in individuals aged 70 years or older is estimated at about 100 to 200 per thousand in countries where surveys have been carried out. Isolated reports of lower incidence of dementia in certain developing countries in Africa merit special attention since they may provide important clues for the etiology and prevention of the condition (6).

Epilepsy

15. The prevalence of epilepsy in the population ranges from 3 to 5 per thousand in the industrialized world to 15 to 20 or even 50 per thousand in some areas of the developing world. This tenfold difference in prevalence provides a measure of what could be accomplished by a comprehensive program of prevention in the developing countries. The extent of social handicap resulting from epilepsy varies with its type, but also with the adequacy of medical management and with community acceptance of or support for the patient with epilepsy. Unfortunately, in many developing countries, the majority of patients with epilepsy receive little or no treatment; in consequence, they suffer from avoidable physical injuries and social handicaps.

Emotional and Conduct Disorders

16. Such disorders (particularly neurotic and personality disorders) are estimated to occur at a frequency of 5% to 15% in the general population. Not all require treatment, but some (e.g., severe anxiety disorders) can

lead to major impairment. Conduct disorders, which are common among schoolchildren and interfere with learning in the classroom and with social adjustment, often respond well to simple treatments (e.g., behavior therapy and parent counseling), although recurrence is common (7). Learning disorders, whether or not they are associated with other psychiatric symptoms, require special help in the classroom in order to avoid secondary emotional problems and occupational handicaps (e.g., those associated with failure to learn to read).

Health-Damaging Behaviors

Psychoactive Substance Abuse and Dependence

17.   **Alcohol-related problems.** Recent decades have witnessed considerable increases in alcohol consumption and in alcohol-related problems (including death from alcohol poisoning) in most parts of the world. Alcohol abuse by the individual has devastating effects on the family. A particularly tragic consequence of drinking during pregnancy is the fetal alcohol syndrome. In the WHO European Region, the number of countries with an annual per capita intake of more than 10 liters of pure alcohol increased from 3 in 1950 to 18 by 1979. Countries in the WHO Western Pacific Region report sharp increases during the 1970s in alcohol-related health damage, in alcohol-related crimes, and in alcohol-related accidents (8).

18. Similar reports have emerged from countries in other WHO regions, including those with long traditions of abstinence from alcohol. Although some countries in Europe and North America are now reporting a leveling off—and even a modest decline in alcohol consumption—the global trend is still that of continuing growth, with particularly sharp increases in commercially produced alcoholic beverages in some developing countries in Africa, Latin America, and the Western Pacific (9). It is notable that in Australia, between 1978 and 1984, a 10% reduction in per capita consumption of alcohol was accompanied by a 30% reduction in deaths caused by alcohol.

19.   In many countries, alcohol use is increasing rapidly among adolescents and among women. These increases in global alcohol consumption

are likely to have serious public health implications, because there is a very substantial body of evidence that a direct relationship generally exists between trends in consumption and trends in alcohol-related problems. As national alcohol consumption increases, so do rates of whatever alcohol-related problems are typical in that country. These can range from cirrhosis of the liver to problems at work and in the home, and, in more and more countries, to alcohol-related traffic accidents.

20. **Drug abuse.** Analysis of trends in the frequency and severity of drug abuse and drug dependence has revealed a general increase in the problem in most countries. It was recently estimated that there is a total of 48 million drug abusers in the world, including 30 million cannabis users, 1.6 million coca leaf chewers, and 1.7 million opium-dependent and 0.7 million heroin-dependent persons (10). Cocaine abuse is known to be widespread and increasing although no reliable figures exist. These figures almost certainly underestimate the magnitude of the problem. Amphetamines, barbiturates, sedatives, and tranquilizers are consumed in most countries and their abuse, as well as multiple drug abuse, is increasing throughout the world, parallel to their increasing availability on both licit and illicit markets. There is a trend to (multiple) drug use in conjunction with alcohol. The sniffing or inhaling of volatile solvents and other inhalants is also spreading in a number of countries, particularly among pre-adolescent and early adolescent urban populations. With an expanding market, large regions have become dependent on the income derived from growing cannabis, the opium poppy, and the coca shrub, which adds to the difficulty of implementing control measures.

21. **Psychotropic drug abuse.** The very considerable benefits from the appropriate use of psychotropic drugs can be offset by their abuse. The ready availability of psychotropic substances sold over the counter without prescription in many countries, insufficient and often misleading information given to the general public, and inappropriate prescribing practices by physicians (who often employ medication instead of counseling in response to the pressures of a busy practice or because of insufficient training) have led to overuse and abuse of psychotropic drugs and a variety of consequent public health problems (11). The magnitude of these problems varies between countries, and epidemiological evidence

is still lacking for most countries where anecdotal reports give rise to serious concern.

22. **Tobacco dependence.** Smoking is a socially induced behavioral pattern which is maintained by the development of dependence on nicotine. One-third of all cases of cancer, at least 80% of all lung cancer, 75% of chronic bronchitis, and 25% of myocardial infarction in the United States of America are due to cigarette smoking (12). Between 1976 and 1980 tobacco consumption decreased at a yearly rate of 1.1% in the industrialized countries, but continued to rise at a yearly rate of 2.1% in the developing countries. Besides premature deaths, which have been estimated at over 1 million per annum, innumerable cases of debilitating diseases (such as chronic obstructive lung disease) are also due to smoking. The proportion of women of reproductive age who smoke regularly, already high in most industrialized countries, has been increasing rapidly in the developing world. There is now evidence of health risks from "passive smoking," (i.e., inhalation of smoke produced by smokers in a confined environment at home or in the workplace). These trends, and possible measures to counter them, are described in the Director-General's report to the 77th session of the Executive Board (see document EB77/1986/REC/1, Annex 3).

Conditions of Life That Lead to Disease

23. Many health-damaging modes of living are the result of factors beyond the control of the individual: homelessness, unemployment, lack of access to health and social services, the loss of social cohesion in slum areas, forced migration, racial and other discrimination, forced idleness in refugee settlements, "conventional" wars, and the threat of nuclear war. These issues will necessarily be of concern to every component of WHO and to other national and international organizations, but they are beyond the scope of this report except to note their impact.

24. In addition to these broad social forces, factors manifested in individual behavior —termed "life-style"—can influence the risk of disease. Although the relative contributions of excess animal fats in the diet, insufficient physical exercise, and psychosocial stress to the pathogenesis of the epidemic of cardiovascular disease in the industrialized world can-

not be specified precisely, most authorities agree that they are important risk factors. The inclusion of "life-style" here does not imply that one or other pattern of eating or exercising is a "psychiatric disorder" (except in extreme instances such as anorexia nervosa and bulimia), but it is intended to emphasize a) the contribution of behavior patterns to disease pathogenesis (e.g., patterns of food preparation as determinants of the risk for cysticercosis, which produces lesions of the central nervous system) and b) the importance of making full use of mental health and psychosocial skills and knowledge in designing interventions aimed at preventing disease secondary to such behavior (e.g., dealing with cultural beliefs in an appropriate manner to improve the acceptability of health measures). In this connection, methods of coping with excessive stress merit further study. "Stress" is an unavoidable part of life; indeed, mild and moderate levels of stress can improve performance under appropriate circumstances. Stress becomes a pathological agent when it is intense, persistent, and generally beyond the coping capacity of the individual exposed to it.

Violence

25. Violence (accidents, homicide, and suicide) is one of the leading causes of death in most countries, and accounts for a high proportion of years of life lost. Psychosocial factors and mental disturbance play an important role in the occurrence of violence which, although not conventionally regarded as a "medical" problem, is an important source of mortality and morbidity (including in particular neuropsychiatric morbidity following damage to the central nervous system). Child abuse and wife battering are among the particularly dramatic indicators of violence in the family. Dealing with the consequences of violence for the victim can be significantly facilitated if mental health care skills are used (13).

Excessive Risk Behavior in Young People

26. Such behavior (e.g., experimenting with drugs and alcohol, sexual activity without precautions against sexually transmitted diseases, adolescent pregnancy, driving at excessive speed, and generally challenging established guidelines for health and safety) results in serious morbidity and mortality. Pregnancy in young teenagers (15 years or less) leads to a cycle of disadvantage. The immature mother is unable to care properly

for her child, while her responsibility for child care is a barrier to the education and employment essential for her own growth. The shortage of child care facilities in most communities compounds the problem. This and other health risks for adolescents have been the subject of previous WHO reports (14).

Family Breakdown

27.   Family breakdown, evident in increasing rates of divorce and separation and in the weakening of ties between generations interferes with the upbringing of children. Households headed by a woman are more likely to be below the poverty threshold, adding to the mother's difficulty in raising a family. Weakened family units also contribute to community disorganization, with a variety of consequent psychosocial and other health problems.

Somatic Symptoms Resulting From Psychosocial Distress

28.   Many patients who consult health staff at the first contact level exhibit no ascertainable organ pathology or complain of discomfort and dysfunction disproportionate to the physical problem. Clinical studies in industrialized countries indicate that such is the case in 30% to 50% of all consultations; in developing countries, such patients make up about 15% to 25% of those coming to the attention of health care personnel, the largest single complaint category in primary care (15, 16). Unfortunately, the narrow biological focus in much of health professional training has resulted in failure to appreciate the importance of recognizing and dealing with distress resulting from psychosocial factors. Unless the psychosocial source of the physical symptoms is recognized by health care personnel, patients will be inappropriately investigated and medicated, will incur excessive expense, and repeatedly seek relief for the symptoms.

III. Proposals for Action

29.   Although the proposals for action in this section have been organized under three headings (relating to the health sector, other social sec-

tors, and the governmental level), intersectoral coordination is essential to their success. For example, action taken against drug abuse through the primary health care system, schools, and the media will be relatively ineffective in the absence of government policy to support and reinforce that action.

Measures to Be Undertaken by the Health Sector

30.   Success in carrying out preventive and therapeutic measures in the health sector depends greatly on the psychosocial skills of primary health care workers (sensitivity, empathy, and ability to communicate) as well as on a thorough knowledge of the community, its culture, and its resources. Therefore, training in generic psychosocial skills is no less essential to the education of these workers than is the customary technical training. In the absence of such skills in clinical practice, diagnostic errors multiply, the patient's adherence to treatment recommendations declines, health workers give up, and the health facility will fail to achieve its goals.

31.   Among specific measures which can be taken by the health sector, the following five groups stand out as being particularly timely and promising.

WHO Initiatives to Be Intensified

32.   **Prenatal and perinatal care.** In view of the need to protect the fetus and the newborn child and to provide optimum conditions for development, and in view of the high mortality and morbidity associated with prematurity and low birth weight:

   1) High priority should be given to a) adequate food, b) education for all pregnant women about nutrition in order to prevent cognitive failure in their children and c) information for all pregnant women about the importance of immunization and the schedules for immunization of their infants.

   2) Direct counseling of pregnant women against smoking and drinking by health workers should be undertaken because it can reduce the

prevalence of developmental anomalies and low birth weight caused by cigarette smoking and alcohol use in pregnancy.

3) In areas where neonatal tetanus is prevalent, pregnant women should receive tetanus toxoid after the first trimester; birth attendants should be trained in techniques for cutting the umbilical cord.[4]

4) In iodine-deficient areas, women of childbearing age should be given iodized oil injections or iodized salt which can prevent the congenital iodine deficiency syndrome (2).

5) Birth attendants should be trained in recognizing the indications for high risk pregnancies in order to refer complicated deliveries to back-up obstetrical facilities since the prevention of obstetrical complications can lead to a significant reduction in the number of children with damage to the central nervous system.

6) The promotion of breast-feeding should be an integral component of primary health care in view of the physiological and psychological benefits that breast-feeding confers.

7) Mental health activities must be integrated into maternal and child health programs.

33.   Scientific advances in the detection of congenital and hereditary diseases and risk factors during pregnancy and the neonatal period have created new possibilities for prevention. However, they require impeccable laboratory technique, careful follow-through, and the provision of appropriate therapeutic interventions. Their use depends upon local decisions about resource allocation and the resolution of attendant ethical issues.

---

[4] Although neonatal tetanus and iodine deficiency are prevalent only in certain areas of the world, where they do occur they have considerable adverse effects on the normal psychological development of children as well as causing high mortality. More importantly, both conditions can be almost totally prevented by relatively simple means.

34. Programs for child nutrition (including the education of mothers about nutrition) are a major component of prevention in view of the role that malnutrition and inadequate child rearing can play in impairing cognitive and social development.

35. Immunization of children against measles, rubella, mumps, poliomyelitis, tetanus, and diphtheria could make an important contribution to the prevention of brain damage caused by these diseases in children.

36. **Family planning**. In view of the strong evidence that child development is adversely affected when the mother has too many children at too short intervals, and when she is under the age of 15, education on family planning and access to effective means of contraception are essential elements of maternal and child care. Appropriate attention should be given to psychological factors in family planning in order to minimize psychosomatic complications from the use of contraceptive methods, once the desired family size has been reached. A multicountry study carried out in 1978–1983 to assess possible psychological effects of tubal ligation showed no negative mental health effects attributable to sterilization (17). Genetic counseling, as part of family planning, can help to minimize hereditary diseases in families known to be at risk.

Measures to Prevent Abuse of and Dependence on Psychoactive Substances in Primary Health Care

37. Health workers should routinely ask about smoking and counsel patients against it. This simple intervention is about as effective as more elaborate measures. Though only 3% to 5% of patients will respond by stopping smoking, this measure has a large public health payoff in view of the prevalence of smoking in the population; if 5% of the many hundred million smokers were to respond to such advice from health workers, millions of individuals would be spared the health hazards of smoking. Moreover, repeated efforts ensure a cumulative rate of success, and low initial response should not discourage the health worker.

38. Health workers can be trained, by the use of an appropriate short set of questions, to identify alcohol and drug abuse early, using manuals and guidelines produced and tested by WHO in a number of countries.

Brief counseling can help a significant number of patients (though not all) to alter their behavior before dependence and irreversible damage result (18).

Crisis Intervention in Primary Health Care

39.   In the event of acute loss (e.g., death of a spouse, which increases the risk of morbidity and mortality among survivors), there is some evidence that group and individual counseling of the bereaved can diminish risk. Self-help and mutual aid groups (e.g., among widows) can improve health status at minimum cost to health services. These measures can be incorporated into health services by short courses of training (19, 20). The acute psychological distress associated with divorce has been shown in a recent controlled clinical trial to be reduced by group counseling, with significant levels of benefit persisting for several years after the intervention (21). Well-trained crisis intervention units have been shown to handle a variety of acute mental health problems effectively, thus preventing more chronic difficulties and social disadvantages to the patients (22).

Prevention of Iatrogenic Damage

40.   Health workers can be trained to inquire routinely about psychosocial problems in the course of evaluating new patients. This will enable them to recognize symptoms which are the expression of psychological distress and to avoid overuse of psychotropic (and other) drugs and the iatrogeny which results from such practices. Brief counseling and, where necessary, referral of patients to social welfare or mental health workers can significantly diminish the burden of repeated clinic visits.

41.   Behavior disorders which are the iatrogenic effect of prolonged or repeated hospitalization can be prevented by minimizing the hospitalization of children, by encouraging family participation when hospital care is unavoidable, and by introducing certain organizational arrangements in hospitals (e.g., assigning a primary nurse to each child). Mental deterioration in the elderly can be prevented by avoiding unnecessary hospitalization.

42.   Although measures to prevent dementia must await the results of further research, cognitive impairment resulting from depression and in-

fection can be reversed by appropriate treatment if it is promptly applied. At present, the distinction between dementia and depression in the elderly is not recognized by the family doctor in four out of five cases (23). Relatively short training can improve physicians' and other health workers' diagnostic skills significantly in this area.

Minimizing Chronic Disability

43. **Education of health workers**. In the recognition of sensory and motor handicaps in children, in the use of prosthetic devices to minimize these handicaps, and in the appreciation of the importance of referring such children to the educational authorities for appropriate educational measures—education of health workers is feasible and can prevent both cognitive underachievement and social maladjustment.

44.   Properly fitted eyeglasses (which can be obtained at very low cost) and hearing aids can reduce the likelihood of mental and social handicaps in children with sensory impairment (24). Community rehabilitation of persons with locomotor handicaps can make it possible for them to work and live independently, thus avoiding the psychological problems of chronic dependency.

45.   Because the incidence of cerebrovascular accidents and consequent brain damage can be reduced by the effective treatment of hypertension, comprehensive programs for the diagnosis and treatment of hypertensive disease should be included in primary health care; in similar fashion, acquired lesions of the central nervous system can be prevented by prompt identification and treatment of infections such as meningitis.

46.   Health workers can and should be trained to manage febrile convulsions, to recognize epilepsy, and to control seizures by low-cost anticonvulsant drugs in order to minimize damage to the central nervous system from prolonged seizures, to reduce accidental injuries (such as burns in epileptics), and to reduce the psychosocial invalidism and isolation which result when treatment is not provided. An uninterrupted supply of drugs of assured quality is of paramount importance. Primary health care workers should take the lead in combating negative attitudes towards epilepsy in their communities (25,26). Care for the mentally ill will be

greatly facilitated if mental health services are provided also in general hospital units and if there is a continuum of care, with assured quality control from primary health care to specialized institutions.

47. Health workers should be trained to recognize schizophrenia and manage it with low-dose antipsychotic drugs, counseling, and support to family members in order to minimize chronicity and to avoid the social breakdown syndrome which leads to severe social disability (27,28).

48. Health workers should be alerted to the need for the treatment of patients thought to be suffering from depression. Patients suffering from depression commonly present multiple somatic symptoms, may be inappropriately investigated and treated for somatic disorders, and are at risk of suicide. Effective treatment can be provided at relatively low cost. The use of lithium salts in appropriate dosage has been shown to reduce recurrence rates in affective disorders.

Action at Community Level in Other Social Sectors

Better Day Care for Children

49. Retarded mental development and behavior disorders among children growing up in families that are unable to provide appropriate stimulation can be minimized by early psychosocial stimulation of infants and by day care programs of good quality, particularly if such programs involve parents as participants (29). However, adequate quality of the day care program is essential; "child minding" in crowded quarters with insufficient numbers of adult caretakers who are often inadequately trained may retard children's development, not facilitate it (30). Among useful measures that countries could take are surveys of existing day care facilities and an assessment of the need for them (particularly pressing in urban areas); establishment of quality standards and appropriate regulatory measures; setting of progressive targets for a) ensuring quality, and b) training staff in the psychosocial development and needs of children.

Better Long-Term Care Institutions

50. While the use of institutions for long-term care (e.g., hospitals, residential institutions, nursing homes) can be minimized by making alter-

natives available in the community, they will remain a necessary part of a full range of services. Whether they care for the young or the old or for the physically or the mentally handicapped, the quality of the institutional environment is a major determinant of the way the inhabitants function. Improvements of architectural design and the content of work programs, and regular evaluations of the quality of long-term care institutions, present important opportunities for preventive interventions.

Self-Help Groups

51. These groups, organized by lay citizens, are effective in a) reducing the chronicity of certain disorders (e.g., Alcoholics Anonymous); b) reducing handicaps (e.g., societies organized to help patients with epilepsy); c) educating the community about the nature of such disorders; and d) playing an advocacy role and facilitating changes in legislation, better resource allocation, and satisfaction of other needs of groups of people with specific disorders. Furthermore, community self-organization for local development has been shown to reduce the psychopathology associated with alienation and helplessness (31).

Role of Schools

52. The progressive extension of obligatory schooling in more countries provides new opportunities to broaden people's understanding of how they can protect their health. At the same time, it leads to the identification of child health problems not previously known to health authorities. Schools also often provide possibilities for preventive measures (32).

53. **Teaching of parenting skills.** A variety of risks to mental health and psychosocial development can result from the lack of parenting skills and from parents' insufficient knowledge of children's needs. Urbanization and other socioeconomic changes (e.g., small families do not offer children opportunities to exercise responsibility with younger siblings) may result in a growing number of young parents not having such skills. Therefore, education for parenthood may well have to become a responsibility of public education. A number of possibilities for such education exist. Creches and nursery schools can, for example, be located next to secondary schools, whose students can be assigned to work in the

nurseries under appropriate supervision and with appropriate classroom exercises. Trained lay group leaders for groups of new mothers (particularly adolescent mothers) to lead discussions on child rearing provide a valuable resource for self-help in the community.

54.   **Health education.** Instruction about premarital counseling, family life, human sexuality, child development, nutrition, accident prevention, and abuse of certain substances are among the subjects that are most frequently recommended for inclusion in school curricula. Evidence of the effectiveness and usefulness of such instruction is still incomplete and evaluation of programs should be incorporated in their design. A particularly promising area of work is the new strategy to prevent abuse of certain substances among young adolescents by equipping them through group work to resist the ubiquitous solicitations to smoke cigarettes and consume drugs and alcohol.

55.   **The role of the teacher.** With appropriate training, teachers can play an important role in identifying children a) with sensory or motor handicaps, and b) with mental health problems that have not been detected by the health sector. Collaboration between teacher, parent, and health worker is central to the identification and rehabilitation of children with chronic handicaps and to the avoidance of their social isolation and other untoward consequences.

Preventing Accidents and Poisoning

56.   In view of the high mortality and morbidity, in particular injury to the central nervous system, resulting from accidents and poisoning, measures for their prevention must have a high public health priority. Measures to prevent traffic accidents have been reviewed by WHO on several occasions. Brain damage through exposure to toxic substances at work can be prevented by imposing strict limits; untoward effects of shift work can be avoided by using the principles of chronobiology; childproof safety caps on medicine bottles and containers of household chemicals can reduce poison ingestion and consequent damage to the central nervous system (33); a ban on re-use of beverage bottles for pesticides and herbicides has been identified as a useful measure; and lead poisoning in children can be prevented by prohibiting paints containing lead for

household use and by decreasing the lead content of gasoline to reduce blood lead levels and lead encephalopathy in children living in urban environments (34).

Role of the Media

57.   Radio, television, newspapers, and comic strips have the potential to play a major role in public health education—for the better (e.g., by explaining why sanitation is essential for health) or for the worse (by advertising cigarettes or making smoking look glamorous because heroes and heroines in television dramas smoke). Studies such as that in Northern Karelia (Finland) and the Stanford Tri-County Studies (USA) directed at changing smoking, exercise, and eating habits have shown that public education campaigns can make a difference to health behavior and consequently to health status. The capabilities of the media for the enhancement of health and the prevention of health-damaging behavior and disease have however hardly begun to be exploited.

Cultural and Religious Influences

58.   Cultural factors are among the principal determinants of human behavior. Knowledge of cultural and religious influences can be utilized by health workers in their efforts to reduce health damaging modes of life (e.g., abuse of certain substances).

Collaboration With Nongovernmental Organizations

59.   A productive alliance with nongovernmental organizations can help to educate the public and to supply care to the victims of disease (e.g., local, national, and international organizations concerned with mental health; Alcoholics Anonymous). Nongovernmental professional organizations can be an important factor in advocating preventive measures among their members and with governments.

Support Services

60.   Support services provided at the community level can enable families to care for members with chronic illnesses (e.g., schizophrenia, senile dementia), who would otherwise require more expensive and less satisfactory institutional care. An excellent example is the organization by the community, on the basis of voluntary efforts by retired workers, of

"home beds" for chronically handicapped mental patients in China: the neighborhood volunteers care for the patients while family members are away at work. To maintain residual function and to avoid institutionalization, chronic mental patients must be provided with housing, opportunities for sheltered employment, and recreation.

Action at the Governmental Level

61. An effective prevention program will be possible only if there is commitment to such a program by the national government and the provision of additional resources for this purpose. Such commitment must find its expression in a policy for the prevention and control of mental, neurological, and psychosocial disorders, a policy which will be an identifiable part of the national health program.

62. The implementation of the policy directives will require intersectoral cooperation and the formulation of at least medium-term program plans developed on a realistic basis. These tasks should be entrusted to a coordinating group on mental health with the authority to lead the activity and to assign specified tasks to the appropriate sectors. Useful experience with such groups has already been obtained and clearly shows that this mechanism can be of crucial importance in program development and evaluation.

63. In an area such as prevention, the work of the national coordinating group must be supported with appropriate information: it would therefore appear important to establish, at the national level, an information center or unit with the resources to collect and feed back data on changes in the nature and trends of problems and the effects of intervention and task performance. A comprehensive review of legislation affecting such matters as mental health, family life, health services, drug control, and schools could be an early task of the center. Such a review would assist the national coordinating group considerably in carrying out its work.

64. In the area of prevention, more so perhaps than in other health work, it is important to recall that government actions in spheres apparently remote from health may have implications for health that were not

taken into account in their formulation; for example, housing projects that worsen mental health because of inappropriate design; industrial development projects that destroy local culture and lead to family disruption, child neglect, and abuse of certain substances; or the widespread use of pesticides which, because of their neurotoxicity, can often lead to brain damage. This makes appropriate intersectoral cooperation, which can be supported by the intersectoral coordinating group, all the more vital.

IV. Research Needs

65.   There is good reason to believe that the preventive measures described in Section I, if applied, would lead to a reduction in the burden which mental, neurological, and psychosocial problems place on health and socioeconomic development. It is therefore highly desirable to apply such measures without delay. It is also clear that there is a need for research into the causes and mechanisms of disease in order to develop new and better means for prevention and control; such research programs have been proposed by WHO and are included in its medium-term mental health programs.

66.   Of immediate importance for action now are the applied research issues of direct relevance to the implementation of preventive programs in each country. Though this report gives data on prevalence and on the effectiveness of interventions where they are available, such data frequently do not exist, particularly in developing countries or for subpopulations within countries. Extrapolation of existing data in country A to the needs of country B may prove entirely misleading. Therefore, it would seem important to foster research programs of two kinds:

1) Studies of the distribution of problems in a specific population and changes in the pattern over time;

2) Investigations to enable member states to assess the value—in their own conditions—of measures which have been proposed for wide-scale application.

67. Both types of study will have to be carried out at the national or subnational level. At the international level, an urgent task—which should be included in programs of technical cooperation between countries—is the development of methods which countries will be able to use effectively in the conduct of such investigations. The past and current work of the organization on the development of cross-culturally applicable assessment instruments, psychosocial indicators, and refined diagnostic criteria will greatly facilitate these efforts.

68. Such research requires an infrastructure in the countries; support to this infrastructure must therefore be given higher priority than is now the case.

69. Involvement of institutions in developing countries in multicenter research, research training courses and grants, more efficient information exchange, and other recommended methods should all be used to create and strengthen the basis for further growth of knowledge in this field.

V. Summary

70. Mental, neurological, and psychosocial disorders constitute an enormous public health burden for both developing and developed nations. Review of the evidence demonstrates that the implementation of a comprehensive program of prevention based on methods currently available could produce a substantial reduction of the suffering, of the destruction of human potential, and of the economic loss they produce. Such a program would attack both the biological and the social causes which underlie these disorders. For success, it requires national commitment and coordinated action in many social sectors.

71. The frequency of these disorders can be reduced, and their consequences for individuals and communities minimized, if, in addition to sustaining and enhancing programs of prenatal and perinatal care, nutrition, immunization, family planning, and accident prevention, countries undertake and emphasize the need for:

1) Action that will prevent occurrence of mental, neurological, and psychosocial disorders and impairment, including:

  i) Measures to reduce risk of social and cognitive failure by
     a) enriching day care for children (para. 49)
     b) providing better long-term care institutions (e.g., nursing homes) (para. 50)
     c) educating for parenthood (para. 53)
     d) introducing health education into school curricula (para. 54)

  ii) Measures to control abuse of certain substances as part of primary health care (paras. 37 and 38) and of education in schools (para. 54)

  iii) Measures to reduce the health consequences of acute stress through crisis intervention in primary health care (para. 39)

  iv) Measures to prevent iatrogenic damage in primary health care by
     a) psychosocial interventions (para. 40), which could reduce excessive psychotropic drug use
     b) minimizing hospitalization (para. 41) by using community alternatives
     c) treatment of depression and infection in the elderly in order to prevent central nervous system damage and suicide (para. 42)

2) Measures that will minimize chronic disability if impairment or disease occurs, including:

  i) Rehabilitation of patients with sensory and motor handicaps (paras. 43 and 44)

  ii) Treatment of hypertension and central nervous system infection (para. 45)

  iii) Control of epilepsy and combating its stigma (para. 46)

iv) Combined drug treatment and family care for patients with schizophrenia (para. 47)

v) Recognition and treatment of depression (para. 48)

72. For full effectiveness, prevention programs must involve self-help groups (para. 51), the media (para. 57), cultural and religious influences (para. 58), nongovernmental organizations (para. 59), and the provision of social support for families (para. 60).

73. At the government level (paras. 61–64), the commitment to dealing with mental, neurological, and psychosocial disorders must be made visible through the introduction of a mental health component into the national health and development policy. An intersectoral coordinating mechanism should be established to assist in program development. It should be able to acquire and distribute information on program performance, have the authority to review national legislation with a view to recommending changes needed to bring it into conformity with policy, and develop agreement among social sectors on their responsibility for and contributions to the program.

74. WHO, in addition to collaborating with countries in these efforts, should help to develop the research infrastructure necessary to study the magnitude and trends of problems and to monitor the impact of interventions or programs.

References

1. World Health Organization: Mental Retardation: Meeting the Challenge (WHO/Offset Publication No. 86). Geneva, World Health Organization, 1985
2. Hetzel B, Orley J: Correcting iodine deficiency: avoiding tragedy. World Health Forum 6(3):260–261, 1985
3. World Health Organization: Peripheral Neuropathies: Report of a WHO/Study Group (WHO Technical Report Series, No 654). Geneva, World Health Organization, 1980

4. Jablensky A, Sartorius N: Culture and schizophrenia. Psychol Med 5:113–124, 1975

5. World Health Organization: Dementia in Later Life: Research and Action: Report of a WHO Scientific Group (WHO Technical Report Series, No 730). Geneva, World Health Organization, 1985

6. World Health Organization: Neuronal Aging and Its Implications in Human Neurological Pathology: Report of a WHO Study Group (WHO Technical Report Series, No 665). Geneva, World Health Organization, 1981

7. World Health Organization: Child Mental Health and Psychosocial Development: Report of a WHO Expert Committee (WHO Technical Report Series, No 613). Geneva, World Health Organization, 1977

8. Report on Regional Workshop on Alcohol-Related Problems, Manila, Philippines, 8–12 August 1983 (unpublished WHO document [WP]MNH/ICP/MNH/004), 1984

9. Walsh B, Grant M: Public Health Implications of Alcohol Production and Trade (WHO Offset Publication No 88). Geneva, World Health Organization, 1985

10. Hughes PH, et al: Extent of drug abuse: an international review with implications for health planners. World Health Statistics Quarterly 36:394–497, 1983

11. Ghodse AH, Khan I (eds): Prescribing Psychoactive Drugs: Approaches to Improve Practices. Geneva, World Health Organization (in press)

12. U.S. Department of Health and Human Services: The Health Consequences of Smoking: Cancer, 1982; Cardiovascular Disease, 1983; Chronic Obstructive Lung Disease, 1984. Rockville, MD, U.S. Department of Health and Human Services, 1982, 1983, 1984

13. Victims of Violence: Proceedings of a WHO Working Group on the Psychosocial Consequences of Violence. Leidschendam, Netherlands, Netherlands Ministry of Health, Welfare and Cultural Affairs, 1983

14. World Health Organization: Young People's Health: A Challenge for Society: Report of a WHO Study Group (WHO Technical Report Series). Geneva, World Health Organization (in press)

15. Harding TW, et al: Mental disorders in primary health care: a study of their frequency and diagnosis in four developing countries. Psychol Med 10:231–241, 1980

16. World Health Organization: Mental Health Care in Developing Countries: A Critical Appraisal of Research Findings: Report of a WHO Study Group (WHO Technical Report Series, No 698). Geneva, World Health Organization, 1984

17. World Health Organization: Mental health and female sterilization (report of a WHO prospective collaborative study). J Biosoc Sci 16:1–21, 1984; 17:1–18, 1985

18. Babor TF, et al: Alcohol-related problems in the primary health care setting: a review of early intervention strategies. Br J Addict (in press)

19. Raphael B: Preventive intervention with the recently bereaved. Arch Gen Psychiatry 34:450–454, 1977
20. Windholz MJ, et al: A review of research on conjugal bereavement. Compr Psychiatry 26:433–447, 1985
21. Bloom BL, et al: A preventive intervention program for the newly separated. Am J Orthopsychiatry 55:9–26, 1985
22. Cooper J: Crisis Admission Units and Emergency Psychiatric Services (Public Health in Europe, No 11). Copenhagen, World Health Organization, 1979
23. Williamson J, et al: Old people at home: their unreported needs. Lancet 1:1117–1120, 1964
24. World Health Organization: The Provision of Spectacles at Low Cost. Geneva, World Health Organization, 1987
25. Robb P: Epilepsy: A Manual for Health Workers. Bethesda, MD, U.S. Department of Health and Human Services, 1981
26. Wig N, Murthy SR: Manual of Mental Disorders for Primary Health Care Personnel. Chandigarh, India, Postgraduate Institute of Medical Education and Research, 1981
27. Falloon RH, Liberman RP: Interactions between drug and psychosocial therapy in schizophrenia. Schizophr Bull 9:543–554, 1983
28. Jablensky A, et al: WHO Collaborative Study on Impairments and Disabilities Associated With Schizophrenic Disorders. Acta Psychiatrica Scandinavica 62 (suppl 285):152–163, 1980
29. Berrueta Clement J, et al: Changed Lives: The Effects of the Perry Pre-School Program on Youths Through Age 19. Ypsilanti, MI, High Scope Press, 1984
30. Tizard B: Evaluation of Early Stimulation Programmes (unpublished WHO report). Geneva, World Health Organization, March 1985
31. Eisenberg C: Honduras: mental health awareness changes a community. World Health Forum 1(1, 2):72–77, 1980
32. Rutter M, et al: Fifteen Thousand Hours: Secondary Schools and Their Effects on Children. Cambridge, MA, Harvard University Press, 1979
33. Walton WW: An evaluation of the Poison Prevention Packaging Act. Pediatrics 69:363–370, 1982
34. Blood lead levels in U.S. population. Morbidity and Mortality Weekly Report 31:132–133, 1982

Annex. List of interventions that can be directed against each problem area

Problem	Intervention
Mental retardation (10)	Prenatal and perinatal care (32–33) Immunization (35) Family planning (36) Epilepsy control (46) Nutrition (34) Day care (49) Accident prevention (56) Family support (27) Teaching of parenting skills (53) Better long-term care institutions (50) Recognition and care of sensory and motor handicaps (43–44)

Acquired lesions of
  the central nervous
  system (11)
	Treatment of hypertension and infection (45)
	Epilepsy control (46)
	Control of abuse of certain substances (37–38, 54)
	Accident prevention (56)

Peripheral neuropathy
  (12)
	Accident prevention (56)
	Recognition and care of sensory and motor handicaps
	    (43–44)
	Health education (54)
	Control of abuse of certain substances (37–38, 54)

Psychoses (13)	Treatment of depression (48) and schizophrenia (13, 47) Family support (27) Better long-term care institutions (50) Dementia control (14) Treatment of anxiety, depression, and infection (42) Support services (60)
Epilepsy (15)	Prenatal and perinatal care (32–33) Immunization (35) Treatment (46) Accident prevention (56) Health education (54)
Emotional and conduct disorders (16)	Family planning (36) Health education (54) Role of teacher (55) Teaching of parenting skills (53) Day care (49) Primary health care (39)

Annex.   List of interventions that can be directed against each problem area *(continued)*

Problem	Intervention
Abuse of certain substances (17–22)	Primary health care (39) Prevention of iatrogeny (40–42) Health education (54)
Conditions of life that lead to disease (23–24)	Psychosocial care (40) Crisis intervention (39) Control of abuse of certain substances (37–38) Health education (54) Teaching of parenting skills (53)
Violence (25)	Accident prevention (56) Control of abuse of certain substances (37–38, 54) Health education (54) Teaching of parenting skills (53)
Excessive risk-taking behavior in young people (26)	Health education (54) Support services (60) Teaching of parenting skills (53) Crisis intervention (39) Accident prevention (56)
Family breakdown (27)	Day care (49) Teaching of parenting skills (53) Support services (60)

Note.   Paragraph numbers in parentheses.

The role of the media (57), cultural and religious influences (58), nongovernmental organizations (59), and intersectoral collaboration and government action (60 and 61–64) apply in greater or lesser degree to *all* problems.

CHAPTER 2

Relationship Between Treatment and Prevention Policies

Leon Eisenberg, M.D.

Is the Prevention of Mental Disorders Possible?

Despite widespread skepticism, effective prevention of some psychiatric disorders is not only possible but is, for certain disorders in some countries, substantially complete; what is not possible now, or in the foreseeable future, is the prevention of all mental disorders.

Pellagra and general paresis provide two telling examples. Patients suffering from pellagra and paresis crowded the wards of mental hospitals of Western countries in the early decades of this century. Pellagra, well before it was shown to result from niacin deficiency but after it was recognized as a nutritional disease (Sydenstricker 1958), was eliminated in most Western countries by improvements in diet (reduction in the dependence on milled corn as a food staple). Paresis was prevented by effective treatment of syphilis, particularly with the introduction of penicillin, after the treponeme was identified as the causal agent.

Neither of these preventive measures is "psychiatric" in the narrow sense of the term. However, what matters is not the mode of action of the agent, the venue in which it is applied, or the academic discipline of the practitioner, but the effectiveness of the measure in preventing diseases manifested by disturbances in mental function (American Psychiatric Association 1990).

As I demonstrate in this chapter, what has been accomplished for pellagra and paresis is now possible for other organic brain disorders; moreover, there are promising interventions for the prevention of functional mental disorders. It is equally important to stress that means are not available for primary prevention of such major diseases as the schizophrenias, the affective disorders, and senile dementia of the Alzheimer's type. Ignorance with respect to neuroses and personality disorders is equally profound; yet these disorders result in enormous morbidity and disability throughout the developing world as well as the developed world. Well-meaning but uninformed advocates for prevention presume that these disorders could be prevented if only parents would follow their advice as "experts." Claims abound; data are entirely absent to support such propositions.

Definitions

The public health approach to prevention distinguishes three levels of disease prevention.

Primary prevention is designed to stop the development of disease among susceptible populations; it uses health promotion (i.e., the teaching of hygienic practices, universal education to promote cognitive development, the provision of optimal nutrition to enhance resistance, social support for family life, peer programs in public schools to increase resistance to solicitations for cigarette smoking and other health-injurious habits, etc.) and specific protection (i.e., immunizations, iodization of salt, crisis intervention following bereavement, etc.).

Secondary prevention is designed to shorten the duration of illness once it occurs, reduce the likelihood of contagion, and limit sequelae by means of early diagnosis and prompt treatment (e.g., the use of psychotropic drugs and psychosocial measures to abort acute psychotic states). Treatment (secondary prevention) of the first disease in a causal series constitutes primary prevention for those conditions that would otherwise follow in its wake (e.g., medical control of hypertension to reduce the likelihood of a cerebrovascular accident or treatment of hypothyroidism to avoid the onset of myxoedematous madness).

Tertiary prevention is directed at individuals with an irreversible disease; its goals are to limit disability (e.g., reform of institutional programs to avert the chronic social breakdown syndrome), minimize exacerbations of the underlying disease (e.g., psychosocial education for the families of schizophrenic patients), and promote rehabilitation (e.g., social skills training, vocational guidance, sheltered workshops for chronic mental patients).

In primary prevention, the goal is to prevent the development of disease; in secondary prevention, to shorten its duration after it has occurred; and in tertiary prevention, to preserve function as far as possible when no effective treatment for the disease itself is available. In this chapter I focus on primary prevention in view of the extensive review of treatment measures provided in the other sections of this book.

Preventive Interventions

In this section I list and describe each of the well-validated means for preventing mental disorders. To organize the discussion, the measures are listed in a life cycle perspective that begins before conception and continues into old age.

Family Planning and Prenatal Care

The more numerous and the more closely spaced the pregnancies in the reproductive lives of women are, the greater are the risks for maternal and infant mortality and the worse are the developmental outcomes for the children. Studies in developed countries have demonstrated that the larger the number of children there are in a family (other variables having been controlled for), the lower their educational attainment is (Blake 1989). Unwanted pregnancies among teenagers are associated with high risk for mother and child (National Research Council 1987). Taken together, these findings indicate the importance of family planning services to reduce the number of offspring and to lengthen interbirth intervals in order to optimize the ability of parents to care for their children. Comprehensive family planning services should include education about contraceptive choices, access to contraceptives, and the availability of safe abortion as a backup for inevitable contraceptive failure.

Inadequate nutrition, cigarette smoking, alcohol consumption, and drug abuse during pregnancy are all associated with increased hazards to the fetus, including higher rates of low–birth weight infants. Low birth weight, in turn, is associated with a disproportionate number of developmentally impaired children. Provision of comprehensive prenatal services, trained birth attendants, and backup hospital services for pregnancies at high risk will reduce psychiatric morbidity among liveborn infants (Institute of Medicine 1985). Most exciting of all, Sosa et al. (1980) and Klaus et al. (1986) have demonstrated that the presence of a supportive female companion during labor and delivery significantly reduced the need for a Caesarean section; in addition, this simple remedy diminished maternal morbidity on an obstetric service in Guatemala (Klaus et al. 1986). Kennell et al. (1991) replicated this striking effect in a randomized trial in Houston, Texas. As those authors stated, "Labor support is centuries old, but its advantages have now been validated in three controlled studies. . . . Its positive effects should not be overlooked in the trend toward more and increasingly complex technology" (p. 2,200).

Where feasible (principally in industrialized countries), screening for elevated blood levels of alpha-fetoprotein, for chromosomal anomalies by cytogenetic methods, and for morphological abnormalities by ultrasonography can permit the detection and abortion of abnormal fetuses carried by mothers at risk. A recently completed randomized prevention trial for women at risk for bearing children with neural tube defects (because of a previously affected pregnancy) revealed a strong protective effect (72%) from folic acid supplementation (Medical Research Council 1991).

Newborn Screening

A number of congenital metabolic abnormalities can be detected by routine screening of newborns. Notable among the correctable conditions are phenylketonuria (PKU), galactosemia, and congenital disorders of thyroid function, all of which result in severe central nervous system pathology if treatment is not instituted in the first weeks of life and maintained thereafter. The clinical manifestations of the first two can be prevented by appropriate diet and the third by extrinsic thyroxine. The fact that these abnormalities occur at low frequency (1/10,000 to 1/25,000 for

PKU, 1/60,000 to 1/80,000 for galactosemia, and 1/3,600 to 1/5,000 for disorders of thyroid function [American Academy of Pediatrics 1989]) makes newborn screening a practicable public health measure only in countries with highly developed health services. Although the cost of case detection is relatively high because the conditions are rare, so are the lifetime costs to the community in caring for severely affected children. Screening programs are, however, of little or no value in the absence of a comprehensive follow-up program to ensure that the infant at risk receives optimal care (Holtzman et al. 1986; Rowley and Huntzinger 1983).

Childhood Immunizations

According to World Health Organization (WHO) data, more than 700,000 deaths in children under age 5 years have been prevented by means of immunization against diphtheria, pertussis, tetanus, measles, polio, and tuberculosis; yet still some 3.5 million deaths occur each year from vaccine-preventable diseases because of the failure to extend the vaccination program to all susceptible children (Galway et al. 1987). At that, mortality data underestimate the magnitude of the public health burden because they do not tabulate the morbidity from central nervous system pathology and from the psychosocial consequences of chronic handicap among survivors. Full implementation of the WHO Expanded Program of Immunization would not only yield enormous gains in further reduction of mortality in childhood (and thus make parents more willing to forgo large family size) but spare compromised brain function and psychosocial disability among survivors.

Preventing Malnutrition

Deficits in the intake of specific micronutrients as well as in overall protein-calorie intake can impair brain development with major consequences for cognitive and emotional function.

Iodine deficiency disorders (IDD) constitute the most pressing instance of micronutrient deficiencies that lead to brain malfunction. IDD affects more than 400 million people in Asia alone (Hetzel 1983). Clinical manifestations include stillbirths, abortions, and congenital anomalies; endemic cretinism, characterized by mental deficiency, deaf mutism, spastic diplegia, and other forms of neurological defect; and impaired mental function associated with goiter. In individuals at risk, IDD can be prevented for 3–5 years with one injection of 2–4 ml of iodized poppy seed oil, a treatment that can be given by primary care workers. To prevent fetal IDD, iodized oil must be administered before conception; treatment even as early as the first trimester of pregnancy is not fully effective. Oil injections are both feasible and practical as an immediate means to control endemic IDD. For reasons of costs and convenience, the long-term goal must be the introduction of an iodized salt program for the entire population (Ramalingaswami 1973). Program success is dependent on the full support of the population, fostered through public education (Hetzel 1983).

Severe protein-calorie malnutrition, life threatening in itself, increases the likelihood that exposure to infectious agents will result in clinical disease because malnutrition impairs host defenses. Furthermore, malnourished persons show increased systemic manifestations of diseases that are more limited in those who are well nourished. Gastrointestinal diseases, made more likely by malnutrition, increase nutritional stresses on the host by increasing caloric requirements at the same time that food intake and absorption are impaired. Traditional "treatments" for diarrhea (i.e., reducing intake of food and fluids) worsen the threat.

The conjoining of chronic malnutrition with disadvantageous family circumstances results in retarded cognitive and social development (Richardson 1976). Studies of malnourished children have indicated that it is the interacting and multiplicative effects of the simultaneous biological and social insults that result in damage (Dobbing 1987). Grantham-McGregor et al. (1978, 1991) showed that nutrition plus social stimulation for hospitalized malnourished children, maintained after hospital discharge by parents who had been educated by home visitors, resulted in greater developmental gains than did a program of renourishment alone. Effective remediation must be targeted at the entire complex of social and nutritional deprivation.

Monitoring the growth of young children, a simple method well within local resources, permits the early detection of developmental failure. It is one of the four components of the United Nation's International Children's Fund (UNICEF) GOBI initiative: Growth monitoring, Oral rehydration, Breast-feeding, and Immunization (Grant 1989).

Injury Prevention

Accidents (more appropriately termed nonintentional injuries) are the leading cause of lost years of potential life (calculated as the number of deaths from a given cause multiplied by the difference in years between age at death and age 65 for each case) in the United States (Centers for Disease Control 1989). Vehicular accidents are a major source of head and spinal cord injuries. Such injuries are preventable by better highway design, traffic regulations, vigorous prosecution of drunk driving, automatic seat belts, child safety seats, and air bags. Among children, cycling is a major cause of hospital admissions for head injuries. In a recent study (Thompson et al. 1989), cyclists wearing helmets had an odds ratio for brain injury after accidents of 0.12 compared with those without helmets (95% confidence interval 0.04 and 0.40).

Poisonings in children can be minimized by mandating childproof safety caps on bottles of medication and toxic chemicals for domestic use (Walton 1982). Blood levels of lead in children can be reduced by effective controls on the lead content of gasoline (Centers for Disease Control 1982a).

Enriched Day Care

There is extensive documentation from both developed and developing countries that children growing up amid psychosocial deprivation exhibit deficits in cognitive development, lower levels of academic achievement, and increased rates of behavioral and antisocial disorders (e.g., see Eisenberg and Earls 1975). The prevention of these disastrous outcomes by means of enriched day care programs that involve parents as participants has been shown in several recent long-term outcome studies to make a significant difference in lowering rates of academic and behavioral pathology (Berrueta-Clement et al. 1984; Jordan et al. 1985; Lazar and Darlington 1982).

Day care programs can facilitate the attainment of a second goal: the teaching of parenting skills to adolescents by having them participate in the supervised care of toddlers. The effectiveness of this strategy has not been formally demonstrated, but its desirability is indicated by the fact that experience in child care within the family, the traditional way these skills have been transmitted, is becoming ever less available. With smaller family size and fragmentation of the family, it can no longer be taken for granted that such naturalistic education is available to all children.

Community and School-Based Programs

An American Psychological Association Task Force on Prevention (Price et al. 1989) has provided a comprehensive survey of model prevention programs for mental disorders that have shown some evidence of effectiveness, at least in the short run. The authors noted that the common features of successful programs include "careful targeting of the population, the capacity to alter life trajectory, the provision of social support and the teaching of social skills, the strengthening of existing family and community supports, and rigorous evaluations of effectiveness" (p. 57).

Prevention in Clinical Settings

Iatrogenic diseases resulting from inappropriate prescription can be reduced by training primary health care workers in the recognition and management of psychosocial disorders. A recent WHO study in four developing countries (Colombia, Philippines, Sudan, and India) demonstrated the high frequency of psychiatric morbidity among clinic attenders as well as the failure of health care workers to recognize more than one in three such cases (Harding et al. 1980). A companion study (Giel et al. 1981) documented the high prevalence of mental disorders in primary child health care in developing countries. Training in the recognition and management of psychiatric disorders in general practice can not only reduce unnecessary diagnostic studies and inappropriate medication but also make effective mental health care available (Gask et al. 1988; Harding et al. 1983).

The prevalence of epilepsy in less developed countries has been estimated to be as high as 15–50 per 1,000 (in contrast to rates of 3–5 per 1,000 in industrialized countries). Improvement in obstetric care, more effective accident prevention, and prompt treatment of central nervous system infections will reduce this prevalence. Untreated epilepsy is associated with progressive neurological compromise and increasing psychosocial impairment, which is made worse by the stigma associated with the disorder. Greater skills in the recognition of the disorder and the appropriate use of anticonvulsant medication can markedly diminish psychosocial handicap (Robb 1981).

Effective treatment of hypertension can reduce the incidence of strokes; thus primary care workers should be trained in the management of hypertension. Carotid endarterectomy is beneficial in patients with recent hemispheric and retinal transient ischemic attacks or disabling strokes and ipsilateral high-grade stenosis (70%–79%) of the internal carotid artery (North American Symptomatic Carotid Endarterectomy Trial Collaborators 1991). Whether surgery reduces the likelihood of stroke in patients with moderate stenosis (30%–69%) is not yet clear and is being assessed in an ongoing randomized trial.

There is evidence that bereavement counseling can reduce the occurrence of depression and somatization among surviving spouses (Rafael 1977; Windholz 1985). Psychosocial stress following marital separation can be reduced by preventive intervention (Bloom et al. 1985).

Although the primary prevention of the schizophrenias eludes present capabilities, secondary prevention, by the use of neuroleptic drugs for patients and psychoeducational training for family members, can reduce the duration of illness episodes and the likelihood of relapse (Brown et al. 1972; Hogarty et al. 1986; Leff et al. 1982; Tarrier et al. 1989). Tertiary prevention, by keeping hospital stays to a minimum, redesigning institutional programs, and providing social skills training and sheltered workshops, can avert chronic social breakdown syndromes among patients with chronic disorders (Gruenberg and Kennedy 1988). However, as Helgason (1990) demonstrated in a 20-year follow-up of all Icelandic schizophrenic patients seen for the first time by a psychiatrist in 1966–1967, outcome remains unsatisfactory because of difficulties in engaging patients and their families in programs of care.

Similar considerations hold in the case of affective disorders. The knowledge base necessary to permit primary prevention is not yet available, but the use of tricyclics, lithium, and interpersonal psychotherapy can shorten morbid episodes and reduce the likelihood of recurrence (Kupfer et al. 1992; National Institute of Mental Health 1985). In view of the long-term morbidity associated with depressive illness (Klerman and

Weissman 1992; Wells et al. 1992) and the rising incidence of depression in recent birth cohorts (Cross-National Collaborative Group 1992), emphasis on the diagnosis and treatment of depression in primary care should have high priority in public health programs.

The prevalence of dementia increases with age, from a rate of less than 1% in those age 60–64 years to a rate as high as 38% in those age 90 years and older (Jorm et al. 1987). Total prevalence is growing both because of an increase in the size of the population at risk (the "graying" of the population) and because of an increase in the survival of patients with chronic disease (Gruenberg 1977). Although primary prevention of the dementias is not yet possible, secondary prevention is feasible by means of treatment of intercurrent physical illness, behavioral management of disruptive symptoms, family support services, treatment of depressive disorders, and appropriate pharmacotherapy for control of symptomatic behaviors (A.S. Henderson 1988).

Is Prevention Always Preferable?

Having shown that prevention of some mental disorders is possible, we must still ask, Is it always preferable? From the standpoint of the individual who would otherwise have become ill, avoidance of illness is almost always more desirable than treatment because it avoids the morbidity associated with illness and its care. However, when prevention requires changing habitual behavior, and particularly when change causes withdrawal symptoms (as in smoking cessation), the "cost" of prevention may deter its acceptance. Moreover, in the instance of smoking, the time lag between risk taking and its pathological consequences is a matter of decades. This reinforces public skepticism because smoking cessation reduces rather than altogether eliminates the probability of disease. Although the risk of lung cancer is far greater among smokers than nonsmokers, not all smokers develop cancer and lung cancer does occur in nonsmokers. Ways of detecting those at greatest risk (presumably because of genetic susceptibility to the carcinogen(s) in cigarette smoke) are being sought but have not yet been discovered. Thus, many who would not develop cancer must be persuaded not to smoke even though cessation of smoking does not guarantee good health. The relatively slow progress of antismoking campaigns attests to the strength of social forces that reinforce cigarette smoking.

From the standpoint of the community, in contrast to that of the individual, decisions about undertaking preventive measures require weighing competing social objectives. To pursue the example of smoking, its elimination involves the loss of jobs in tobacco farming and cigarette production, the loss of revenues from taxation, and the loss of foreign exchange from exports. These factors do not gainsay the extraordinary benefits from smoking cessation: significant reductions in rates for cancer, ischemic heart disease, chronic obstructive pulmonary disease, prematurity, and other health hazards. But they do highlight the magnitude of the political challenge (World Health Assembly 1986).

If the incidence of the disease targeted for prevention is low, the ratio between benefit to the individual and cost to the community shifts markedly. Consider the case of maple syrup urine disease (MSUD; also known as branched-chain ketoaciduria). The incidence of MSUD in newborns is between 1/250,000 and 1/300,000 (American Academy of Pediatrics 1989). When untreated, MSUD is associated with mental retardation, convulsions, repeated infections, and, in the classic form of the disease, early death. Treatment with diets low in branched-chain amino acids can improve the prognosis for the patient if the disorder is detected in the newborn period and if treatment is begun promptly. However, the costs of screening, low yield of confirmed cases, and complexity of the dietary regimen combine to make prevention of MSUD a public health measure feasible only where health care systems are highly developed.

Cost-Benefit Analysis

Advocates for prevention commonly assert that it is cheaper than treatment. However, this is not true in many instances. In addition, reliance on cost savings as the primary justification for prevention undermines public support for measures that yield better health at increased costs. Therefore, it is important at the outset of this discussion to examine costs in relation to benefits.

Cost-benefit analysis is designed to determine whether an investment in a specific preventive measure will produce a net savings for the health budget by lowering the costs that would have been incurred had the targeted disease not been intercepted. The first technical decision the analyst must make is whether the calculation is to be limited to the direct costs from a disease (i.e., the costs for clinic visits, drugs, hospital care, special schooling, and/or long-term institutionalization) or whether it will also include the indirect costs resulting from a disease and its sequelae (wages lost from work missed and earnings lost over a lifetime because of incapacity or death). A further and more difficult question is whether to attempt to translate pain and suffering from disease into monetary terms so that these components can be factored into the calculation (Russell 1986).

Incorporating indirect costs into the cost-benefit equation permits a more inclusive assessment, but it does not take into account basic bookkeeping practices in government agencies. Specifically, the increased expenditures from a new preventive initiative are immediately evident as additional costs in the health budget; in contrast, the direct health care costs averted by preventing disease will be reflected only by a smaller demand on later budgets. Furthermore, savings in indirect costs do not appear in the health budget at all; in fact, to make the political problem more difficult, such savings accrue to other department budgets (i.e., income tax revenues) over a longer time period; moreover, the savings are not readily attributable to a preventive measure undertaken some years earlier. The promise of long-term savings may not be compelling to an official preoccupied with this year's budget, the one by which taxpayers will judge him or her.

Money saved even by a spectacularly successful prevention campaign is not an identifiable item in the national budget. For example, the total U.S. contribution to the WHO campaign against smallpox is less than the savings to the United States each month because vaccination against smallpox is no longer necessary (D.A. Henderson 1987). Yet, because other health care costs have continued to escalate, the national health budget grows larger each year; nowhere to be found is an item headed "savings resulting from investment in the worldwide elimination of smallpox."

Because accurate morbidity and mortality data are often unavailable in less developed countries, examples of cost-benefit analysis have been limited to industrialized nations. As an illustration of its application, consider the impact of measles vaccination for the 3.5 million infants born in the United States in 1981, 95% of whom would have been infected before adulthood in the absence of immunization (Gruenberg et al. 1986). The total cost for the program was $51 million (including vaccine side effects and vaccine failures); without vaccination, direct plus indirect costs from measles would have totaled $745 million; the benefit-to-cost ratio is 14.6:1. If the calculation is restricted to direct costs alone, the benefit-to-cost ratio is still 3:1, a considerable bargain. Measured by health effects, the gains to those 3.5 million infants are even more impressive: 360 deaths, 1,100 cases of measles encephalitis, and 30 cases of subacute sclerosing panencephalitis were prevented.

Health benefits from a measles vaccination program in less developed countries would be greater because measles is much more of a deadly disease in these countries. In Africa, the death rate from measles in infants less than 1 year old is as high as 10% because of comorbidity. However, the U.S. economic cost-benefit analysis cannot be extrapolated to less developed countries because of marked differences in costs, the limited availability of health care services, and the lack of an existing infrastructure for vaccination (including means to maintain the cold-chain). For many impoverished nations, a populationwide immunization campaign would consume the entire health care budget, thus precluding treatment services altogether. External funds supplied by international organizations such as UNICEF are necessary to enable immunization programs to be undertaken.

Cost-benefit analysis serves to define the circumstances under which monetary costs exceed monetary benefits. A telling example is provided by screening for lead toxicity by means of the free erythrocyte protoporphyrin (FEP) assay. FEP permits the detection of asymptomatic lead intoxication. It is only when the prevalence of elevated blood levels of lead among preschool children in a community is 7% or higher that total dollar costs for FEP screening and appropriate intervention for children at risk are less than the cost of treating children after they become symptomatic (Berwick and Komaroff 1982). If prevalence is lower than 7%, it is monetarily "cheaper" to provide care after clinical illness appears. Clearly, it is not cheaper for the poisoned children and their families, whose personal costs from encephalopathy, learning disorders, mental retardation, and personal suffering are not weighed in the formal analysis.

Cost-benefit analysis can be a useful and informative exercise. There is, for every prevention program, a point at which the magnitude of the investment may not be warranted if disease prevalence is less than "x" and if the program can only be undertaken at the cost of other more effective measures. However, it is morally unacceptable to base decisions on economic considerations alone, without taking into account human costs and the differential distribution of benefits in the various sectors of the population.

Furthermore, it is possible to argue that, taken together, measures that prevent premature mortality will create an ever greater drain on state funds in the long term. As more citizens survive past the age of retirement into their 70s, 80s, and even 90s (the most rapidly growing segments of the population in industrialized nations), they deplete social security reserves and incur disproportionate medical care costs because of the cumulative burden of degenerative diseases (Gori and Richter 1979). This contention, it should be noted, applies no less to treatment than to prevention. Few may be willing to endorse the draconian recommendation that disease be welcomed as a zealous guardian of the national treasury. But this argument does caution against ready recourse to "cost saving" as the major justification for measures to prolong life. The fundamental goal of health policy must be better health outcomes!

Weighing Risks and Benefits

Prevention is so attractive a concept that, all too often, little thought is given to the potential for "toxicity" that may be associated with implementing putative preventive programs. Methods to identify at-risk individuals can harm those incorrectly labeled. Programs can fail. They can cause disease in those who are not enrolled as well as harm in those who are included. Paradoxically, they can have an overall negative effect on health in the community even when they benefit target groups.

Population screening to identify individuals at increased risk for disease inescapably carries with it dual hazards: that of being incorrectly labeled as being at risk (false positives) and that of being incorrectly reassured of safety (false negatives). The likelihood of error is a function of test sensitivity (the proportion of affected persons who test positive), test specificity (the proportion of unaffected persons who test negative), and the *a priori* probability of being affected (the proportion of individuals in the population with the condition). Even so remarkable a screening test as the enzyme immunoassay (EIA) for antibodies to human immunodeficiency virus (HIV), which has a sensitivity somewhat greater than 98% and a specificity somewhat greater than 99%, would yield more than two false positives for every true positive if it were to be applied to a population with a seroprevalence of 0.5%, the current estimate for the U.S. population as a whole (Eisenberg 1989). Confirmatory testing of EIA-positive sera by a Western blot (WB) would markedly reduce, but not eliminate, false positives and would leave false negatives undetected. Moreover, the status of those who are EIA positive but WB negative would remain ambiguous since the Western blot has a sensitivity of 92% and a specificity of 95% on EIA-screened sera. Given the ominous medical prognosis for HIV infection and the social discrimination HIV-infected persons face, the individual falsely labeled as HIV positive would be at serious hazard for harm. At the same time, that small number of infected individuals who had been falsely reassured they were uninfected would continue to transmit the disease unwittingly.

Thelin (1985) has tracked the negative psychological consequences of a Swedish pilot program for the early identification of children with alpha-1-antitrypsin deficiency, an inherited disorder that leads to a greatly increased risk for chronic obstructive lung disease in adulthood. Because the onset of lung disease can be considerably postponed if the individual with the disorder avoids exposure to tobacco smoke, Swedish authorities authorized a pilot screening program for newborns. Wisely, the Swedish Medical Board required a follow-up study of the psychological consequences for the family before authorizing a populationwide program. Despite counseling about the meaning of a positive test finding, mothers of the identified children reported great distress and considerable misunderstanding of its implications. Moreover, despite emphasis on the risk for the child from exposure to cigarette smoke, there was no change in parental smoking, itself a precursor of later decisions by children to smoke. The evidence led to a decision not to implement screening as a public health program.

Ineffective measures carry two kinds of costs: first, the waste of resources that could have been used to provide other services and second, a negative impact on public opinion. When unrealistic promises are made in the name of prevention, the failure to redeem those promises makes the public cynical about other public health proposals.

An effective measure can be counterproductive when it does not reach a sufficient proportion of the population. If the uptake of rubella vaccine among susceptible children is less than 90% (the level necessary for herd immunity), an immunization program can lead to an increase in rates for congenital rubella syndrome (CRS) in the next generation because it postpones the age at natural infection among unvaccinated persons. Even though CRS rates among the vaccinated population will be close to zero, rates will increase disproportionately among the offspring of those who are unvaccinated (Knox 1984).

An incompletely implemented prevention program can harm those it is designed to benefit. Newborn screening for sickle cell anemia poses risks for the infants positive for the disease and those positive for the trait. The infant with sickle cell anemia will benefit only if the parents are thoroughly informed about the significance of the finding and if appropriate medical care is available from physicians knowledgeable about managing the disease (Rowley and Huntzinger 1983). The infant at greatest risk for harm without offsetting benefit is the one with sickle cell trait. Undue parental apprehension may lead to a vulnerable child syndrome (Green and Solnit 1964); as an adult, the individual may be denied employment or insurance if the trait is mistaken for the disease. Further, as in the case of every recessive genetic disorder, testing parents carries the risk of discovering that the husband is not the father of the child, information that can compromise the relationship between the parents.

A preventive measure can be on target for those it enrolls and nonetheless increase the public health hazard. For example, high school driver education courses produce a modest but real reduction in crashes per licensed driver. Yet because driver education courses increase the number of teenage drivers on the road, they result in an overall increase in fatal motor vehicle accidents (Robertson and Zador 1978).

That premature introduction of programs said to prevent disease can be hazardous to health is not an argument against prevention; however, it does emphasize the need for careful review of potential hazards before undertaking new initiatives and rigorous evaluation to assess negative as well as positive effects after programs are introduced.

Setting Priorities

Given the fact that the resources available for health programs are finite and that assigning them to one use precludes their availability for another, the challenge is to assess the competing claims of various proposals for prevention and to decide on the proper balance between prevention and treatment. Decisions must be based on a close analysis of the extent and distribution of disease on a country-by-country basis and the resources, both internal and external, available to each country for public health measures. The most that one can do is to outline the general criteria that should guide decision makers. It would be absurd, not to say arrogant, to imply that a set of generic policies will be applicable to the varied health problems that face member states.

The criteria to be used in weighing competing options include the following:

- Illness burden produced by the disease
- Effectiveness of the intervention
- Toxicity
- Feasibility
- Opportunity cost

The *illness burden* resulting from a specific disease (e.g., senile dementia of the Alzheimer type) or a category of diseases (e.g., mental disorders) is a function of 1) the prevalence of the disease or diseases, 2) the severity of the morbidity and mortality resulting therefrom, and 3) the distribution of the ages at onset. That burden includes the cost of providing medical and social services for the ill person, the losses to economic productivity resulting from sickness and death, the encumbrance on the family from caring for the sick member, and the pain and suffering experienced by sick persons and their families. Because they are more easily measured, the first two indicators (health care costs and output losses) are the ones used when attempts are made to quantitate illness burden.

Black and Pole (1975), in a pioneering study in the United Kingdom, measured burden in terms of inpatient days, outpatient referrals, sickness benefits, and mortality. On the basis of 1972 data, they reported that mental illness accounted for 31% of all inpatient days (and mental handicap for an additional 15%), 4% of outpatient referrals, almost 8% of general physician consultations, and almost 10% of sickness benefit days; just over 1% of life years lost was attributable to suicide.

Rice et al. (1976), in a pioneering study of illness burden in the United States (a study that was replicated by the same authors 10 years later [Rice et al. 1985]), used an analogous set of measures to those used by Black and Pole. In addition, they computed direct (costs for care) and indirect (losses of output from sickness or premature death) economic costs of illness. As in the U.K. study, mental disorders accounted for the largest proportion of inpatient days, and were ranked third as a cause of disability, sixth in contributing to total economic costs, and twelfth as a cause of life years lost. In a more recent assessment based on 1980 data, the Board on Mental Health and Behavioral Medicine of the Institute of Medicine (IOM; 1984) noted that mental illness accounted for about $20 billion in direct health care costs in the United States, which amounted to about 8% of all direct health care expenditures in that year. Indirect expenditures were estimated as eight times as great. Hay and Ernst (1987) computed the aggregate net social costs for caring for all persons diagnosed with Alzheimer's disease over those patients' remaining lifetimes in that single year to be $30 billion. An IOM study (1989) of child and adolescent mental disorders estimated that about 16% of inpatient and 23% of outpatient pediatric insurance costs incurred by dependents were attributable to psychiatric problems.

Clearly, mental disorders place a severe burden on the resources of the community. That their prevention would be highly desirable, however, does not establish that it is possible. Decisions to proceed with specific preventive programs have to be based on data demonstrating *effectiveness*; that is, the evidence that the measures will reduce the incidence or the prevalence of the disease at which they are targeted. Data exist to validate measures such as family planning, newborn screening, childhood immunizations, iodine supplementation, injury prevention, hypertension control, and combined pharmacological and psychosocial therapies for schizophrenia and the affective disorders. Although, as noted earlier, the benefit-to-cost ratio has been precisely computed for immunization programs, such economic analyses are available for few preventive measures. Reifman and Wyatt (1980) estimated that, from 1969 through 1979, lithium prophylaxis of manic depressive illness in the United States yielded savings of $2.9 billion in direct and $1.3 billion in indirect costs. An unpublished study by Wyatt et al. (F.K. Goodwin, personal communication, 1989), has found a $12 billion savings in direct, and a $28 billion in indirect, costs from lithium use in the two decades since 1969.

The potential *toxicity* of an intervention must be weighed against its efficacy in reducing the risks posed by the disease to be prevented; that is, although every effort must be made to minimize toxicity, even substantial side effects are tolerable if the intervention is highly effective in averting serious morbidity and mortality. The decision, however, cannot rest on expert opinion alone. The public must have accurate information about benefits and risks set before it and must be persuaded that the one outweighs the other. Distorted publicity on side effects can lead to an increase in avoidable morbidity and mortality. Such has been the case with pertussis immunization in the United Kingdom (Centers for Disease Control 1982b); concern about vaccine side effects reduced parental compliance and resulted in a substantial increase in cases of pertussis.

The *feasibility* of a program depends on whether the necessary infrastructure for implementation is in place; there must be adequate personnel with the requisite competence to administer it, appropriate geographic distribution of such personnel, and a health system able to coordinate their activities. Thus even a potentially effective intervention may not make sense for a particular community if it requires a level of skill and an administrative system that does not exist in that community. The simpler the method and the more compatible it is for use by primary health care workers, the more likely that it can be implemented in a less developed country.

Finally, it is necessary to take into account the *opportunity cost*, that is, those other programs forgone because funding and energy have been committed to the program under review. Because health care resources are finite, a decision to embark on a prevention program will entail diversion of resources from other health programs. The allure of cost savings from prevention is so attractive to governments that treatment facilities may be closed down on the mere assumption that disease will be avoided. Such has been the case in the United Kingdom and the United States where the illusory promise of community mental health, with its claim of averting iatrogenic illnesses arising from hospitalization, has led to the wholesale closing of psychiatric hospitals, leaving many chronically ill mental patients without any care because the intended community treatment alternatives were not available (Weller 1989).

Even when such spurious logic is not used to rationalize denial of needed care, choices between prevention and treatment, especially in developing countries, create difficult dilemmas. Indeed, when the disease is devastating and the treatment for it costly and of limited value, efforts at prevention may well be the only appropriate response, as exemplified by the current epidemic of acquired immunodeficiency syndrome (AIDS) in Africa. Yet, although attempting to prevent HIV infection makes more sense than providing treatment with current methods, the quandary for health policy officials goes beyond decisions about AIDS itself. To what extent, the health minister must ask, should resources, whether they are derived from internal budgets or external contributions, be devoted to this disease in the face of the burden of illness from other infectious and parasitic diseases? This question becomes all the more problematic because external funds are dedicated funds; their use is directed by external agencies. It would seem foolhardy to refuse them simply because they will not be made available for other purposes; yet such funds come with an internal cost in that they divert highly skilled personnel, few in number, from other essential programs.

The Need for Epidemiological Intelligence

It is clear is that policy decisions can be no better than the quality of the information on which they are based. In the absence of reliable data on the extent, distribution, and social burden of mental disorders in the population and of time trends in prevalence, decisions on the allocation of resources can be no better than guesses in the dark. Essential is the development of information centers capable of collecting and feeding back data on the nature and magnitude of the health problems in each country and on the results from treatment and prevention programs. Thus every new public health initiative should include a mandatory set-aside for epidemiological surveillance by the least expensive methods available in order to facilitate periodic reassessments of effectiveness and to permit midcourse corrections in resource allocation when they are warranted.

References

American Academy of Pediatrics, Committee on Genetics: Newborn screening fact sheets. Pediatrics 83:449–464, 1989

American Psychiatric Association, Task Force on Prevention Research: Report of the task force. Am J Psychiatry 147:1701–1704, 1990

Berrueta-Clement JR, Schweinhart LJ, Barnett WS, et al: Changed Lives: The Effects of the Perry Preschool Program on Youths Through Age 19. Ypsilanti, MI, High Scope Press, 1984

Berwick DM, Komaroff AL: Cost effectiveness of lead screening. New Engl J Med 306:1392–1398, 1982

Black DAK, Pole JD: Priorities in biomedical research: indices of burden. Brit J Prev Soc Med 29:222–227, 1975

Blake J: Number of siblings and educational attainment. Science 245:32–36, 1989

Bloom BL, Hodges WF, Kern MB, et al: A preventive intervention program for the newly separated. Am J Orthopsychiatry 55:9–26, 1985

Brown GW, Birley JLT, Wing JK: Influence of family life on the course of schizophrenic disorders: a replication. Br J Psychiatry 121:241–258, 1972

Centers for Disease Control: Blood lead levels in U.S. population. Morbid Mort Wkly Report 31:132–133, 1982a

Centers for Disease Control: Pertussis—England and Wales. Morbid Mort Wkly Report 31:629–632, 1982b

Centers for Disease Control: Years of potential life lost before age 65, U.S., 1987. Morbid Mort Wkly Report 38:27, 1989

Cross-National Collaborative Group: The changing rate of major depression: cross-national comparisons. JAMA 268:3098–3105, 1992

Dobbing J (ed): Early Nutrition and Later Achievement. London, Academic Press, 1987

Eisenberg L: Health education and the AIDS epidemic. Br J Psychiatry 154:754–767, 1989

Eisenberg L, Earls FJ: Poverty, social depreciation and child development, in American Handbook of Psychiatry, Vol 6. Edited by Hamburg DA. New York, Basic Books, 1975, pp 275–291

Galway K, Wolff B, Sturgis R: Child Survival: Risks and the Road to Health. Washington, DC, Institute for Resource Development/Westinghouse, 1987

Gask L, Goldberg D, Lesser AL, et al: Improving the psychiatric skills of the general practice trainee: an evaluation of a group training course. Medical Education 22:132–138, 1988

Giel R, de Arango MV, Climent CE, et al: Childhood mental disorders in primary health care: results of observations in four developing countries. Pediatrics 68:677–683, 1981

Gori GB, Richter BJ: Macroeconomics of disease prevention in the United States. Science 200:1124–1130, 1979

Grant JP: The State of the World's Children. United Nations Children's Fund, Oxford, UK, Oxford University Press, 1989

Grantham-McGregor SM, Stewart ME, Desai P: A new look at the assessment of mental development in young children recovering from severe malnutrition. Dev Med Child Neurol 20:773–778, 1978

Grantham-McGregor SM, Powell CA, Walker SP, et al: Nutritional supplementation, psychosocial stimulation and mental development of stunted children. Lancet 338:1–5, 1991

Green M, Solnit A: Reactions to the threatened loss of a child: a vulnerable child syndrome. Pediatrics 34:58–66, 1964

Gruenberg EM: The failures of success. Milbank Mem Fund Quart 55:3–24, 1977

Gruenberg EM, Kennedy C: Some determinants of social disability, in Handbook of Social Psychiatry. Edited by Henderson AS, Burrows GD. Amsterdam, Elsevier, 1988

Gruenberg EM, Lewis C, Goldston SE (eds): Vaccinating Against Brain Syndromes: The Campaign Against Measles and Rubella. New York, Oxford University Press, 1986

Harding TW, De Arango MV, Baltazar J: Mental disorders in primary care: a study of their frequency and diagnosis in four developing countries. Psychol Med 10:231–241, 1980

Harding TW, Busnello ED, Climent CE: The WHO collaborative study on strategies for extending mental health care: evaluative design and illustrative results. Am J Psychiatry 140:1481–1485, 1983

Hay JW, Ernst RL: The economic costs of Alzheimer's disease. Am J Public Health 77:1169–1175, 1987

Helgason L: Twenty years follow-up of first psychiatric presentation for schizophrenia: what could have been prevented? Acta Psychiatr Scand 81:231–235, 1990

Henderson AS: An Introduction to Social Psychiatry. Oxford, UK, Oxford University Press, 1988

Henderson DA: Smallpox eradication: a WHO success story. World Health Forum 8:283–292, 1987

Hetzel BS: Iodine deficiency disorders (IDD) and their eradication. Lancet ii:1126–1129, 1983

Hogarty GE, Anderson CM, Reiss DJ, et al: Family psychoeducation, social skills training and maintenance chemotherapy in the after care of schizophrenic patients. Arch Gen Psychiatry 43:633–642, 1986

Holtzman C, Slazyk WE, Cordero JF, et al: Descriptive epidemiology of missed cases of phenylketonuria and congenital hypothyroidism. Pediatrics 78:553–558, 1986

Institute of Medicine: Research on Mental Illness and Addictive Disorders. Report of the Board on Mental Health and Behavioral Medicine. Washington, DC, National Academy Press, 1984

Institute of Medicine: Preventing low birth weight. Washington, DC, National Academy Press, 1985

Institute of Medicine: Research on Children and Adolescents With Mental, Behavioral, and Developmental Disorders. Washington, DC, National Academy Press, 1989

Jordan TJ, Grallo R, Deutsch M: Long-term effects of early enrichment: a twenty year perspective on persistence and change. Am J Community Psychol 13:393–415, 1985

Jorm AF, Korten A, Henderson AS: The prevalence of dementia: a quantitative integration of the literature. Acta Psychiatr Scand 76:465–479, 1987

Kennell J, Klaus M, McGrath S: Continuous emotional support during labor in a U.S. hospital: a randomized controlled trial. JAMA 265:2197–2201, 1991

Klaus MH, Kennell JH, Robertson SS, et al: Effects of social support during parturition on maternal and infant morbidity. BMJ 293:585–587, 1986

Klerman GL, Weissman MM: The course, morbidity, and costs of depression. Arch Gen Psychiatry 49:831–834, 1992

Knox EG: Theoretical aspects of rubella vaccination strategies. Int J Infect Dis 7:194–197, 1984

Kupfer DJ, Frank E, Perel JM, et al: Five-year outcome for maintenance therapies in recurrent depression. Arch Gen Psychiatry 49:769–773, 1992

Lazar I, Darlington R: Lasting Effects of Early Education. Monographs of the Society for Research in Child Development 47, 1–2, Serial No 194, 1982

Leff J, Kuipers L, Berkowitz R, et al: A controlled trial of social intervention in the families of schizophrenic patients. Br J Psychiatry 141:121–134, 1982

Medical Research Council, Vitamin Study Research Group: Prevention of neural tube defects: results of a Medical Research Council vitamin study. Lancet 338:131–137, 1991

National Institute of Mental Health: Mood disorders: pharmacologic prevention of recurrences. NIMH Consensus Development Conference Statement. Am J Psychiatry 142:469–476, 1985

National Research Council: Risking the Future: Adolescent Sexuality, Pregnancy and Childbearing. Washington, DC, National Academy Press, 1987

North American Symptomatic Carotid Endarterectomy Trial Collaborators: Beneficial effect of carotid endarterectomy in symptomatic patients with high grade carotid stenosis. N Engl J Med 325:445–453, 1991

Price RH, Cowen EL, Lorion RP, et al: The search for effective programs: what we learned on the way. Am J Orthopsychiatry 59:49–58, 1989

Rafael B: Preventive intervention with the recently bereaved. Arch Gen Psychiatry 34:450–454, 1977

Ramalingaswami V: Endemic goiter in Southeast Asia: new clothes on an old body. Ann Int Med 78:277–283, 1973

Reifman A, Wyatt RJ: Lithium: a brake in the rising cost of mental illness. Arch Gen Psychiatry 37:385–388, 1980

Rice DP, Feldman JJ, White KL: The Current Burden of Illness in the United States. Washington, DC, Institute of Medicine, National Academy of Sciences, 1976

Rice DP, Hodgson TA, Kopstein AN: The economic costs of illness: a replication and update. Health Care Financing Review 7:61–80, 1985

Richardson SA: The relation of severe malnutrition in infancy to the intelligence of children with different life histories. Pediatric Res 10:57–61, 1976

Robb P: Epilepsy: A Manual for Health Workers. Bethesda, MD, U.S. Department of Health and Human Services, 1981

Robertson LS, Zador PL: Driver education and fatal crash involvement of teen-aged drivers. Am J Public Health 68:959–965, 1978

Rowley PT, Huntzinger DJ: Newborn sickle cell screening: benefits and burdens realized. Am J Dis Child 137:341–345, 1983

Russell LB: Is Prevention Better Than Cure? Washington, DC, The Brookings Institution, 1986

Sosa R, Kennell J, Klaus M, et al: The effect of a supportive companion on perinatal problems, length of labor and mother-infant interaction. N Engl J Med 303:597–600, 1980

Sydenstricker VP: The history of pellagra, its recognition as a disorder of nutrition and its conquest. Am J Clin Nutrition 6:409–414, 1958

Tarrier N, Barrowclough C, Vaughn C, et al: Community management of schizophrenia: a two year follow up of a behavioral intervention with families. Br J Psychiatry 154:625–628, 1989

Thelin T: Psychological Effects of Neonatal Screening. Studentlitteratur, University of Lund, Sweden, 1985

Thompson RS, Rivara FP, Thompson DC: A case-control study of the effectiveness of bicycle helmets. N Engl J Med 320:1361–1367, 1989

Walton WW: An evaluation of the Poison Prevention Packaging Act. Pediatrics 69:363–370, 1982

Weller MPI: Mental illness—who cares? Nature 339:249–252, 1989

Wells KB, Burnham MA, Rogers W, et al: The course of depression in adult outpatients: results from the medical outcomes study. Arch Gen Psychiatry 49:788–794, 1992

Windholz MJ: A review of research on conjugal bereavement. Compr Psychiatry 26:433–447, 1985

World Health Assembly: Tobacco or Health. Director General's Report. Geneva, Switzerland, World Health Assembly, Executive Board Document No. 77, 1986

Section II

Biological Treatments

Introduction to Section II

The following two chapters deal with biological modes of treatments. The first chapter, by Saraceno, Tognoni, and Garattini, raises a number of relevant critical questions about psychotropic drugs. A plethora of books and articles on psychopharmacology have been published since the introduction of chlorpromazine in 1957. Many of them serve the need for training or educational update by mental health professionals and we felt that it would have been redundant to provide another didactic account of the main drugs available in psychiatry. Instead the authors have concentrated on some critical questions about psychopharmacology that have general implications for the entire field of psychiatry. This approach is pertinent in the area of psychopharmacology where the random controlled trials were first introduced, for many researchers doubt that any significant breakthrough has occurred since the introduction of the main prototypical drugs (chlorpromazine, imipramine, lithium, and diazepam). Although the introduction of the psychotropic drugs has undoubtedly helped in the revolution in psychiatric care by giving an essential impulse to community-based treatments, it is still unclear what the overall impact of the main psychopharmacological treatment methods has been on the natural history of the most important psychiatric disorders.

Despite the lack of significant recent breakthroughs in this field, two unexpected developments are noteworthy: they are represented by the belated recognition of the effectiveness of clozapine in the management of severely psychotic patients and of the effectiveness of clomipramine in the treatment of obsessive-compulsive disorder. Although these drugs were already established, it has been possible, thanks to the methodology of the random controlled trial, to prove that in these selected conditions that they can be of significant benefit.

The chapter by Bolwig provides a comprehensive evaluation of electroconvulsive therapy (ECT), which to date is the most ancient biological form of psychiatric treatment. Although in the past ECT was sometimes used nonspecifically without proper indication, carefully controlled studies have shown that this treatment method can be helpful for the management of severely depressed patients, especially those with delusions and severe retardation. At the same time, new nonpharmacological methods, such as light therapy, have been introduced, and it will be of interest to see whether they prove to be of value.

CHAPTER 3

Critical Questions in Clinical Psychopharmacology

Benedetto Saraceno, M.D.
Gianni Tognoni, M.D.
Silvio Garattini, M.D.

Introduction

A review of psychotropic drugs can hardly appear to be an original undertaking. The field is so well covered that the selection of a few good references as a proof of the existing substantial consensus should suffice (Avery 1980; Bellantuono and Tansella 1989; Bellantuono et al. 1980; Lader and Petursson 1983; MacKay 1982; Rudorfer and Potter 1989). However, a focus on the context of the problems for which psychotropic drugs are prescribed is seldom encountered. From the point of view adopted in this paper the scenario seems particularly controversial with respect to

1. The contents, tools, and prognostic implications of diagnosis (by definition the critical variable in the assessment of drugs) (Ciompi 1980; Guimon 1989; Paykel 1972)
2. The context of care as a determinant, rather than a confounding variable of outcome (Tognoni and Bignami 1981)
3. The choice of the most appropriate paradigm for describing biochemical and/or functional correlates of behaviors and drug actions (Garattini and Samanin 1988)

This paper attempts to explore some implications of the contradictory situation sketched above. In the first part of the text, a therapeutics-oriented synopsis derived from some recent reviews is presented; in the second part the focus is on the uncertainties and challenges facing the physician in the current clinical practice of psychiatry. While in the first section a classical frame of reference (i.e., drug classes) is assumed, the second section refers to the problems for which and the settings in which the same drugs are used. The core of the first part is knowledge on the efficacy and safety of the available treatments and the alleged capacity of treatments to provide a framework for interpretation of the problems susceptible to successful treatment. The core of the second part is the inefficacy of drugs. This makes them a poor starting point in the search for better treatments; also, because of their inefficacy it cannot be suggested that poor understanding of disease processes is the limiting factor in the failure of therapeutic developments.

The Art of Clinical Psychopharmacology

That there is stagnation in this area does not need demonstration; it stands out in most reviews (Klerman 1986) of the three classical subgroups of psychiatric drugs. The addition of new molecules has not produced therapeutic breakthroughs.

Antipsychotic Drugs

(For reviews see Appleton 1988; Bradley 1986; Jain et al. 1988; Johnson 1985; Kane 1989; Kessler and Waletsky 1981; Lader 1980; MacKay 1982.) Antipsychotic drugs have been shown to be effective in the control of many psychotic symptoms. Antipsychotic drugs induce a sensible reduction of symptoms such as disturbed thinking (delusions) and hallucinations, of manic symptoms, and of agitation, a common symptom in the acute phase of many psychoses. The efficacy of these compounds in controlling *positive* schizophrenic symptoms has been well documented, while the evidence of their effect on *negative* symptoms (e.g., attention deficit, learning disturbances, affective blunting, catatonia, and pervasive autism) is still controversial (Breier et al. 1987; MacKay and Crow

1980). In fact, in some cases negative symptoms may be a consequence of positive symptoms (e.g., social withdrawal might be a consequence of persecutory ideation); therefore, an improvement in positive symptoms should entail some improvement in the negative ones.

With respect to chronic treatment for the prevention of relapses, it has been documented that antipsychotic drugs are more effective than placebo in preventing rehospitalization of schizophrenic patients (Hartmann et al. 1980; Johnson 1982); however, the appropriateness of such an indicator in defining relapse is highly debatable. As shown by Leff and Vaughn (1981), the prevention of relapse is dependent on the setting: schizophrenic patients living in highly conflictive, emotively threatening families appear to require more antipsychotic drugs to avoid relapse compared with patients in less conflictive family contexts. The statements listed in Table 3–1 summarize the existing consensus about the therapeutic profile of this group of drugs.

The many drug utilization reviews published during the last 10 years demonstrated that the broad dosage ranges attributed to each molecule are not so much the result of well-documented pharmacological titrations as a reflection of the empirical behavior of clinicians with differing preferences for upper or lower doses (Baldessarini et al. 1988; Kane 1985) (see Table 3–2). Along the same line, the recurrent suggestion of adopting *targeted* and *low dose* strategies to reduce behavioral and extrapyramidal side effects appears a sensible attitude (dictated by

Table 3–1. The clinical profile of antipsychotic drugs

Problem	Activity	Notes
Acute "positive" symptoms of psychosis	+++	Efficacy limited to delusions, hallucinations, manic crises, agitation
Chronic treatment for prevention of relapse	++	Efficacy is highly setting dependent and counterbalanced by the unpredictable appearance of side effects
Acute and chronic "negative" symptoms of psychosis	±	

Note. +++ = very active; ++ = less active; ± = no definite proof of activity.

common sense and documented in small series of patients), rather than the result of formal testing of a hypothesis of optimization of the benefit/risk profile in a priori definable populations.

The failure of population pharmacokinetics to substantiate the importance for clinical practice of plasma level monitoring (Bollini et al. 1984a; Simpson and Yadalam 1985; Van Putten et al. 1985) further stresses the key characteristic of antipsychotic drugs, namely, their relative ineffectiveness in controlling negative symptoms.

Short of showing innovative strength in the direction of higher efficacy, research has produced its most useful results with respect to the safety profile of these drugs. Table 3–3 is a suggestive account of where knowledge stands today. Although at first glance the picture may appear

Table 3–2.　Classification and dosage profile of antipsychotic drugs

Drugs (by class)	Daily dose (mg)
Butyrophenones	
Haloperidol	4–30
Trifluperidol	4–30
Phenothiazines	
Chlorpromazine	100–800
Fluphenazine	4–40
Levomepromazine	120–800
Perphenazine	12–60
Propericiazine	25–190
Thioridazine	100–800
Trifluoperazine	6–50
Thioxanthenes	
Clopenthixol	4–30
Flupenthixol	4–30
Thiothixene	4–30
Diphenyl-butylpiperidines	
Pimozide	4–30
Dibenzo-X-azepines	
Clothiapine	16–120
Clozapine	150–450
Substitute benzamides	
Sulpiride	400–1200

comprehensive and detailed, it reveals many unknowns, despite the long and intensive use of these compounds (Bergen et al. 1989; Kane et al. 1985; Marsden et al. 1986; Stahl 1986).

Table 3–3. Clinical-epidemiological profile of main adverse effects of antipsychotic drugs (APDs)

Clinical manifestations	APD	Lag time	Estimated incidence (%)
Extrapyramidal[a]			
Acute dystonias	B, PhPz	2–5 days	2.5–5
Akathisia	B, PhPz	2–8 weeks	5–50
Parkinsonism	B, PhPz	within 3 months	20–40
Tardive dyskinesia[b]	All	2 years	5–56
Other CNS effects			
Behavioral disturbances	All	1–2 weeks	?
Excessive sedation[c]	PhA, PhPi, Ct, Cz	1–2 days	?
Grand mal seizures	Cz	?	4
Autonomic disturbances			
Anticholinergic effects	Ch, Ct, Cz, T	1–2 days	?
Antiadrenergic effects	Ch, Ct, Cz, T	1–2 days	?
Endocrine problems			
Amenorrhea, galactorrhea	S	4–8 weeks	?
Gynecomastia, impotence	S	4–8 weeks	?
Weight gain	All	4–6 months	50–70
Arrhythmias	Ch, T	?	?
Dermatologic reactions	Ch (Ph?)	?	5 (?)
Idiosyncratic effects			
Agranulocytosis	Ph, Cz	< 4 weeks (?)	0.1–1
Jaundice	Ph (Ch?)	4–8 weeks	?
Degenerative retinitis	T (> 800 mg/d)	? long	? rare
Corneal and lens deposits	Ph	? long	? rare

Note. Molecules most often, not exclusively, implicated: B = butyrophenones; Ch = chlorpromazine; Ct = clothiapine; Cz = clozapine; Ph = phenothiazines; PhA = aliphatic; PhPi = piperidines; PhPz = piperazines; S = sulpiride and congeners; T = thioridazine. CNS = central nervous system.

[a]A classic distinction is made (? mechanism) between antipsychotic drugs with high (haloperidol, flupenthixol, perphenazine, fluphenazine, and pimozide) and low (chlorpromazine, levomepromazine, clotiapine, clozapine, and thioridazine) induction potential.

[b]Higher (? how much) reported risk for females, and age greater than 50 years.

[c]Higher risk (with hypotension) for those scored low under *a* above.

Antidepressants

(For reviews see Blackwell 1987; Hollister 1981; Rudorfer and Potter 1989.) The drugs listed in Table 3–4 must be considered in the context of their recommended indications (Table 3–5) in order to fully appreciate both expectations and existing ambiguities (Baldessarini 1989; Biziere et al. 1987; Bollini et al. 1984b; Klerman 1986; "Treatment of depression in medical patients" 1986):

1. All listed antidepressant drugs can claim, on the basis of published controlled trials, an efficacy of the order of 60%–70% patients recruited.
2. The classification of depression has substantially evolved in the last few years. Some degree of consensus has been reached on the benefit of confining antidepressant drugs to major depressions (i.e., to those cases presenting markedly lowered mood, sleep disturbances, psychomotor retardation or agitation, guilt or worthlessness, and occasionally suicidal ideation) (Bellantuono and Tansella 1989). With respect to the conditions defined as *neurotic depressions* (or *dysthy-*

Table 3–4. Classification of antidepressant drugs

Tricyclic antidepressants	Nontricyclic antidepressants	Benzodiazepines
Amineptine	1 ring:	Alprazolam
Amitriptyline	Bupropion	Adinazolam
Butriptyline	Fluvoxamine	
Chlorimipramine		
Desipramine	2 rings:	
Doxepin	Fluoxetine	
Imipramine	Viloxazine	
Minaprine		
Nortriptyline		
Trimipramine	4 rings:	
	Amoxapine	
	Maprotiline	
	Mianserin	
	Trazodone	

mia according to DSM-III [American Psychiatric Association 1980])
or ill-defined depressive disorders other than bipolar disorders or
major depression, the efficacy of antidepressant drugs is still highly
controversial (Muscettola and Barbato 1987; Paykel 1987).

3. The restriction of the use of these drugs to episodes of major depression is not paralleled by the epidemiology of their actual use, which
   reflects looser prescription habits for a wide variety of depressive
   symptoms.

4. The notion of equivalent efficacy applies to the whole range of old
   and new molecules, irrespective of the differences in their expected
   mechanism(s) of action; nothing new has been added to the original
   tricyclic molecules, thus confirming the clinical perception of a substantial gap between pharmacological research, biochemical explanations, and models of depressive disorders (Garattini and Samanin
   1988). However, some new antidepressants that are selective serotonin reuptake inhibitors (e.g., fluoxetine) seem useful in the case of
   concurrent obsessive-compulsive disorders, and are broadly used as
   initial treatment in patients with minor depression or dysthymia (Pot-

Table 3–5. Guidelines for the clinical use of antidepressant drugs

1. The prescription of an antidepressant drug should result from a thoughtful
   decision, and should be considered only for major depression disorders
   (although tricyclic antidepressants and monoamine oxidase inhibitors have
   been suggested for obsessive-compulsive and panic disorders, their
   efficacy in these conditions is still controversial, and not enough
   experimental evidence is available in this respect).

2. A clinical condition of depression may be labeled as major if
   - On the basis of a consistent anamnestic record it can be qualified as an
     episode of affective psychosis, bipolar disorder, or major depression
   - It is characterized by severe symptoms and a long duration (several
     consecutive weeks)

3. Patients who do not satisfy the above criteria should be considered
   candidates for other therapeutic interventions (anxiolytics, psychological
   support, and psychotherapy).

4. Patients correctly prescribed antidepressant drugs should always also be
   considered for other therapeutic interventions.

ter et al. 1991); however, these indications require further study.

5. A relation between plasma levels and efficacy has been proven with fair certainty only for nortriptyline for which a curvilinear response profile has been proposed—a therapeutic window below or above which no effect is expected and observed. This puzzling finding and the variation in recommended dosage ranges raise serious doubts about the strength of the quantitative criteria proposed to guide prescriptive behavior, requiring careful titration at the start and in phasing out, at least with respect to the search for optimal efficacy profiles (Quitkin 1985).

6. As with antipsychotic drugs, the adverse reaction side of antidepressant drugs is better established. These side effects are included in Table 3–6; however, it should be kept in mind that a specific epidemiological profile of adverse reactions is available only for tricyclic antidepressants (TCAs) (Beaumont 1989; Committee on Safety of Medicines Update 1985; Schmidt et al. 1986).

7. Virtually no attention has been given to systematic direct clinical comparisons of different molecules; every new drug in the field needs to aim merely at proving itself as effective as its progenitors in order to be accepted. No systematic evaluation is available about the size of benefits expected when switching from one molecule to another following a first choice failure due to side effects or to the persistence of depressive symptoms.

8. Eventually the physician is again left to rely on personal preferences, personal beliefs, or market pressure as guides to the existing menu of molecules.

The older TCAs may still be the first choice drugs for episodes of significant depression; however, the new benzodiazepines might eventually prove to be a better choice if they do have, as claimed, a more rapid onset of action and a safer pharmacological profile. The fact that such a decisive shift in clinical practice has not yet taken place may have different explanations: either the evidence is not sufficiently compelling or old expectations connecting depression with monoamine abnormality are so deeply rooted that few are willing to confront these prejudices directly by using molecules with a pharmacological profile linked to other mediators. The extrapolation from pharmacological response to etiology is such a widespread notion that it must be assumed as an implicit tenet of prescribing attitudes.

Monoamine oxidase inhibitors (MAOIs), developed as antidepressants in the 1950s, had been almost completely supplemented by tricyclic drugs until recently, when their possible advantage in some types of de-

Table 3–6. A comparative profile of side effects in old[a] and new antidepressants[b]

Antidepressant	Sedation	Anticholinergic effects[c]	Specific toxicities
TCAs			Cardiotoxicity, skin rash, anxiety,
Amitriptyline	++++	++++	insomnia, tremor, seizures, nausea
Maprotiline	++	++	
Desipramine	+	+	
Amineptine	−	+	

			Expected frequency		
			Frequent	Less frequent	Rare
Non-TCAs					
Fluoxetine	−	−	Nausea, insomnia, irritability	Headache, sweating, diarrhea	
Mianserin	+++	−	Drowsiness		Blood dyscrasias, transaminase alterations
Trazodone	+++	+	Weakness, drowsiness	Dizziness, gastralgias, headache, hypotension	Priapism, impotence, ejaculation inhibition
Viloxazine	+	+	Nausea, vomiting	Dizziness, headache, drowsiness, weight loss	Migraine, seizures
Alprazolam	+++	−			

Notes. + = slightly active; ++ = fairly active; +++ = active; ++++ = very active; − = inactive.
[a]Old antidepressants = tricyclic antidepressants (TCAs).
[b]All old and new antidepressant drugs can induce hypomania.
[c]Anticholinergic effects: dryness of mouth, constipation, visual accommodation disturbances, urinary retention, and hyperexcitability are the most frequent side effects in 10%–40% of the patients receiving antidepressant drugs. Confusion is a "central anticholinergic" side effect, particularly important in elderly patients.

pression, including atypical, refractory, and bipolar depression was noted (Potter et al. 1991). Even at therapeutic doses, MAOIs can induce important side effects and negative interactions with other drugs or foods; therefore they are best managed by specialists. It should be noted that the proposed "new" indications of some MAOIs in other clinical entities (e.g., compulsive behavior, panic attacks) are potentially interesting areas of research that are in need of further evaluation (Adami et al. 1987; Judd et al. 1986; Robinson and Kurtz 1987).

Lithium

(For reviews see Dickson and Kendell 1986; Gitlin et al. 1989; Waller and Edwards 1989; Wood and Goodwin 1987.) Lithium has been used for many years in the treatment of affective psychoses; its efficacy in the control of the acute manic phase has been well documented (although, because its therapeutic action appears after about 10 days of treatment, an antipsychotic drug is indicated in the first few days). On the other hand, lithium does not seem to be effective in the treatment of an acute depressive phase. The main advantage of lithium lies in the prevention of relapses and in the attenuation of their intensity, both in the manic and in the depressive phase. Maintenance therapy with lithium is currently recommended for the prevention of recurrent manic and bipolar episodes, while TCAs are generally used in the prevention of recurrent major depressions (American Psychiatric Association 1975). A pharmacological and clinical profile of lithium is summarized in Table 3–7.

Lithium produces a number of adverse effects, although some, particularly cardiotoxicity and skin reactions, have been overestimated in the past. The most common adverse effects concern the kidney (a diuresis increase is observed, with secondary polydipsia), thyroid (hypothyroidism and goiter), and central nervous system (CNS; memory and attention deficits, fine tremors, and muscular asthenia).

The range between therapeutic and toxic concentrations of lithium is quite narrow; the first overdose symptoms (vomiting, diarrhea, gross hand tremor, dysarthria, ataxia, and drowsiness) appear just above 1.4 mEq/L; at 3 mEq/L these symptoms worsen and are accompanied by severe CNS alterations (nystagmus, hyperreflexia, muscular fasciculations, seizures, sopor, or coma).

Table 3–7. Pharmacological and clinical profile of lithium (Li+)

Pharmacological titration and monitoring
- Gradual increase of a starting schedule of 300 mg of Li+ carbonate, to reach a therapeutic regimen of 300 mg × 4–6 times a day over 10 days
- Therapeutic levels: acute phase, 0.8–1.2 mEq/L; maintenance 0.6–0.8 mEq/L. To be checked weekly for the first month, monthly for the first 6 months, then every 3–4 months
- Toxic levels: greater than 1.3–1.4 mEq/L

Clinical monitoring
- Before starting: hematologic profile and serum electrolytes; renal and thyroid functions; neurological and cardiological examination (with electroencephalogram and electrocardiogram); pregnancy test
- Risk factors for lithiemia increase: 1) decreasing renal function; 2) sodium-depleting diuretics; 3) excessive sodium loss (e.g., vomiting)

Finally, it should be mentioned that carbamazepine has been suggested as an alternative to lithium salts in those who do not respond to the latter. Apparently *rapid-cycle* patients (i.e., those subjects in whom mood changes intervene almost without intervals and last a few weeks) often do not respond to lithium. However, the controlled clinical trials carried out so far on carbamazepine do not provide sufficient evidence to definitively establish its efficacy (Balestrieri et al. 1987).

Benzodiazepines

(For reviews see Bellantuono et al. 1980; Benzodiazepines on trial 1984; Lader, 1986, 1987a; Lader and Petursson 1983; Nicholson 1986; Rosenbaum 1982.) Given the history of their development and their current spectrum of indications (see Table 3–8), it would be tempting to avoid a specific discussion of benzodiazepines in a psychiatric context. That the recent literature concerning these drugs has focused almost exclusively on their potential to produce dependence is an important, though indirect, confirmation of this statement. Their prescription is widespread in general practice, and an important fraction of long-term consumers start off with symptomatic treatment irrespective of formal diagnoses of mental disorder and eventually become "cases" of formal psychiatric interest precisely on the grounds of their developing dependence. On the other hand, drug utilization studies show that benzodiazepines play an important role in the management of psychiatric patients, being more extensively used in primary care than antipsychotic drugs and antidepressants. Their two main targets (anxiety and insomnia) are common features of many psychiatric conditions—either as intrinsic components or as secondary products of the disorder.

Benzodiazepines, however, are used mainly as an accompanying treatment. The absence of any specific consideration in the psychiatric literature of their role in terms of efficacy is an interesting phenomenon, as is the mostly pharmacological emphasis and lack of psychiatry-oriented curiosity in periodic updates on benzodiazepines and in standard educational programs. In fact this point could be framed in a more appropriate perspective by saying that general symptoms of anxiety and insomnia are not given the "dignity" of psychiatric disorders, and that benzodiazepines—the drugs targeted to these conditions—quite consistently share this ambiguity.

The recent qualification of one of the newest members of this class, alprazolam, as a treatment of choice for one of the most fashionable ob-

Table 3–8.   Spectrum of activities and reported clinical uses of benzodiazepines

Activities
  Relief of anxiety
  Sleep induction
  Anticonvulsant
  Muscle relaxation

Clinical indications
  Anxiety (due to any cause and with any concomitant cardiovascular, gastrointestinal, dermatologic disorder)
  Anxious depression
  Panic disorders
  Insomnia
  Alcohol withdrawal
  Muscle disorders
  Seizures
  Preanesthesia
  Sedation before invasive diagnostic procedures

jects of psychiatric research—panic disorders (Aronson 1987)—may appear an exception to the scenario outlined above (particularly because alprazolam has often been proposed more broadly as an antidepressant) (Ballenger et al. 1988; Soderpalm 1987). In the ambiguity perspective suggested earlier, however, this indeed appears to obey rather than violate the rules, with panic attacks probably being a model case of diagnostic, clinical, and epidemiological ambiguity that attracts many heterogeneous treatments, including prescription of a benzodiazepine.

The high specificity of action claimed for psychotropic drugs is in fact a historical replay: years ago many trials (Feighner 1982; Rudorfer and Potter 1989; Schatzberg and Cole 1981) supported an equivalence of some benzodiazepines and antidepressants in formally defined depressive episodes. The prevalent interest of research on the biochemical correlates of depression, increasingly directed to a world of mediators, could hardly fit the biochemical pharmacological profile of benzodiazepines. In clinical practice, however, benzodiazepines disappeared from the treatment of formally defined depression, and were confined to the relief of minor symptoms. Alprazolam may follow the same path, with some help from trials of poor methodological quality (due to their size and to problems related to diagnostic uncertainty, unsatisfactory follow-up criteria, and variability in the proportion of those responding to the drug) (Mattick et al. 1990). To identify a specific target for a drug is a quite useful step in creating a market whence broader, less specific, uses are likely to ensue.

Benzodiazepines therefore continue to be of pharmacological interest. In Table 3–9 are listed the most commonly available benzodiazepine molecules, classified according to their metabolic and kinetic characteristics, which over the years have provided a wonderful, endless focus for descriptive research for clinical pharmacologists.

The currently accepted guidelines for rational use of benzodiazepines (see Table 3–10)—largely based on accumulated kinetic and metabolic evidence—provide a reasonable basis for prescribing behavior, together with the cautionary notes drawn from the safety profile (see Table 3–11 for guidelines for spotting and preventing dependence) and from the potency of the compounds and the main aim of the prescription (see Table 3–12) (Higgitt et al. 1985; Lader 1987b; Tyrer et al. 1989).

The evidence concerning the "new" nonbenzodiazepine anxiolytics (listed in Table 3–13) is still too scanty to regard these diverse compounds as a substantial step forward from a clinical point of view, although at present they seem to be free of dependence-inducing capacity. The better studied molecule, buspirone, is undoubtedly interesting (Buspirone: a radical advance 1988; Goa and Ward 1986). However, although it appears to be as effective as a benzodiazepine, its activity seems to be minimal in patients already exposed to benzodiazepines. Whether buspirone has the potential of becoming a first-choice drug, followed by benzodiazepine in those who do not respond, remains an open question.

Table 3–9.   Structural, metabolic, and kinetic classification of benzodiazepines

Pronordiazepam-like[a]	
Long half-life (> 40 hours)	Chlordiazepoxide
	Medazepam
	Clorazepate
	Diazepam
	Flurazepam
	Pinazepam
	Prazepam
	Desmethyldiazepam
Short half-life (< 24 hours)	Bromazepam
Nitrobenzodiazepines	
Medium half-life (24–48 hours)	Flunitrazepam
	Nitrazepam
Oxazepam-like[b]	
Short half-life (< 24 hours)	Camazepam
	Lorazepam
	Lormetazepam
	Oxazepam
	Temazepam
Tienodiazepines	
Short half-life (< 24 hours)	Clotiazepam
Triazolobenzodiazepines[c]	
Ultrashort half-life (2–5 hours)	Alprazolam
	Estazolam
	Triazolam

[a]Active metabolites with long half-life. Accumulation over long-term daily dosages.
[b]Elimination via direct glucuronization.
[c]Active metabolites with similarly ultrashort half-life.

Intermediate Conclusions

Reductive as it may seem, the preceding section could be summarized in the following statement: experimental, clinical, and epidemiological research on psychotropic drugs during the last 30 years has produced very limited additional therapeutic knowledge. The few molecules developed display relatively little specificity and have not proved capable of extending their role, beyond symptom control, to the cure of the target disorder. The apparent austerity of the World Health Organization (WHO)

Table 3–10. Guidelines for use of benzodiazepines

1. The anxiolytic or hypnotic role of benzodiazepines is a dose-dependent characteristic, therefore the existence of two separate markets has no rational foundation.

2. Kinetic differences may be useful.
   - Choose a benzodiazepine with a short half-life and no metabolites when an hypnotic effect is sought and in elderly patients (to avoid the effects of a reduced metabolic clearance).
   - Choose a benzodiazepine with medium-to-long half-life when the main target symptom is anxiety.

3. Oral administration is the rule; the intravenous route (slow injection to avoid hypotensive and respiratory complications) is preferred for emergency situations and in status epilepticus. Intramuscular administration is discouraged, as the amount absorbed by this route is highly unpredictable.

4. The very high interindividual variability in benzodiazepine disposition means that it is not possible to accurately determine recommended dosages. A low-dosage approach should be adopted, starting with an evening dose, to reach an acceptable "individual" effect. The optimal dosage should be recorded in the clinical notes, to be easily retrieved if benzodiazepine therapy appears again indicated.

5. The prescriber should personally adopt a restricted selection of two to three molecules, to learn their optimal use.

6. The patient should be clearly informed on the expected benefit-risk profile of benzodiazepine treatments, with special focus on
   - Association with alcohol
   - Reduced performance in skillful activities
   - Criteria for duration of use (and withdrawal)

list of essential drugs (World Health Organization 1977, 1988) still illustrates, after over 10 years, the necessary baseline reference. Reliable criteria allowing for the a priori selection of a molecule to provide a higher likelihood of response for individual patients are not yet available. Once certain choices are ruled out on the basis of clear-cut contraindications, clinical wisdom (be it bias or empiricism) prevails. Curiously, these features apply equally well to each of the three main drug classes (lithium may be a partial exception) despite widely different target problems, ranging from the hard core of psychiatry to the fluctuating reality of depression, to the increasingly social—as opposed to medical—conditions for which benzodiazepines are prescribed.

Table 3–11. Pharmacological, clinical, and epidemiological profile of benzodiazepine dependence

1. All benzodiazepines may be associated with dependence.

2. Epidemiological evidence does not provide reliable indications on dosage thresholds or on personality traits that could facilitate the development of dependence.

3. A proportional increase of the risk of developing dependence with increasing duration of exposure has been described (from a 0 incidence for an exposure for less than 4 months, to a 5%–10% for 5–12 months, 25%–45% for 2–4 years, and about 75% for 6–8 years).

4. Withdrawal reactions include
   - Frequently
     Anxiety
     Insomnia
     Irritability
     Nausea
     Headache
     Tremors
     Sweating
   - Less frequently
     Muscle pain
     Vomiting
     Decrease of perception threshold
   - Exceptionally
     Seizures
     Psychotic symptoms

The psychopharmacological knowledge developed for each drug class has undoubtedly focused attention on, and sharpened the understanding of, the relevant target problems and diseases. Furthermore, that drug treatments are the component of care with the highest degree of diffusion at all levels of psychiatric care and in the management of psychiatric-like disorders in general practice can hardly be disputed. It is

Table 3–12. Suggested dosage equivalences for common benzodiazepines (in mg)

	Expected effect on	
Drug	**Anxiety**	**Sleep**
Alprazolam	0.50	*
Bromazepam	1	6
Chlordesmethyldiazepam	1	5
Chlordiazepoxide	10	75
Diazepam	5	20
Flunitrazepam	*	4
Flurazepam	*	30
Lorazepam	1	3.5
Oxazepam	15	60
Triazolam	*	0.5

Note. * = Not proposed for this indication.

Table 3–13. Spectrum of expected clinical activities of nonbenzodiazepine anxiolytics versus diazepam

Drug	Anxiety	Sedation	Hypnotic effect	Muscular relaxation	Anti-convulsant	Withdrawal
Diazepam	+++	+++	+++	+++	+++	yes
Zolpidem	+++	+	+++	+	–	*
Alpidem	+++	+	+++	+	–	*
Zopiclone	+	+++	+++	+	–	*
Buspirone	+++	+	+	–	–	*
Ritanserin	+++	+	+	–	–	*

Note. + = active; +++ = very active; – = inactive; * = no data.

also clear that if so many drugs have been introduced on the market, they are probably meeting an existing need, albeit somewhat encouraged by the promotional activities of the industry.

Clinical psychopharmacology, rather than being a necessary discipline to master an updated wealth of knowledge, is evidence of our being in a borderland of ambiguity: defined, on the one hand, by the confidence that available achievements guarantee further achievements along the same lines, and, on the other hand, by the sobering awareness that dramatically innovative findings are chance events. Nor could it be otherwise, in the absence of models or paradigms fostering the exploration of innovative hypotheses based on better understood biochemical targets (A critique of biological psychiatry 1990; Klerman 1986).

Psychiatric Practice and Psychopharmacology

The three further questions considered under this heading relate to the three major challenges (Sternai et al. 1985–1991; Tognoni 1987) that confront clinical psychopharmacology.

1. What happens to nonresponsive patients?   This question addresses two complementary issues and populations. Clinical evaluation of drugs focuses mainly on the assessment of relative degrees of response (to treatments) by means of randomized clinical trials (RCTs). Patients who do not respond merely compose the "expected" proportions of nonresponsive patients, as no drug is claimed to be the perfect treatment. The proportions of nonresponsive patients have remained by and large the same over the years and across drug classes, showing substantial variations only when evaluated across those different contexts in which drugs appear to play a secondary role (Leff and Vaughn 1980; Tognoni et al. 1981).

What can the cases of nonresponsive patients teach, remind, or propose to psychopharmacology? Nonresponsive patients in RCTs should be formally and systematically followed up, either by randomization to other treatments or by clinical monitoring focused on whether, how, and to what extent they do respond. This attitude should be widespread in routine care; nonresponsive patients should be granted more conspicuous visibility compared with that given to responsive patients, for from them we may glimpse the unknown face of the drug and the disease model. Patients who do not respond to one drug but do respond to another, non-biochemically equivalent one, or patients who respond to no treatment cannot be forever confined to the realm of anecdotal reports or of epidemiological studies retrospectively documenting ineffectiveness. We would suggest that cases of patients who are nonresponsive be handled as follows:

a. In order to provoke more thought it would be interesting to conceptualize drugs with different mechanisms of action and roughly the same proportion of responsive patients as follows: "The persistence of a substantial fraction of nonresponsive patients, largely unpredictable on the basis of individual characteristics or inclusion criteria, confirms that the problem we are dealing with cannot be considered a well-defined target disease. The prescriber is provided another tool for empirical behavior, as no prognostic indicator is available favoring either compound as first choice [...]" (Saraceno et al. 1986). The adoption of realistic attitudes such as the above might modify treatment and research behaviors. General practitioners and psychiatrists might more readily recognize their position as being at the frontier amidst illusory innovation, overt fraud, and challenging clues to a better understanding of the complexity underlying the diagnostic entities.

b. The routine care setting could be recognized as an experimental laboratory (Goldberg 1985; Mollica and Jalbert 1989; Saraceno et al. 1988; Skuse and Williams 1984; Spagnoli et al. 1986). The naturally presenting large cohorts of patients are allocated to different treatments to allow comparative evaluation to be carried out periodically. The comparative burden of responsive patients, nonresponsive patients, and patients who relapse could be evaluated—for example, after 1 year—to obtain quantitative estimates. On the other hand, quantitative estimates could initiate an epidemiologically framed focus on individual or subgroup histories. In practice this could translate into choosing to recruit nonresponsive patients and patients who relapse and matched control subjects for qualitative in-depth comparative evaluation. The formal definition of the strategy could be that of a prospective case-control surveillance trial nested into an observational longitudinal study of randomly allocated or naturally occurring cohorts (Bollini et al. 1986; Susser 1991).

Some interest in this kind of approach is already present in the literature, although such studies are for the most part occasional and small, thereby providing only limited information. A large-scale, multicenter observation of routine clinical care would not only provide reassuring statistical power, but it would also allow an intrusion into the wide heterogeneity of many patients' disease histories, as opposed to traditional evaluations often focused on repetitive drugs. Such strategies need to be given priority in that they establish research as a necessary part of clinical care.

2. Of what relevance are the patient's context, life, or surroundings?
This question stems from a landmark study, curiously seldom recalled in the general psychiatric literature (and practically ignored by psychopharmacology). The WHO Pilot Study on Schizophrenia (World Health Organization 1979) showed that carefully controlled diagnostic and therapeutic comparability of cases does not necessarily entail comparability of outcomes, which seem to be more setting dependent. This finding, though not particularly new in itself, has added an important experimental—as well as institutional—weight to the diffuse, consistent, albeit fragmented, evidence.

The question is clearly related to the previous one; however, it underscores another conceptual and operational aspect of psychopharmacological research and care. Let us assume for the sake of discussion that psychotropic drugs are a central feature of the scene, if only because they are the most common and ubiquitous component of treatment. With respect to outcome, drugs will certainly continue to have an important function, albeit not a privileged status; they belong to the basket of "dirty" variables, the role of which often eludes straightforward evaluation (regardless of the degree of precision with which they may be formally defined). Their role and impact should be appreciated within the same frame of expectations generally adopted in etiological case-control studies of diseases, which defy a priori formulations of linear or quasi-causal explanations. Patients are in fact exposed to psychotropic drugs as they are exposed to other protective or risk factors; consequently, the weight attributed to the recommended pharmacological behaviors (dosage, compliance, and so on) should equal the explanatory importance assigned to other variables (e.g., time allowed to the patient, expressed emotions, social support).

Not only could retrospective case-control studies evaluate the yield of this approach across different categories of patients and settings, but prospective case-control strategies, including formal RCTs, could be planned with two specific goals: to explore the features characterizing clinically relevant subpopulations, and to favor the transformation of psychotropic drugs into one of the many environmental variables—methodologically handled and treated as such not only in research, but likewise apprehended in the psychiatric culture and care.

The need for such a research/care bridge can be further highlighted by concluding the answer to this second question—introduced by a reference to the macro-framework of the WHO study—with an explicit reference to the micro-contexts of one of the most thought-provoking lines of investigation in the area of interplay between settings and treatments: namely, the consistent findings of the research on expressed emotions (Leff and Vaughn 1980; Vaughn and Leff 1976). What the macro approach discovered via the evidence on the differences in outcomes, the micro results have linked (through well-controlled observational and experimental study designs) with identifiable causal pathways. The reproducibility of the substance of the findings with such different approaches has provided sound evidence that serves as the necessary basis for therapeutic recommendations.

Thus diagnosis is still the term of reference for therapeutic decision making and for outcome evaluation. Prospective, multicenter, service-based clinical and epidemiological investigations taking seriously the macro-micro consistency could prove illuminating as a corroboration of research findings and highly effective in improving the quality of care of important subgroups of patients currently considered "orphans" with respect to the available knowledge.

3. Can drugs originally developed for one category of disease be properly applied to the care of a newly established category of disease using the same criteria? The changing field of diagnosis was earlier singled out as probably the most important factor indicating that a re-evaluation of the role of psychotropic drugs has become due. The question can be split into two: what is the efficacy (the benefit/risk) profile of drugs experimentally tested at the time of their first introduction on carefully categorized diseases, and subsequently used for the increasingly sizable "gray" areas of psychiatry? Can psychotropic drugs be bestowed their "old" role (i.e., can they be prescribed and evaluated with unchanging criteria) among the "new" populations entering psychiatry, such as those burdened, for instance, by different kinds of posttraumatic stress disorders (Jackson 1991)?

An obvious answer could follow a positive, though reductionist, line of thought: psychotropic drugs are traditionally considered symptomatic tools; provided we do not ask too much of them, their function holds true across the board. The case of benzodiazepines and the never-ending story of antidepressants (Bollini et al. 1984b; Garattini and Samanin 1988) represent concrete examples of this attitude. Their case could also be seen, however, as suggesting the adoption of a more prospective strategy; that is, a strategy that assumes any "new" situation as an occasion for further challenge in drug assessment (of the biological, clinical, epidemiological expected profile) and as a favorable context for exploring the direction and the implications of the differences, rather than the potential similarities. What has been said for the former questions remains valid: the latter, however, points to a more substantial challenge.

The paradigm of drug development could be formally, rather than just empirically, reversed. Psychotropic drugs provide a model case for a notion that ideal drugs lack specificity but are capable of modifying favorably, albeit unpredictably, undefined components of the background noise from which "diseased" behaviors arise. Study designs, variables, and expectations again need to be carefully thought out to fit the new conceptual framework.

Concluding Remarks

Psychotropic drugs and psychopharmacology have been widely commended as a "revolution" in the control of psychiatric behaviors. Although the degree of enthusiasm might well be a matter for discussion, psychiatry, both in the specialist and in the general practice settings, could hardly be conceived of today in the absence of psychotropic drugs. For years, drug treatments have been advertised and promoted as evidence for the power of research with respect to patients and diseases. Perhaps the time has come to consider the opposite proposition—namely, the limits of current knowledge, with the significant proportion of patients and problems beyond the reach of drug treatments serving as a concrete reminder.

However, the main point is largely conceptual: contentment lies in the adoption of substantially repetitive strategies in research and care. Far from causing a sense of inadequacy and powerlessness, such a course may lead to a season of creativity in clinical and evaluative epidemiology. Unanswered needs require prolonged and sympathetic attention in order to become visible, thereby producing favorable cultural conditions in which radically innovative methodological choices may thrive (Saraceno and Tognoni 1989).

References

A critique of biological psychiatry. Psychol Med 20:3–6, 1990

Adami M, Balestrieri M, Fiorio R, et al: Il trattamento farmacologico del disturbo da attacchi di panico. Rivista di Psichiatria 22:267–279, 1987

American Psychiatric Association: Report of the Task Force on Lithium Therapy: the current status of lithium therapy. Am J Psychiatry 133:997–1001, 1975

American Psychiatric Association: Diagnostic and Statistical Manual of Mental Disorders, 3rd Edition. Washington, DC, American Psychiatric Association, 1980

Appleton WS: Principles of prescribing antipsychotics, in Practical Clinical Psychopharmacology. Edited by Appleton W. Baltimore: Williams & Wilkins, 1988

Aronson TA: Is panic disorder a distinct diagnostic entity? a critical review of the borders of a syndrome. J Nerv Ment Dis 175:584–594, 1987

Avery GS (ed): Drug Treatment, Principles and Practice of Clinical Pharmacology and Therapeutics, 3rd Edition. Sydney, Australia, Adis Press, 1980

Baldessarini RJ: Current status of antidepressants: clinical, pharmacology and therapy. J Clin Psychiatry 50:117–126, 1989

Baldessarini RJ, Cohen BM, Teicher MH: Significance of neuroleptic dose and plasma level in the pharmacological treatment of psychoses. Arch Gen Psychiatry 45:79–91, 1988

Balestrieri M, Marino S, Bellantuono C: La carbamazepina nel trattamento delle psicosi affettive. Rivista Sperimentale di Freniatria 61:1153–1164, 1987

Ballenger JC, Burrows GD, DuPont RL Jr, et al: Alprazolam in panic disorder and agoraphobia: results of a multicenter trial. Arch Gen Psychiatry 45:413–422, 1988

Beaumont G: The toxicity of antidepressants. Br J Psychiatry 154:454–458, 1989

Bellantuono C, Tansella M: Gli Psicofarmaci Nella Pratica Terapeutica, 2d Edition. Rome, Italy, Il Pensiero Scientifico Editore, 1989

Bellantuono C, Reggi V, Tognoni G, et al: Benzodiazepines: clinical pharmacology and therapeutic use. Drugs 19:195–219, 1980

Benzodiazepines on trial. BMJ 288:1101–1102, 1984

Bergen JA, Eyland EA, Campbell JA, et al: The course of tardive dyskinesia in patients on long-term neuroleptics. Br J Psychiatry 154:523–528, 1989

Biziere K, Garattini S, Simon P (eds): Diagnostic et traitement de la depression: quo vadis? Montpellier, France, Groupe Sanofi, 1987

Blackwell B: Newer antidepressant drugs, in Psychopharmacology: The Third Generation of Progress. Edited by Meltzer HY. New York, Raven Press, 1987

Bollini P, Andreani A, Colombo F, et al: High-dose neuroleptics: uncontrolled clinical practice confirms controlled clinical trials. Br J Psychiatry 144:25–27, 1984a

Bollini P, Cotecchia S, De Blasi A, et al: Drugs: guide and caveats to explanatory and descriptive approaches, II: drugs in psychiatric research. J Psychiatr Res 18:391–400, 1984b

Bollini P, Muscettola G, Piazza A, et al: Mental health care in Southern Italy: application of case-control methodology for the evaluation of the impact of the 1978 psychiatric reform. Psychol Med 16:701–707, 1986

Bradley PB: Pharmacology of antipsychotic drugs, in The Psychopharmacology and Treatment of Schizophrenia. Edited by Bradley PB, Hirsch SR. Oxford, England, Oxford University Press, 1986

Breier A, Wolkowitz OM, Doran AR, et al: Neuroleptic responsivity of negative and positive symptoms in schizophrenia. Am J Psychiatry 144:1549–1555, 1987

Buspirone: a radical advance in the treatment of anxiety? Lancet i:804–806, 1988

Ciompi L: The natural history of schizophrenia in the long term. Br J Psychiatry 136:413–420, 1980

Committee on Safety of Medicines Update. Adverse reactions to antidepressants. BMJ 291:1638, 1985

Dickson WE, Kendell RE: Does maintenance lithium therapy prevent recurrences of mania under ordinary clinical conditions? Psychol Med 16:521–530, 1986

Feighner JP: Benzodiazepines as antidepressants, in Modern Problems of Pharmacopsychiatry. Edited by Ban TA. Basel, Switzerland, Karger, 1982

Garattini S, Samanin R: Biochemical hypotheses on antidepressant drugs: a guide for clinicians or a toy for pharmacologists? Psychol Med 18:287–304, 1988

Gitlin MJ, Cochran SD, Redfield-Jamson K: Maintenance lithium treatment: side effects and compliance. J Clin Psychiatry 50:127–131, 1989

Goa KL, Ward A: Buspirone: a preliminary review of its pharmacological properties and therapeutic efficacy as an anxiolytic. Drugs 32:114–129, 1986

Goldberg D: Identifying psychiatric illness among general medical patients. BMJ 291:161–162, 1985

Guimon J: The biases of psychiatric diagnosis. Br J Psychiatry 154:33–36, 1989

Hartmann W, Kind J, Meyer JE, et al: Neuroleptic drugs and the prevention of relapse in schizophrenia: a workshop report. Schizophr Bull 6:536–541, 1980

Higgitt AC, Lader MH, Fonagy P: Clinical management of benzodiazepine dependence. BMJ 291:688–690, 1985

Hollister LE: Current antidepressant drugs: their clinical use. Drugs 22:129–152, 1981

Jackson G: The rise of post-traumatic stress disorders. BMJ 303:533–534, 1991

Jain AK, Kelwala S, Gershon S: Antipsychotic drugs in schizophrenia: current issues. Int Clin Psychopharmacol 3:1–30, 1988

Johnson DAW: Treatment of chronic schizophrenia, in Haloperidol Decanoate and Treatment of Chronic Schizophrenia. Edited by Johnson DAW. Auckland, New Zealand, Adis Press, 1982

Johnson DAW: Antipsychotic medication: clinical guidelines for maintenance therapy. J Clin Psychiatry 46:6–15, 1985

Judd FK, Normann TR, Burrows GD: Pharmacological treatment of panic disorder. Int Clin Psychopharmacol 1:3–16, 1986

Kane JM: Antipsychotic drug side effects: their relationship to dose. J Clin Psychiatry 46:16–21, 1985

Kane JM: The current status of neuroleptic therapy. J Clin Psychiatry 50:322–328, 1989

Kane JM, Woerner M, Lieberman JA: The prevalence of tardive dyskinesia. Psychopharmacol Bull 21:136–139, 1985

Kessler KA, Waletsky JP: Clinical use of the antipsychotics. Am J Psychiatry 138:202–209, 1981

Klerman G: Future prospects for clinical psychopharmacology, in Psychopharmacology: The Third Generation of Progress. Edited by Meltzer HY. New York, Raven Press, 1986

Lader M: Antipsychotic drugs, in Introduction to Psychopharmacology. Kalamazoo, MI, The Upjohn Company, 1980

Lader M: A practical guide to prescribing hypnotic benzodiazepines. BMJ 293:1048–1049, 1986

Lader M: Clinical pharmacology of benzodiazepines. Ann Rev Med 38:19–28, 1987a

Lader M: The biological basis of benzodiazepine dependence. Psychol Med 17:539–547, 1987b

Lader M, Petursson H: Rational use of anxiolytic/sedative drugs. Drugs 25:514–528, 1983

Leff J, Vaughn C: The interaction of life events and relative expressed emotion in schizophrenia and depressive neurosis. Br J Psychiatry 136:146–153, 1980

Leff J, Vaughn C: The role of maintenance therapy and relatives' expressed emotions in relapse of schizophrenia: a two-year follow-up. Br J Psychiatry 139:102–104, 1981

MacKay AVP: Antischizophrenic drugs, in Drugs in Psychiatric Practice. Edited by Tyrer PJ. London, Butterworths, 1982

MacKay AVP, Crow IJ: Positive and negative schizophrenic symptoms and the role of dopamine. Br J Psychiatry 137:379–386, 1980

Marsden CD, Mindham RH, MacKay AV: Extrapiramidal movement disorders produced by antipsychotic drugs, in The Psychopharmacology and Treatment of Schizophrenia. Edited by Bradley PB, Hirsch SR. Oxford, England, Oxford University Press, 1986

Mattick RP, Andrews G, Hadzi-Pavlovic D, Christensen H: Treatment of panic and agoraphobia: an integrative review. J Nerv Ment Dis 178:567–576, 1990

Mollica RF, Jalbert RR: Community of Confinement: The Mental Health Crisis in Site Two (Displaced Persons Camps on the Thai-Kampuchean Border). World Federation for Mental Health, 1989

Muscettola G, Barbato G: Similarities and dissimilarities in the action of antidepressant drugs, in Diagnosis and Treatment of Depression: Quo Vadis? Edited by Biziere K, Garattini S, Simon P. Montpellier, France, Groupe Sanofi, 1987

Nicholson AN: Hypnotics: their place in therapeutics. Drugs 31:164–176, 1986

Paykel ES: Depressive typologies and response to amitriptyline. Br J Psychiatry 120:147–156, 1972

Paykel ES: Classification of depression and response to treatment, in Diagnosis and Treatment of Depression: Quo Vadis? Edited by Biziere K, Garattini S, Simon P. Montpellier, France, Groupe Sanofi, 1987

Potter WZ, Rudorfer MV, Manji H: Drug therapy: the pharmacologic treatment of depression. New Engl J Med 325:633–642, 1991

Quitkin FM: The importance of dosage in prescribing antidepressants. Br J Psychiatry 147:593–597, 1985

Robinson DS, Kurtz NM: Monoamine oxidase inhibiting drugs: pharmacological and therapeutic issue, in Psychopharmacology: The Third Generation of Progress. Edited by Meltzer HY. New York, Raven Press, 1987

Rosenbaum JF: The drug treatment of anxiety. New Engl J Med 306:401–404, 1982

Rudorfer MV, Potter WZ: Antidepressants: a comparative review of the clinical pharmacology and therapeutic use of the "newer" versus the "older" drugs. Drugs 37:713–738, 1989

Saraceno B, Tognoni G: Methodological lessons from the Italian psychiatric experience. Int J Soc Psychiatry 35:98–109, 1989

Saraceno B, Asioli F, Tognoni G: Manual de Salud Mental Guia Basica Para Atencion Primaria. Milano, Italy, Ministerio de Salud de Nicaragua-OPS/OMS, 1986

Saraceno B, Asioli F, Tognoni G, et al: Laying foundations for improved care of mentally ill. World Health Forum 9:542–545, 1988

Schatzberg AF, Cole JO: Benzodiazepines in the treatment of depressive borderline personality and schizophrenia disorders. Br J Clin Pharmacol 11:17S–22S, 1981

Schmidt LG, Grohmann R, Muller-Oerlinghausen B, et al: Adverse drug reactions to first and second generation antidepressants: a critical evaluation of drug surveillance data. Br J Psychiatry 148:38–43, 1986

Simpson GM, Yadalam K: Blood levels of neuroleptics: state of art. J Clin Psychiatry 46:22–28, 1985

Skuse D, and Williams P: Screening for psychiatric disorders in general practice. Psychol Med 14:365–377, 1984

Soderpalm B: Pharmacology of the benzodiazepines; with special emphasis on alprazolam. Acta Psychiatr Scand 76(suppl 335): 39–46, 1987

Spagnoli A, Foresti G, MacDonald A, et al: Dementia and depression in Italian geriatric institutions. International Journal of Geriatric Psychiatry 1:15–23, 1986

Stahl SM: Tardive dyskinesia: natural history studies assist the pursuit of preventive therapies. Psychol Med 16:491–494, 1986

Sternai E, Bolongaro G, Bressi S, et al: Lettera Percorsi Bibliografici in Psichiatria, I-XI. Milano, Italy, Istituto "Mario Negri," 1985–1991

Susser M: What is a cause and how do we know one? A grammar for pragmatic epidemiology. Am J Epidemiol 133:635–648, 1991

Tognoni G: Per una definizione dell'oggetto (revisione della letteratura psicofarmacologica: 1981–1986), in Lettera IV Percorsi Bibliografici in Psichiatria. Milan, Italy, Istituto "Mario Negri," 1987

Tognoni G, Bignami G: The confounding role of institution in scientific evaluation, in Epidemiological Impact of Psychotropic Drugs. Edited by Tognoni G, Bellantuono C, Lader M. Amsterdam, Netherlands, Elsevier North-Holland, 1981

Tognoni G, Bellantuono C, Lader M (eds): Epidemiological Impact of Psychotropic Drugs. Amsterdam, Netherlands, Elsevier North-Holland, 1981

Treatment of depression in medical patients. Lancet i:949–950, 1986

Tyrer P, Ashton H, Rubin P: Risks of dependence on benzodiazepine drugs. BMJ 298:102–105, 1989

Van Putten T, Marder S, May RA, et al: Plasma levels of haloperidol and clinical response. Psychopharmacol Bull 21:69–72, 1985

Vaughn CE, Leff JP: The influence of family and social factors on the course of psychiatric illness: a comparison of schizophrenic and depressed neurotic patients. Br J Psychiatry 129:125–137, 1976

Waller DG, Edwards G: Lithium and the kidney: an update. Psychol Med 19:825–833, 1989

Wood AJ, Goodwin GM: A review of the biochemical and neuropharmacological actions of lithium. Psychol Med 17:579–600, 1987

World Health Organization: The Selection of Essential Drugs. Report of a WHO Expert Committee. Technical Report Series 615. Geneva, Switzerland, World Health Organization, 1977

World Health Organization: Schizophrenia: An International Follow-Up Study. New York, John Wiley, 1979

World Health Organization: The Use of Essential Drugs. Report of a WHO Expert Committee. Technical Report Series 770. Geneva, Switzerland, World Health Organization, 1988

CHAPTER 4

Biological Treatments Other Than Drugs

(Electroconvulsive Therapy, Brain Surgery, Insulin Therapy, and Phototherapy)

Thomas G. Bolwig, M.D.

Electroconvulsive Therapy

Background and Development

Convulsive therapy was originally introduced by Meduna (1937), who induced seizures in schizophrenic patients with camphor. The introduction of electroconvulsive therapy (ECT) should be attributed to Cerletti and Bini (1938). Kalinowsky (1939) had the first publication in the English language.

To prevent distortions and fractures due to convulsive movements, the use of curare was introduced (Bennett 1940). As used in most countries today, ECT is modified by brief anesthesia, relaxation with succinylcholine, and artificial ventilation with oxygen (Holmberg and Tesleff 1952).

A further development in ECT has been the placement of both electrodes over the right hemisphere (Lancaster et al. 1958). Using this unilateral electrode placement, Lancaster et al., and later Valentine et al. (1968), d'Elia (1970), Strömgren (1973), and Heshe et al. (1978), found that the difference between bilateral and unilateral electrode placement with respect to therapeutic outcome was small, whereas the original bilateral electrode placement produced greater cognitive impairment. In recent years these findings have been challenged in studies by Abrams et al. (1983), Abrams (1986), and Sackeim et al. (1987). With respect to both clinical considerations and neurobiological findings, the unilateral-bilateral controversy has given rise to a number of unanswered questions. Because the cognitive effects following ECT are partially due to the intensity of the electrical stimulus, a modification of the electrical stimulation has been made substituting the sine-wave stimulation with short, discrete pulses (Liberson 1953; Weaver et al. 1974).

Careful estimation of the seizure threshold (Sackeim et al. 1986) is a method whereby a more precise administration of ECT can lead to safer clinical results with fewer unwanted effects on cognitive functions.

Indications

Convulsive therapy was first introduced for the treatment of schizophrenia, but clinical experience soon showed that it was more effective for depressive illness (melancholia) in particular and affective disorders in general. Because of modification of ECT with the use of anesthesia and short-acting muscle relaxant, this treatment has been widely accepted by psychiatrists on the grounds that it is effective, seems to give better and quicker results than antidepressant drugs, is safe, has very few contraindications, and finally, side effects are usually only minor (see critical evaluation in the discussion of the efficacy of ECT in treating depression, below). The most important indications are reviewed in the section on efficacy, below.

Depression

It has been generally accepted that among the various subtypes of depression the endogenous one has a very good response. Through the 1950s and 1960s a number of studies suggested that endogenous-like symptoms may predict ECT outcome. The search over the last 20 years, however, has consistently indicated that with samples being restricted to major depressive disorder, these symptoms (or the subtypes of endogenous or melancholic depression) no longer have predictive value (Abrams 1988; Hamilton 1986).

There is general agreement that ECT is especially efficacious when delusions are present in a depressive syndrome (Chodoff et al. 1950; Hamilton and White 1960; Johnstone et al. 1980). The distinctions among the subtypes of depressive disorders listed in the DSM-III (American Psychiatric Association 1980) and of the Research Diagnostic Criteria (Spitzer et al. 1978) are not related to outcome (Rich et al. 1984). This applies also to the subtypes distinguished by Paykel (see Paykel et al. 1974) and the more important distinction between unipolar and bipolar depression (Abrams and Taylor 1974).

Mania

Before the introduction of neuroleptics, the treatment for mania was convulsive therapy. ECT has a rapid effect on mania (Fink 1979; Kalinowsky and Hoch 1952; Small 1985a, 1985b). Today ECT is used for mania only occasionally, primarily in therapy-resistant patients or patients who cannot tolerate medication. ECT and lithium, with or without antipsychotic drugs, have been found to be equivalent in efficacy (Alexander et al. 1988; Black et al. 1987). Recent controlled prospective studies found ECT as effective or more so than pharmacotherapy (Milstein et al. 1987; Mukherjee et al. 1986; Small et al. 1988). In the light of these data ECT should be considered in a number of cases, particularly because up to 30% of manic patients respond poorly to medication. In pregnant manic patients ECT is often the only effective treatment alternative.

Schizophrenia

In the first decades of its use, convulsive therapy was seen as an effective treatment for psychotic manifestations in patients whose duration of illness was relatively brief (Kalinowsky and Hoch 1952; Meduna 1937). Today ECT is mainly used for schizophrenic patients who are drug refractory or intolerant of medication, especially when catatonic or affective symptoms or a history of a positive response to ECT is evident. Some schizophrenic episodes recently have been found to respond rapidly to ECT, especially when there is affective symptomatology (Brandon et al. 1984; Gregory et al. 1985; Taylor and Fleminger 1980). Further, good results have been found in patients with schizoaffective or schizophreniform disorder (Black et al. 1987; Tsuang et al. 1979). Schizophrenic patients with a chronic course respond less favorably, especially when there are no affective or catatonic symptoms (Salzman 1980).

Other Indications

Delirious conditions. Delirious conditions often respond extremely well to one or a very few ECT treatments (Heshe and Röder 1976; Kramp and Bolwig 1981). This is an acknowledged clinical condition in the Scandinavian countries (Heshe and Röder 1976), and case reports have indicated the usefulness of ECT in delirium with clouded consciousness.

Epilepsy. ECT has a major effect on seizure threshold and duration, and this anticonvulsant effect can be used in the treatment of epileptic patients with and without psychiatric symptoms (Caplan 1946; Kalinowsky and Kennedy 1943; Sackeim et al. 1983).

Parkinson's disease. A large number of clinical observations and controlled studies have shown a solid effect of ECT in Parkinson's disease, whether or not it is complicated by depression. Virtually all case reports of patients with Parkinson's disease receiving ECT describe a favorable effect on both depression and Parkinsonian motor symptoms (Asnis 1977; Balldin et al. 1981; Dysken et al. 1976; Young et al. 1985). The major indication is Parkinson's disease with on-off phenomena (Balldin et al. 1981).

Tardive dyskinesia. Some reports point to a beneficial effect of ECT in some cases of tardive dyskinesia (for review, see Abrams 1988).

Neuroleptic malignant syndrome. For this condition, the background of which is not fully understood, but which may involve adrenergic blockade or hypoactivity in striatal and hypothalamic neurons, there are several recent reports pointing to a successful outcome using ECT. Davis et al. (1991) recently published a review of 734 published cases of neuroleptic malignant syndrome (NMS). Forty-eight of those subjects received ECT either during or shortly after an episode of NMS and were compared to control subjects who received no specific treatment for their episode. The authors found a better outcome in the drug-treated or ECT-treated groups compared to the group receiving no specific treatment, and concluded that ECT is safe to use shortly after an episode of acute

NMS and further that ECT is probably safe in the actual treatment of NMS provided concomitant neuroleptics are discontinued.

Relative Contraindications

ECT normally will give rise to increased blood pressure and pulse rate and increased cerebral blood flow (CBF). Special caution should be observed in the presence of cerebral or aortic aneurysms or raised intracranial pressure, and when there is a history of cerebral hemorrhage. Recent myocardial infarction and cardiac arrhythmia should be considered relative contraindications to ECT. Pregnancy, pulmonary tuberculosis, diabetes mellitus, and bone fractures are not contraindications. In the presence of cerebral infections or inflammatory states, ECT should only be given when life-threatening delirium, which cannot be controlled with drugs, is developing. In this rare situation each treatment should be considered separately and administered only in an intensive care unit.

In conclusion, no contraindication to ECT is absolute, and even relative contraindications are few. It is more pertinent to talk in terms of level of risk rather than in terms of contraindication (American Psychiatric Association 1990).

Efficacy of ECT

Following the classic work of Ottosson (1960) it was assumed that elicitation of a generalized seizure is essential to the therapeutic process (d'Elia et al. 1983) and that there was a relation between stimulus intensity and unwanted side effects.

Over the last decade, Robin and de Tissera (1982) and Sackeim et al. (1991) showed that the relationships between seizure and efficacy and stimulus intensity in cognitive disturbance are not as simple as had been assumed. In their study, Robin and de Tissera (1982) suggested that the quantity of current, as well as the induction of the convulsion, is relevant to the therapeutic outcome with ECT; furthermore, in two random-assignment, double-blind studies, Sackeim et al. (1991) showed that unilateral ECT administered with an electrical dose just above seizure threshold had a response rate of approximately 20% versus a rate of about 70% for comparison bilateral ECT-conditions. The speed of clinical response with both unilateral and bilateral ECT was sensitive to electrical dose. Both the efficacy and efficiency (speed) of unilateral and bilateral ECT were associated with the degree to which the stimulus dose exceeded the seizure threshold and not with the absolute electrical dose administered, with the former determining dosing effects on clinical outcome and on the magnitude of cognitive deficits. Thus generalized seizures that lack therapeutic properties can be reliably produced. Based on these results from carefully conducted studies, the practice of administering the same absolute electrical dose to all patients is no longer tenable. Electrical dosage should be adjusted to meet the needs of individual patients, a recommendation that is consistent with the guidelines of the American Psychiatric Association task force report on ECT (American Psychiatric Association 1990).

In the following sections, a number of studies dealing with the relative efficacy of ECT in depression, mania, schizophrenia, and other disorders will be reviewed.

Depression

The chief use of ECT is in patients with major depression. In general, controlled studies investigating the effects of ECT on depressive disorders can be separated into retrospective and prospective categories, with the latter being broken down further into groups that compare ECT either with sham ECT (the use of general anesthesia to convince patients that they have received ECT) or with tricyclic antidepressant drugs (TCAs), monoamine oxidase inhibitors (MAOIs), and placebo.

Controlled studies of ECT.   In the 1960s, two trials established the efficacy of ECT for treating depression relative to the then-recently introduced antidepressant drugs: a trial in the United States by Greenblatt et al. (1964) and one in the United Kingdom (Cawley et al. 1965). Each group examined ECT relative to imipramine, a MAOI, and placebo in a series of at least 250 inpatients with depression. The results of these two studies were remarkably similar. At the end of the first trial (Greenblatt et al. 1964), 91% were judged at least moderately improved and 76% markedly improved with ECT, and in the second trial (Cawley et al. 1965) 84% were judged improved and 71% had no or only slight symptoms. The comparisons with the percentage of patients improved on placebo showed advantages for ECT significant at the 1% level.

Together, data from these trials indicated that ECT is at least as effective as antidepressant medication and perhaps more rapid in its action. Neither of these trials was conducted blind with respect to ECT. Clinicians as well as patients knew who had received ECT. Thus these two trials did not eliminate the possibility that some aspect of the treatment procedure other than the induction of the convulsion was responsible for the therapeutic effect.

Earlier studies did attempt to cast light on the role of convulsion in the efficacy of ECT by comparing ECT with simulated (sham) ECT or other treatments in such a way that this pertinent problem could be elucidated. Crow and Johnstone (1986) reviewed ECT trials undertaken between 1953 and 1966 and six more recent trials conducted mainly in the United Kingdom between 1978 and 1985 (the essential data from these latter studies are summarized in Table 4–1). In the six latest studies, only Lambourn and Gill (1978) found no difference between sham and real ECT. These authors used for their real ECT condition a form of low-dose, right unilateral ECT subsequently found to be ineffective. The other studies showed superior efficacy for real versus sham ECT. Thus, five out of six methodologically sound studies of simulated versus real ECT in the treatment of depressive illness found both a statistically significant and clinically substantial advantage for real ECT in the depression scale scores during and immediately following the treatment course.

In summary, the strong effect of ECT in the treatment of depressive illness of sufficient severity to require inpatient admission was established in the controlled but nonblind trial of Greenblatt et al. (1964) and in the study by Cawley et al. (1965). Controlled studies of simulated versus real ECT clearly point to ECT being highly efficacious in the treatment of depressive illness and significantly more so than sham ECT.

ECT versus antidepressant medication. Among a number of retrospective studies on the effectiveness of ECT versus antidepressant medication, two should be mentioned. Avery and Winokur (1976) reviewed an investigation including a total of 609 separate psychiatric hospitalizations meeting rigorous diagnostic criteria for major depressive episode. Groups of subjects were assigned to the following treatment conditions: ECT, adequate antidepressant drug dosage (at least 4 weeks of inpatient use, with at least 150 mg/day imipramine equivalent for 2 weeks or

Table 4–1. Studies comparing real and simulated electroconvulsive therapy

Study	Sample assessed for entry	Selection criteria	Comparison groups	Blind procedure adopted
Freeman et al. 1978	Not stated	Primary depression (Hamilton and Beck >15)	2 sham + 2 real ECT	Yes
Lambourn and Gill 1978	38 patients referred for ECT	Depressive psychoses	6 sham ECT 6 real ECT	Yes
West 1981	Not stated	Primary depression (Feighner criteria)	6 sham ECT 6 real ECT	No details given
Northwick Park ECT Trial (Johnstone et al. 1980)	128 depressed inpatients	MRC 1965 (Newcastle and Feighner criteria)	8 sham ECT 8 sham ECT	Yes
Leicestershire Trial (Brandon et al. 1984)	143 depressed inpatients	Patients referred for ECT including those with retardation, delusions, and neurotic depression	Up to 8 sham ECT Up to 8 real ECT	Yes
The Nottingham ECT Study (Gregory et al. 1985)	69 depressed inpatients	Primary depression (MRC criteria)	Up to 8 sham ECT Up to 8 real ECT	Yes

Note. ECT = electroconvulsive therapy; MRC = Medical Research Council. *Source.* Adapted in part from Crow and Johnstone 1986.

more), inadequate antidepressant drug dosage, and no somatic treatment. They found that ECT produced marked improvement at a significantly higher rate (90%) than any of the other treatments (74% [adequate antidepressant drug dosage], 60% [inadequate antidepressant drug dosage], and 60% [no somatic treatment]). Coryell (1978) studied patients who received ECT for depression in the pre-antidepressant era (1920–1959) and who later received tricyclic antidepressants from 1961–1975 for different episodes. In 94% of the episodes treated with ECT there was complete recovery compared to only 53% of those treated with antidepressants.

A number of studies have provided interesting and useful insights into special aspects of the relative efficacy of the two treatment methods (i.e., ECT or antidepressant medication); these have been carefully reviewed by Abrams and Essman (1982), Janicak et al. (1985), and Rifkin (1988). All authors listed the methodological flaws of the published comparisons of ECT and antidepressant drugs in the treatment of depressive illness. Almost half of the studies could be excluded from consideration because of a retrospective design. Nonblind evaluation and faulty data analyses accounted for most of the remainder of studies discounted. In several studies patients had not been randomly assigned to treatment, there was no sure way to equate the groups for psychopathology or illness severity, the reason for physicians or patients choosing one or the other treatment could have constituted a major source of bias, there was no control of drug dosage or numbers of ECT treatments administered, and the assessment of outcome was necessarily based on the nonsystematic observations recorded at the time by nonblind clinicians with their unknown biases.

The most convincing report in the literature of ECT versus medication is the work of Janicak et al. (1985). These authors reported the only meta-analysis of the literature concerning the relative efficacy of ECT versus drug therapy, and they documented a superior response rate to ECT relative to both tricyclic antidepressants and MAOIs, with the magnitude of the differences clinically meaningful.

ECT in the medication-resistant patient. This crucial issue has been carefully reviewed by Sackeim et al. (1990a, 1990b). The work by Sackeim and colleagues (Prudic et al. 1990; Sackeim et al. 1990a, 1990b) showed that the rate of relapse following ECT treatment was substantially higher in patients who had failed adequate antidepressant medication trials prior to ECT treatment than in patients not found to be resistant to medication. The authors concluded that in patients with major depressive disorder who have not failed an adequate medication trial, 80%–90% respond to bilateral ECT. In medication-resistant depressed patients this rate may be closer to 50%. British studies from the 1960s (e.g., Medical Research Council 1965) found that post-ECT continuation with tricyclic antidepressants reduced relapse rates from 50% to 20%. Recent data (Devanand et al. 1991) are interesting because they suggest that relapse rates following ECT are high in medication-resistant patients, and during the first 4 months following clinical response. Medication resistance during the index episode seems to predict a higher rate of relapse, while patients who have not received an adequate medication trial prior to ECT seem less likely to relapse. The work of Sackeim and colleagues suggests the possibility that patients who fail an antidepressant trial with no response to ECT may be considered for alternative pharmacological strategies or maintenance ECT. Replication of this work is needed before too strong conclusions can be drawn.

Mania

ECT in the treatment of mania has been studied much less than in the treatment of either depression or schizophrenia. Surveys of practicing psychiatrists and task force reports (American Psychiatric Association 1990) indicate that ECT is still widely accepted as a treatment for mania, and mania is the third most common indication cited for ECT (American Psychiatric Association 1978; Fink 1979; Frederiksen and d'Elia 1979; Heshe and Röder 1976; Royal College of Psychiatrists 1977).

Retrospective studies have been made comparing ECT with neuroleptic medication and with no definitive treatment, showing that both somatic therapies were superior to no treatment, with minimal differences between ECT and neuroleptic medication (Alexander et al. 1988; McCabe 1976; Thomas and Reddy 1982).

Two prospective controlled trials have been conducted (Mukherjee et al. 1988; Small et al. 1988). The Small et al. study mainly compared lithium to ECT in the treatment of mania and found ECT superior; the Mukherjee et al. study group comprised patients who failed adequate treatment with lithium or neuroleptic medication. Both studies found ECT to be as effective or more so than pharmacotherapy.

Schizophrenia

Although there have been many retrospective claims suggesting that ECT is effective in treating acute schizophrenia, there is a paucity of adequate clinical trials testing those claims. May (1968) found that, in the short term, ECT used alone was significantly more effective than psychological forms of therapy, though not as effective as phenothiazines. In a double-blind trial, Taylor and Fleminger (1980) studied 20 patients who, according to the Present State Examination (PSE) criteria (Wing et al. 1974), were diagnosed as being paranoid schizophrenic. All patients received standard doses of neuroleptic medication, were randomly allocated to either real or simulated ECT, and received a maximum of 12 treatments. The group receiving real ECT treatments showed significantly greater improvement compared to the controls at the end of the trial, while during the follow-up period there was no difference between the groups. The Leicester ECT trial (Brandon et al. 1984) studied 19 patients fulfilling the PSE criteria for schizophrenia. Patients were randomly allocated to 8 real ECT or 8 simulated ECT treatments. At the end of the 4-week trial period, patients receiving real ECT showed a significantly greater improvement when measured on the Montgomery-Åsberg Schizophrenia Scale. At 12- and 28-week follow-up, the superiority of real ECT could not be demonstrated.

Predictors of Outcome

Clinical Indexes

A number of scales devised to predict response to ECT have yielded conflicting results (Abrams et al. 1973; Hamilton and White 1960; Roberts 1959). Nyström (1964) selected a number of variables correlated with the outcome and calculated individual prognostic value for each patient based on the partial regression coefficients of the items. The favorable features should be mentioned: early waking, retardation, and a profound depressed mood; unfavorable ones included inclusiveness, ideas of reference, depersonalization, obsessionality, and histrionic behavior. In the Newcastle Scale Predictive Index (Carney et al. 1965), five favorable features (weight loss, pyknic physique, early waking, somatic delusions, and paranoid delusions) and five unfavorable ones (anxiety, worsening of mood in the evening, self-pity, hypochondriasis, and hysterical traits) were shown to have a predictive accuracy of 76%.

Coryell and Zimmerman (1983) showed the presence of delusions to be the most favorable predictor variable followed by increasing age and female gender.

In the Northwick Park Trial (reported in Clinical Research Center Division of Psychiatry 1984; Johnstone et al. 1980) an attempt was made to examine some of the above-mentioned scales, and in general the outcome was disappointing. In this study the presence of delusions turned out to be the critical factor, and if this finding can be replicated it will confirm a general clinical impression and may delineate delusional depression as a distinct entity that responds especially to ECT.

Neuroendocrine Tests

During the last 15 years information linking depression and neuroendocrine abnormalities has been published. Unlike conventional pharmacotherapy, ECT links itself well to the study of both acute and chronic neuroendocrine changes. Investigations have been directed at documenting specific neuroendocrine abnormalities and also at attempting to understand whether these represent trait or state markers for depressive illness. Kamil and Joffe (1991) published a review of various neuroendocrine tests applied, subdividing them into five categories: 1) the hypothalamic-pituitary-adrenal axis, 2) the hypothalamic-pituitary-thyroid axis, 3) prolactin, 4) growth hormone, and 5) neurophysins.

Hypothalamic-pituitary-adrenal axis. The authors emphasized early data relating depression to changes in plasma cortisol and its response to oral dexamethasone (as determined by the dexamethasone suppression test [DST]). The value of the DST following the course of ECT remains controversial. It is justifiable to say that the DST remains a soft state-specific marker for major depressive illness, and that there is no clear evidence for its value as a serial test for following the course of ECT or for predicting outcome. The corticotropin-releasing factor (CRF) stimulation test may hold promise as a more reliable state marker in depression treated with ECT.

Hypothalamic-pituitary-thyroid axis. It is well documented that ECT has an effect on thyroid-stimulating hormone (TSH); further, there are findings that TSH response to thyrotropin-releasing hormone (TRH) is reduced in many patients with endogenous depression. The original work by Kirkegaard et al. (1975) has stimulated a number of investigations, among which the work of Decina et al. (1987) on the effects of ECT on the TRH stimulation test should be mentioned. Unlike Kirkegaard et al. (1975), Decina et al. (1987) found that TSH values were unable to predict prognosis of ECT in their study. Although TRH-stimulation tests show some promise as a state-dependent marker for depression treated with ECT, there are recent studies that have questioned the robustness of the finding that there is a normalization of the blunted TSH-response to TRH following successful treatment with ECT.

Prolactin. Production of the hormone prolactin has been found to increase following a convulsion; in addition, bilateral ECT yields significantly higher prolactin (PRL) levels than unilateral ECT, suggesting that bilateral ECT may demonstrate a greater hypothalamic-stimulating effect than unilateral ECT. Devanand et al. (1989) studied the possible significance of other monoamine systems mediating the rise in PRL seen with ECT. As they could not find a relationship between the acute PRL serum level increase and the rise in the dopamine metabolite homovanillic acid (HVA) following six ECT treatments, they suggested that the changes induced in PRL levels by ECT are independent of dopamine metabolism. It must be concluded that the therapeutic significance of the rise in serum-prolactin so far is unknown.

Growth hormone. Several studies have been conducted on growth hormone, and while provocative challenges with insulin-induced hypoglycemia have been reported to be associated with a blunted growth hormone response in depressed patients, this finding has not been studied adequately in patients treated with ECT and must, to date, be considered without major clinical importance in relation to ECT.

Neurophysins. Both oxytocin and vasopressin (AVP) are released in equivalent amounts as their respective carrier peptides (neurophysins). Neurophysins are easier to assay in the serum because their half-lives are longer than those of AVP and oxytocin. AVP rises following a convulsive stimulus (Sørensen et al. 1982) and oxytocin likewise is increased following a series of ECT treatments as studied in 25 patients. Only in those responding to ECT was there a significant increase in oxytocin (Bendsen et al., unpublished manuscript, 1993). The work by Scott et al. (1989) suggested that measurement of neurophysins in the plasma following an ECT series may have a clinical value in predicting a therapeutic outcome.

Concluding Remarks

From the earliest days of convulsive therapy attempts have been made to improve the selection of suitable cases (i.e., to predict which ones would show a good response to treatment). Both the clinical indexes, a number of predictive scales, and the promising area of research in neuroendocrine tests have so far not given a single test to predict the outcome of ECT. Further research, not least in the area of biological measures, should be encouraged.

Side Effects to ECT Treatment

Behavioral Morbidity With ECT

The behavioral morbidity linked with ECT is mainly associated with confusion and amnesia. The former is clearly more transient than the latter (Daniel and Crovitz 1986; Sackeim et al. 1986). Amnesia following a course of ECT varies considerably across patients both idiopathically and as function of certain treatment parameters.

The memory deficit consists of three types: 1) difficulty in remembering newly learned material (anterograde amnesia); 2) difficulty in remembering material learned prior to the initiation of the ECT (retrograde amnesia); and 3) difficulty in remembering material learned during the course of ECT. Cognitive changes associated with ECT have been the focus of intense investigation (Squire 1986), and the nature of ECT-related amnesia has been reviewed in recent years by Fink (1979), Harper and Wiens (1975), Weiner (1984), and Squire (1986). Memory impairment is a weighty issue because it is central to all discussions of adverse effects of ECT. From a patient's point of view, memory impairment is the most prominent and troublesome adverse effect of ECT.

Anterograde amnesia. This type of amnesia diminishes between ECT treatments and accumulates across treatments. It is difficult to identify exactly the point at which new learning ability reaches normal levels. Patients with anterograde amnesia following bilateral ECT in a number of studies seem to have recovered by 6 months after treatment and there is no good evidence that new learning ability is still deficient at this time (Squire and Chace 1975). Presumably, once treatment is completed recovery occurs gradually in a negative accelerated fashion over a period of many weeks.

Retrograde amnesia. This type of amnesia was studied by Janis (1950). He estimated remote memory for events that occurred before ECT, asking questions about public events that were verifiable or by asking about past autobiographical events. It was found that retrograde amnesia was present 4 weeks after the treatment course and was still present 10 to 14 weeks after treatment. In a study by Squire et al. (1981), patients treated with bilateral ECT were asked about their personal history covering the period from elementary school to the period just prior to hospitalization. Most patients given ECT and controlled patients recorded a large number of details on their first testing sessions. After ECT, patients showed a sharp reduction in the number of facts that could be recalled, while at the follow-up period 7 months later the ECT and control patients once again performed similarly. Thus, when all questions were considered together there was no indication of a persisting deficit in remote memory. In a later study, Squire and Slater (1983) found an anterograde amnesia of 2 months and a retrograde amnesia of 6 months in patients when they were questioned years after having received bilateral ECT. The authors concluded that the anterograde amnesia presumably was related to the ECT, and appeared to be an accurate assessment of missing memory. The retrograde amnesia may also have been accurate, but it was not clear how much of it should be related to ECT and how much to the depression that led up to ECT. (For further review of cognitive measurements see Squire 1986.)

Difficulty in remembering material learned during the course of ECT. The specific cognitive difficulties occurring during the course of ECT have been carefully studied by Daniel and Crovitz (1986). These investigators focused on the study of disorientation during a course of ECT. They classified the ECT-induced central nervous system dysfunction as delirium rather than as an amnestic syndrome.

It may be concluded that the results of numerous studies of memory performance after ECT still have not provided a definitive answer to the question of whether, and, if so, to what degree, ECT is associated with persistent memory loss. Fink (1979) has estimated the incidence of such a phenomenon at 0.5%, while the Royal College of Psychiatrists' survey (Pippard and Ellam 1982) showed that British psychiatrists estimated a 1% incidence for persistent deficits with unilateral ECT and 2% with bilateral ECT. The only reliable way to consider such a low-incidence phenomenon is to study large numbers of ECT and control subjects with sufficient measures, and to focus on individual responses in addition to group means.

Neuropathological Changes

ECT is controversial because of its inherent involvement with electrical stimulation of the brain and seizure production, its cognitive side effect, and its effect on cerebral physiology and metabolism (Weiner 1984). These factors have raised the concern that ECT may produce structural brain damage, an issue that continues to have a major impact on the acceptance of ECT as a therapeutic modality, within both the medical community and among the public at large.

The question of whether ECT causes damage to cerebral structures has been examined experimentally in animals and with correlative autopsy and radiological studies in humans. A great number of animal studies previously performed have been reviewed by Weiner (1984). Many of those in which structural changes following epileptic seizures were reported were performed under conditions quite dissimilar to the seizures induced by ECT in humans, partly because the seizures induced were long-lasting, often lasting more than 1 hour, or because brief seizures were repeated in large numbers, sometimes without oxygenation and muscle relaxation. In studies of neuropathology in animals, including cell counts in regions thought to be at the highest risk, there has been no evidence of brain damage when the seizures are induced under conditions that approximate standard clinical practice (i.e., when the seizures are spaced, relatively brief, and modified by oxygenation and muscle relaxation) (Dam and Dam 1986; Meldrum 1986). Study of the pathophysiology of seizure-induced structural brain damage in animals has indicated that the conditions necessary for injury do not apply to the modern practice of ECT (Ingvar 1986; Siesjö et al. 1991). These animal studies are important, as they allow a closer look at both cellular and subcellular consequences in such a way that it is possible to draw conclusions concerning the effect of seizures, and the results are not impeded by coexisting age- or illness-related cerebral impairment.

It is, however, necessary to look closely at research in humans because of the possibility that the more complex human brain may be more vulnerable to seizure-induced brain injury. There are only few studies of humans dying during a course of ECT (reviewed in Abrams 1988), and in those the interpretations of the findings were confounded by the effects of agonal changes as most such patients sustained cardiovascular deaths. A number of studies applying pneumoencephalography and computed tomography (CT) have been used to examine premortem anatomic effects of ECT in humans, but the investigations have been severely limited by retrospective methods and a lack of systematic approach in identifying possible ECT-related changes (Menken et al. 1979; Weinberger et al. 1979; Weiner 1984).

In a recent carefully conducted prospective study of the effects of ECT on brain structures using magnetic resonance imaging (MRI), Coffey et al. (1991) looked at 35 inpatients with depression who completed a course of brief-pulse bilateral ECT. The MRI images were analyzed blindly for evidence of changes in brain structure using two approaches: measurement of regional brain volumes and a pairwise global comparison. The result was that the course of ECT produced no acute or delayed (6 months) change in brain structures, and the findings confirmed previous imaging studies that also found no relationship between ECT and brain damage. The data of the Coffey et al. (1991) study also failed to support earlier suggestions, based on retrospective studies, pointing to ECT courses resulting in lateral ventricular enlargements or frontal lobe atrophy (Andreasen et al. 1990; Calloway et al. 1981). The Coffey et al. (1991) study underlines the serious limitations that may be inherent in retrospective studies that report associations between previous forms of treatment (e.g., ECT) and later brain imaging abnormalities, because such abnormalities may have been present before the therapy, as was also evidenced by the prevalence of pre-ECT brain MRI abnormalities noted in the Coffey et al. (1991) study. In that investigation it was also interesting to note, that these abnormalities did not change during the 6-month follow-up period. Because the majority of the patients improved clinically the abnormalities can hardly be considered state markers for affective illness.

Concluding Remarks

Evidence that ECT given in a contemporary fashion should lead to the development of brain damage and its lasting physiological and cognitive correlates is weak. However, in light of data from studies that have suggested possible ECT-related effects on autobiographical memory for recent events and in light of subjective complaints, there should be further definitive research. Even with these weak doubts, when considering ECT it should be remembered that patients for whom such a treatment modality is considered are typically profoundly ill, not uncommonly with debilitating if not life-threatening manifestations, and alternatives to ECT often display a wide range of risks and side effects, some affecting central nervous system function. These adverse effects in many cases may well represent a greater overall risk than that associated with ECT.

Technical Applications of ECT

Interest in the physical characteristics of the electrical stimulus for ECT has been biphasic: an initial peak in research interest from 1940 to 1955 was followed by 20 years in which no research in this area was done, again followed by a rise in interest around 1975, which has increased to the present. Recent investigations into the nature of the electrical stimulus for ECT have built upon many of the principles elaborated during the early years, but with more precise quantification of their relation to cognitive and electroencephalographic (EEG) effects.

Stimulus Waveform

The electrical stimulus in ECT treatment can be delivered in an infinite variety of forms, of which the two most common are the sine-wave and brief-pulse. (For further details, see Weaver and Williams 1982.)

Sine-wave current is now considered obsolete for ECT (Weaver and Williams 1982) and the British Government has ordered the replacement of all sine-wave devices in its National Health Service Hospitals with brief-pulse instruments (Health Service Management 1982).

Unilateral and Bilateral Electrode Placement

As mentioned earlier, it is still an unresolved issue whether right unilateral ECT should be considered equal to bilateral ECT. A great number of studies have recently been reviewed and discussed by Ottosson (1991) and Sackeim et al. (1991).

The controversy over the comparative efficacy of unilateral versus bilateral ECT has not been laid to rest despite over 30 comparative trials. This points to future studies in which bilateral and unilateral modalities will be considered under conditions predetermined to be most favorable to ECT (e.g., low-dosage bilateral versus high-dosage unilateral).

Concluding Remarks

To obtain grand mal activity it is necessary to give a suprathreshold amount of electrical energy and to diminish confusion and memory disturbances to avoid excess dosage of electricity. Therefore ECT should be given with brief-pulses and not with sine-wave current.

In its recent task force report on ECT treatment, the American Psychiatric Association (1990) pointed to the combination of bilateral electrode placement and high stimulus intensity being likely to maximize cognitive deficits without conferring additional therapeutic advantage. The report recommended that the determination of which electrode placement to use should, therefore, be made in concert with stimulus intensity considerations.

ECT and the High-Risk Patient

ECT is a low-risk procedure. Recent mortality statistics of 2 deaths per 100,000 treatments (Kramer 1985) places it at the low end of the range reported for anesthesia induction alone—less risky, in fact, than childbirth. There seems to have been an improvement over the previous decade's best estimate for 4 deaths per 100,000 treatments (Heshe and

Röder 1976). The safety of ECT combined with an increasingly precise understanding of its medical physiology and the widespread availability of advanced monitoring techniques (e.g., EEG, electrocardiography [ECG]) now enables its routine and successful application in a population of patients hitherto believed to be too old or physically ill to undergo the stress of induced convulsions—the *high-risk patient*.

Recent reviews of the use of ECT in high-risk patients (Abrams 1988; 1989) reported a number of measures—often sophisticated—that can be used in patients with physical conditions that would have made ECT impossible during its earlier use. The most severe complications included acute myocardial infarction, coronary insufficiency, ventricular fibrillation, myocardial rupture, cardiac arrest, cardiovascular collapse, stroke, and ruptured cerebral or aortic aneurysm. Although their occurrence is extremely rare, such complications constitute the primary mortality risk with ECT (Hurwitz 1974; Ungerleider 1960).

As mentioned above, there are relative contraindications for ECT, but in well-equipped modern hospitals there are today possibilities to counteract the increased risk of patients with both cardiovascular problems and other severe medical conditions, especially through the prevention of the sympathoadrenal cardiovascular effects of ECT with ganglionic-blocking agents such as trimethaphan, nitroprusside, diazoxide as well as with lidocaine and propranolol.

Basic Research in ECT

It is outside the scope of this review to discuss the working action of ECT. However, it should be mentioned that with the explosion of knowledge within the area of neuroscience, hundreds of papers concerning basic research issues related to ECT have appeared over the last two decades. Studies have concentrated on neurotransmitter and receptor mechanisms and neuroendocrine aspects. Among many theories for the working action of seizures a few have concentrated on neurochemical events going on in deep brain structures (see Bolwig 1984; Bolwig and Jørgensen 1986; Fink 1986).

During the last 5 years two multi-authored books have appeared covering both basic and clinic research aspects of ECT: Lerer et al. (1984) and Malitz et al. (1986).

The advancement in brain imaging techniques (computerized EEG, regional cerebral blood flow [single photon emission computed tomography], metabolism [positron emission tomography], MRI) goes hand in hand with experimental studies using the most sophisticated methods to investigate events taking place in and about the synapse. Further, it does not seem unlikely that by the turn of the century ECT may be the best understood treatment modality in psychiatry.

The Public Image of ECT

ECT generally has had bad press. This is due to a variety of factors. Before the days of modern ECT the treatment was dramatic and not infrequently followed by fractures and subluxation. There has been abuse of ECT, and the treatment has been described in a very negative way in popular movies such as *One Flew Over the Cuckoo's Nest* and *Frances*. Especially in the United States an anti-ECT lobby with occasional support from members of the medical profession has been operating successfully. In Europe ECT to many has been linked to something old-fashioned, brutal, and brain-damaging, which was created in a politically dark period. Also, it is difficult for the clinician who wants to treat a melancholic patient with ECT to make the relatives understand that the symptoms of the disease, often experienced by friends and family as exaggerated manifestations of normal "crisis" phenomena, should be treated with induced seizures in the unconscious patient. However, recent public surveys have revealed an unexpectedly overall positive attitude toward ECT (Baxter et al. 1986; Kalayam and Steinhart 1981).

Patients' attitudes toward ECT were studied by Freeman and Kendell (1980); the authors found that almost one-half of 166 patients who had received ECT from 1 to 6 years earlier had no particular feelings prior to receiving their first ECT. More than 80% of the patients said that having ECT was no worse than a visit to the dentist, but nonetheless only 65% reported that they would be willing to have it again. Half of the patients felt that memory impairment was the worst side effect, and 30% felt that their memory had never returned to normal afterward. A review by Freeman and Cheshire (1986) showed that most patients having had ECT did not find the treatment especially frightening, upsetting, painful, or unpleasant.

Although there seems to be a slight change in the attitude of the public toward ECT, it should be considered important that further research be done, both in the basic and the clinical issues concerning this treatment modality.

Summary

ECT has been in use for a little more than 50 years. During this period the indications for its use have changed from being a therapy for schizophrenic patients to mainly an antidepressant therapy. Concerning the efficacy of ECT, the indications for the use of ECT, the risks and adverse effects, the administration of ECT, and the directions for future research, the reader is referred to the important statement developed at the National Institutes of Health (1985) regarding ECT.

Psychosurgery

Background and Present Status

Psychosurgery performed in the 1940s and 1950s were radical frontal leukotomies in which a large section of white matter was severed between the frontal lobes and the rest of the brain. A review is given by Tooth and Newton (1961).

Standard frontal leukotomy is now viewed with clinical revulsion, and a number of psychosurgical operations have declined considerably. A variety of technical modifications have been developed; taken together they could be named stereotactic limbic leukotomy. Numerous anecdotal reports point to psychosurgery being effective in certain groups of patients, especially those with chronic depressive illness and obsessive-compulsive disorder.

Controlled studies are impossible to perform. Among careful clinical descriptions, those of Göktepe et al. (1975) and Mitchell-Heggs et al. (1976) should be mentioned. These investigators found that affective symptoms and anxiety were most effectively relieved in operated schizophrenic patients. Kelly (1980) reported an overall improvement rate of 63% in schizophrenic patients with "distressing psychotic symptoms or high levels of anxiety, depression or obsessions."

Using the PSE, Curson et al. (1983) conducted a careful study of the outcome of stereotactic limbic leukotomy. The interviews were done by two specially trained research assistants who were blind to the independent assessments of outcome. In a sample of 34 patients with intractable depression, anxiety, tension, and obsessional states who were interviewed prior to the operation and again one year postoperatively, the authors found an overall improvement. No patients were significantly worse, and the symptoms that improved were nervous tension, depressed mood, and somatic anxiety. The investigators could not identify symptomatic predictors of outcome.

In a retrospective Danish study by Hansen et al. (1982), the authors concluded that 60% to 80% of the depressive patients were cured or improved as a result of the operation. A few investigations even found an improvement percentage approaching 100. Improvement was found in 40%–60% of anxiety states and in 50%–60% of obsessional states, while more than 80% of the patients with obsessional symptoms were found improved or cured by limbic leukotomy.

Jenike et al. (1991) made a long-term follow-up of 33 patients who had undergone one or more cingulotomy operations as a treatment of intractable obsessive-compulsive disorder. Six patients were deceased, four of whom took their own lives. Among the remainder of the patients 9% had easily controlled seizures and 6% transient mania. Using very conservative criteria the authors estimated that at least 25%–30% of the patients benefited substantially from this procedure.

There are no reports of studies conducted under circumstances reasonably comparable to the studies reported for the evaluation of outcome of psychotropic drugs or ECT.

Concluding Remarks

Psychosurgery is the term at present used to denote the treatment of certain psychiatric disorders by the destruction of apparently normal brain tissue. One of the best reviews of the current situation in psychosurgery is the position endorsed by the Canadian Psychiatric Association (Earp 1979). This review summarizes the evidence for the effectiveness of psychosurgery and also delineates the main strands of opinion that have influenced professional and public attitudes about this treatment.

The indiscriminate use of this type of therapy is a major factor that has led to disquiet, so that the procedure has been abandoned or made illegal in many parts of the world (Snaith et al. 1984). The best results seem to come in the treatment of chronic depression and obsessive-compulsive disorder.

The recommendations given in the 1983 British Mental Health Act should be considered. Section 57 of the act requires that a medical practitioner, other than the responsible medical officer, appointed by the secretary of state, shall, together with two other people who are not medical practitioners, certify in writing that the patient is capable of understanding the nature, purpose, and likely effects of the operation and has consented to it. The appointed medical practitioner must then consult with two other persons who have been concerned with the patient's treatment, one of whom must be a nurse and the other neither a nurse nor a medical practitioner, and the medical practitioner must then certify in writing that, having regard to the likelihood of the treatment alleviating or preventing a deterioration of the patient's condition, the operation should be carried out. These requirements point to the need for close liaison between members of the psychosurgical team and the hospital staff who have been concerned with the treatment of the patient. This requirement will impose problems if large distances separate the two locations.

Insulin Therapy

Techniques

Treatment with insulin was introduced in Vienna by Manfred Sakel (1935), who found that the withdrawal or deprivation symptoms in morphine addicts did not occur if limited doses of insulin were given. Before that time, small doses of insulin had been used, for example, by Klemperer (1926) in the treatment of delirium tremens. It was also used to overcome refusal of food and to build up run-down patients, but the dosage in these treatments was small, and only mild hypoglycemia was produced.

Before the introduction of ECT and neuroleptics, insulin was used extensively, having spread to most European countries, particularly

Switzerland, as well as to Japan and the United States. Very favorable responses were reported by numerous authors (for a review see Kalinowsky and Hippius 1969).

The original form of insulin treatment was the induction of coma following the injection of crystalline insulin, but subcoma (ambulatory) insulin therapy has been widely applied.

Efficacy

Data from before the introduction of neuroleptics will not be considered in this review. One of the few comparative studies between neuroleptics and insulin (Boardman et al. 1956) concluded that the methods are equally effective in a group of previously untreated schizophrenic patients. Markowe et al. (1967) found no difference between insulin and chlorpromazine in treatment of schizophrenia. Visotsky (1968) reviewed the treatment system in Russian psychiatry and described the widespread use of insulin treatment especially in schizophrenia. Most of the positive reports of Russian or Eastern European research groups are anecdotal, and only a few controlled studies exist.

Side Effects

Apart from the risk of death due to prolonged coma, the risk of permanent damage of the temporal lobes should be considered as the hippocampal region is highly susceptible to neuronal damage following hypoglycemia. It should be emphasized that prolonged coma is one of the serious complications of insulin treatment, whether this be coma or subcoma. The result may be a persisting anterograde amnesia.

The Future of Insulin Therapy

The majority of studies concerning efficacy and side effects of insulin therapy are not scientifically well conducted, and in spite of the fact that insulin coma has been recommended by clinicians in the former Soviet Union and the Peoples' Republic of China, the increase in the worldwide practice of treating psychosis with modern neuroleptic and other psychotropic drugs should make insulin treatment a form of therapy considered only in the rare cases of otherwise intractable illness.

Phototherapy

Background

In the past decade there has been a rapid expansion of interest in phototherapy in the treatment of seasonally occurring mood disorders, termed seasonal affective disorder (SAD) (Blehar and Rosenthal 1989; Rosenthal et al. 1984). For more than 2,000 years seasonal and environmental influences have been enduring themes in writings on depression and mania and have played a significant role in theories of pathogenesis and treatment (for a review see Wehr and Rosenthal 1989).

Indications for Phototherapy

In a recent report of a National Institute of Mental Health (NIMH)–sponsored workshop (Blehar and Rosenthal 1989), phototherapy was reviewed; the following conclusions can be drawn: 1) Phototherapy is efficient in treating winter depression with an atypical depressive picture consisting of fatigue, overeating, carbohydrate craving, weight gain, and oversleeping. 2) While bright-light treatment works well with patients with SAD, its therapeutic value in the treatment of other forms of depression is as yet an open issue. Before looking at some critical issues regarding phototherapy, it should be noted that even in carefully conducted studies of light therapy there is a considerable placebo problem, as no credible placebo seems to exist.

Critical Issues in the Use of Phototherapy

Most studies indicate that bright light (2,500 lux) is more of an antidepressant than dim light ≤ 400 lux, which is frequently used as control (Rosenthal et al. 1985). Terman (1988) found 10,000 lux significantly superior to 2,500 lux.

The response to phototherapy is proportional to its total daily duration. Terman (1988) found that 4 hours are superior to 2, and that 2 hours are superior to 1 when 2,500 lux is used, while one-half of an hour of 10,000 lux was as effective as 2 hours of 2,500 lux, suggesting that there may be a reciprocal interaction of duration and intensity in patients' response to phototherapy.

It is as yet unclear how important it is to treat patients with winter depression at a particular time of day. Several investigations (Jacobsen et al. 1987; Lewy et al. 1987; Terman et al. 1987) suggested morning treatments were superior to evening treatments. Terman et al. (1987), in a cross-center analysis, concluded that adding evening to morning light treatment did not improve efficacy.

The biological effects of light and the mechanism of action in phototherapy contain some crucial problems that are so far unresolved. Undoubtedly the relationships between light, timing, and its effect on circadian rhythms play an important role. It has been hypothesized by Lewy et al. (1987) that phototherapy exerts its antidepressant effect, at least in part, by phase advancing patients with SAD, most of whom are, according to this theoretical framework, phase delayed.

Conclusions and Recommendations

The seasonal influences on depression and mania appear to attract the attention of psychiatrists who treat affective disorders. There still seem to be problems concerning the validity of SAD. It is not yet clear whether it is an atypical form of bipolar illness. Seasonal affective disorder thus does not appear to be uncommon in clinics specializing in the treatment of affective disorders. Further, it is unknown whether factors that trigger summer and winter depressions may also be risk factors for suicide and depression.

Based on the report from the NIMH-sponsored workshop (Blehar and Rosenthal 1989), there does appear to be scientific evidence to support phototherapy as an effective treatment for SAD. However, the mechanism by which its antidepressant effect is achieved is not understood.

With the uncertainties mentioned, phototherapy so far cannot be recommended as first-choice treatment in patients with severe symptomatology, especially if there is even the slightest risk of suicide.

References

Abrams R: Is unilateral electroconvulsive therapy really the treatment of choice in endogenous depression? in Electroconvulsive Therapy. Edited by Malitz S, Sackeim HA. Ann N Y Acad Sci 462:50–55, 1986

Abrams R: Electroconvulsive Therapy. Oxford and New York, Oxford University Press, 1988

Abrams R (guest ed): ECT in the High-Risk Patient (special issue). Convulsive Therapy 5:1–122, 1989

Abrams R, Essman WB: Electroconvulsive Therapy: Biological Foundations and Clinical Application. New York, Spectrum Publications, 1982

Abrams R, Taylor MA: Unipolar and bipolar depressive illness: phenomenology and response to electro-convulsive therapy. Arch Gen Psychiatry 30:320–321, 1974

Abrams R, Volavka J, Fink M: EEG seizure patterns during multiple unilateral and bilateral ECT. Compr Psychiatry 14:25–28, 1973

Abrams R, Taylor MA, Faber R, et al: Bilateral versus unilateral electroconvulsive therapy: efficacy in melancholia. Am J Psychiatry 140:463–465, 1983

Alexander RC, Solomon M, Ionescu-Pioggia, et al: Convulsive therapy in the treatment of mania: McLean Hospital 1973–1986. Convulsive Therapy 4:115–125, 1988

American Psychiatric Association: Electroconvulsive Therapy. Task Force Report No 14. Washington, DC, American Psychiatric Association, 1978

American Psychiatric Association: Diagnostic and Statistical Manual of Mental Disorders, 3rd Edition (DSM-III). Washington, DC, American Psychiatric Association, 1980

American Psychiatric Association: The practice of electroconvulsive therapy: recommendations for treatment, training, and privileging. A task force report. Washington, DC, American Psychiatric Association, 1990

Andreasen NC, Ernhardt JC, Swayze VW, et al: Magnetic resonance imaging of the brain in schizophrenia. Arch Gen Psychiatry 47:35–44, 1990

Asnis G: Parkinson's disease, depression and ECT: a review and case study. Am J Psychiatry 134:191–195, 1977

Avery D, Winokur G: Mortality in depressed patients treated with electroconvulsive therapy and antidepressants. Arch Gen Psychiatry 33:1029–1037, 1976

Balldin J, Granerus AK, Lindstedt G, et al: Predictors for improvement after electroconvulsive therapy in Parkinsonian patients with on-off symptoms. J Neural Transm 52:199–211, 1981

Baxter LR, Roy-Byrne P, Liston EH, et al: Informing patients about electroconvulsive therapy: effects of a videotape presentation. Convulsive Therapy 2:25–29, 1986

Bennett AE: Preventing traumatic complications in convulsive shock therapy by curare. JAMA 141:322, 1940

Black DW, Winokur G, Nasrallah A: Treatment of mania: a naturalistic study of electroconvulsive therapy versus lithium in 438 patients. J Clin Psychiatry 48:132–139, 1987

Blehar MC, Rosenthal NE: Seasonal affective disorders and phototherapy: report of a National Institute of Mental Health–sponsored workshop. Arch Gen Psychiatry 46:469–474, 1989

Boardman RH, Lomas J, Markowe W: Insulin and chlorpromazine in schizophrenia. Lancet 2:487, 1956

Bolwig TG: The influence of electrically induced seizures on deep brain structures, in Biological Psychiatry—New Prospects, Vol 1. ECT: Basic Mechanisms. Edited by Lerer B, Weiner RD, Belmaker RD. London and Paris, John Libbey, 1984, pp 132–138

Bolwig TG, Jørgensen OS: Electroconvulsive therapy effects on synaptic protein, in Electroconvulsive Therapeutic, Clinical and Basic Research Issues. Edited by Malitz S, Sackeim HA. Ann N Y Acad Sci 462:140–146, 1986

Brandon S, Cowley P, McDonald C, et al: Electroconvulsive therapy: results in depressive illness from the Leicestershire trial. BMJ 288:22–25, 1984

Calloway SP, Dolan RJ, Jacoby RJ, et al: ECT and cerebral atrophy: a computed tomographic study. Acta Psychiatr Scand 64:442–445, 1981

Caplan G: Electrical convulsion therapy in the treatment of epilepsy. J Ment Sci 92:784, 1946

Carney MWP, Roth M, Garside RF: The diagnosis of depressive syndromes and the prediction of ECT response. Br J Psychiatry 111:659–674, 1965

Cawley RH, et al: Clinical trial in the treatment of depressive illness (Medical Research Council). BMJ 5439:881–886, 1965

Cerletti U, Bini L: L'elettroshock. Arch Gen Neuro Psichiat Psicoanal 19:266, 1938

Chodoff PD, Legault D, Freeman W: Ambulatory shock therapy. Dis Nerv Syst 11:1–8, 1950

Clinical Research Center Division of Psychiatry: The Northwick Park ECT trial: predictors of response to real and simulated ECT. Br J Psychiatry 144:227–237, 1984

Coffey CE, Weiner RD, Djang WT, et al: Brain anatomic effects of electroconvulsive therapy. Arch Gen Psychiatry 48:1013–1021, 1991

Coryell W: Intrapatient responses to ECT and tricyclic antidepressants. Am J Psychiatry 135:1108–1110, 1978

Coryell W, Zimmerman M: The dexamethasone suppression test and ECT outcome: a six month follow-up. Biol Psychiatry 18:21–27, 1983

Crow TJ, Johnstone EC: Controlled trials of electroconvulsive therapy, in Electroconvulsive Therapy. Edited by Malitz S, Sackeim HA. Ann N Y Acad Sci 462:12–29, 1986

Curson DA, Trauer T, Bridges PK, et al: Assessment of outcome after psychosurgery using the present state examination. Br J Psychiatry 143:118–123, 1983

Dam AM, Dam M: Quantitative neuropathology in electrically induced generalized convulsions. Convulsive Ther 2:77–89, 1986

Daniel WF, Crovitz HF: Disorientation during electroconvulsive therapy: technical, theoretical, and neuropsychological issues. Ann N Y Acad Sci 462:293–306, 1986

Davis JM, Janicak PG, Sakkas P, et al: Electroconvulsive therapy in the treatment of the neuroleptic malignant syndrome. Convulsive Ther 7:111–120, 1991

Decina P, Guthrie EB, Sackeim HA, et al: Continuation ECT in the management of relapses of major affective episodes. Acta Psychiatr Scand 75:559–562, 1987

d'Elia G: Unilateral electroconvulsive therapy. Acta Psychiatr Scand 215 (suppl):5–98, 1970

d'Elia G, Ottosson J-O, Strömgren LS: Present practice of electroconvulsive therapy in Scandinavia. Arch Gen Psychiatry 40:577–581, 1983

Devanand DP, Bowers MB, Hoffman FJ, et al: Acute and subacute effects of ECT on plasma HVA, MHPG and prolactin. Biol Psychiatry 26:408–412, 1989

Devanand DP, Sackeim HA, Prudic J: Electroconvulsive therapy in the treatment-resistant patient. Electroconvulsive Therapy 14:905–923, 1991

Dysken M, Evans HM, Chan CH, et al: Improvement of depression and Parkinsonism during ECT: a case study. Neuropsychobiology ___:281–286, 1976

Earp JD: Psychosurgery: the position of the Canadian Psychiatric Association. Can J Psychiatry 24:353–365, 1979

Fink MF: Convulsive Therapy: Theory and Practice. New York, Raven, 1979

Fink M: Neuroendocrine predictors of electroconvulsive therapy outcome, in Electroconvulsive Therapy. Clinical and Basic Research Issues. Edited by Malitz S, Sackeim HA. Ann NY Acad Sci 462:30–36, 1986

Frederiksen S-O, d'Elia G: Electroconvulsive therapy in Sweden. Br J Psychiatry 134:283–287, 1979

Freeman CPL, Basson J, Crighton A: Double-blind controlled trial of ECT and simulated ECT in depressive illness. Lancet 2:738–740, 1978

Freeman CPL, Cheshire KE: Attitude studies on electroconvulsive therapy. Convulsive Therapy 2:31–42, 1986

Freeman CP, Kendell RE: ECT: patients' experiences and attitudes. Br J Psychiatry 137:8–16, 1980

Göktepe EO, Young LB, Bridges PK: A further review of the results of stereotactic subcaudate tractotomy. Br J Psychiatry 126:270–280, 1975

Greenblatt M, Grosser GH, Wechsler H: Differential response of hospitalized depressed patients to somatic therapy. Am J Psychiatry 120:935–943, 1964

Gregory S, Shawcross CR, Gill D: The Nottingham ECT study: a double-blind comparison of bilateral, unilateral and simulated ECT in depressive illness. Br J Psychiatry 146:520–524, 1985

Hamilton M: Electroconvulsive therapy: indications and contraindications. Ann NY Acad Sci 462:5–11, 1986

Hamilton M, White J: Factors related to outcome of depression treated with ECT. J Ment Sci 106:1030–1040, 1960

Hansen H, Andersen R, Theilgaard A, et al: Stereotactic psychosurgery: a psychiatric and psychological investigation of the effects and side effects of the interventions. Acta Psychiatr Scand 66 (suppl 301), 1982

Harper RG, Wiens AN: Electroconvulsive therapy and memory. J Nerv Ment Dis 161:245–254, 1975

Health Service Management, Psychiatric Services: Electro-Convulsive Therapy: Equipment. Health Notice HN(82)18. HSS Store, Health Publications Unit, May 1982

Heshe J, Röder E: Electroconvulsive therapy in Denmark. Br J Psychiatry 128:241–245, 1976

Heshe J, Röder E, Theilgaard A: Unilateral and bilateral ECT. A psychiatric and psychological study of therapeutic effect and side effects. Acta Psychiatr Scand Suppl 275:1–180, 1978

Holmberg G, Tesleff S: Succinylcholine iodide as a muscular relaxant in electroshock therapy. Am J Psychiatry 108:842–848, 1952

Hurwitz TD: Electroconvulsive therapy: a review. Compr Psychiatry 15:303–314, 1974

Ingvar M: Cerebral blood flow and metabolic rate during seizures. Ann NY Acad Sci 462:194–206, 1986

Jacobsen FM, Weht TA, Skwerer RA, et al: Morning versus midday phototherapy of seasonal affective disorder. Am J Psychiatry 144:1301–1305, 1987

Janicak PG, Davis JM, Gibbons RD, et al: Efficacy of ECT: a meta-analysis. Am J Psychiatry 142:297–302, 1985

Janis IL: Psychologic effects of electric convulsive treatments (post-treatment amnesias). J Nerv Ment Dis 111:359–382, 1950

Jenike MA, Baer L, Ballantine HT, et al: Cingulotomy for refractory obsessive-compulsive disorder. Arch Gen Psychiatry 48:548–555, 1991

Johnstone EC, Deakin JF, Lawler P, et al: The Northwick Park electroconvulsive therapy trial. Lancet ii:1317–1320, 1980

Kalayam B, Steinhart MJ: A survey of attitudes on the use of electroconvulsive therapy. Hosp Community Psychiatry 32:185–188, 1981

Kalinowsky LB: Electric-convulsion therapy in schizophrenia. Lancet 2:1232–1233, 1939

Kalinowsky LB, Hippius H: Pharmacological, Convulsive and Other Somatic Treatments in Psychiatry. New York and London, Grune & Stratton, 1969

Kalinowsky LB, Hoch PH: Shock Treatment, Psychosurgery, and Other Somatic Treatments in Psychiatry. New York, Grune and Stratton, 1952

Kalinowsky LB, Kennedy F: Observations in electric shock therapy applied to problems of epilepsy. J Nerv Ment Dis 98:56–67, 1943

Kamil R, Joffe RT: Neuroendocrine testing in electroconvulsive therapy. Psychiatr Clin North Am 14:961–970, 1991

Kelly D: Anxiety and Emotions: Physiological Basis and Treatment. Springfield, IL, Charles C Thomas, 1980

Kirkegaard C, Norlem N, Lauritsen UB, et al: Prognostic values of thyrotropin releasing hormone stimulation test in endogenous depression. Acta Psychiatr Scand 52:170–177, 1975

Klemperer E: Versuch einer Behandlung des Delirium tremens mit Insulin. Psychiatr Neurol Wehnschr 50:549, 1926

Kramer BA: Use of ECT in California, 1977–1983. Am J Psychiatry 142:1190–1192, 1985

Kramp P, Bolwig TG: Electroconvulsive therapy of acute delirious conditions. Compr Psychiatr 12:368–371, 1981

Lambourn J, Gill D: A controlled comparison of simulated and real ECT. Br J Psychiatry 133:514–519, 1978

Lancaster NP, Steinert RR, Frost I: Unilateral electro-convulsive therapy. J Ment Sci 104:221–227, 1958

Lerer B, Weiner RD, Belmaker RH: ECT: Biological Psychiatry—New Prospects: 1. ECT: Basic Mechanisms. London and Paris, John Libbey, 1984

Lewy AJ, Sack RL, Miller LS, et al: Antidepressant and circadian phase-shifting effects of light. Science 235:352–354, 1987

Liberson WT: Current evaluation of electric convulsive therapy. correlations of the parameters of electric current with physiologic and psychologic changes. Res Publ Assoc Res Nerv Ment Dis 31:199–231, 1953

Malitz S, Sackeim HA, Decina P, et al: The efficacy of electroconvulsive therapy: dose-response interactions with modality. Ann NY Acad Sci 462:56–64, 1986

Markowe M, Steinert J, Heyworth-Davis F: Insulin and chlorpromazine in schizophrenia: a ten year comparative survey. Br J Psychiatry 113:1101–1106, 1967

May PR: Treatment of Schizophrenia: A Comparative Study of Five Treatment Methods. New York, Science House, 1968

McCabe MS: ECT in the treatment of mania: a controlled study. Am J Psychiatry 133:688–691, 1976

Medical Research Council, Clinical Psychiatry Committee: Clinical Trial of Treatment of Depressive Illness. BMJ 1:881–886, 1965

Meduna LJ: Die Konvulsionstherapie der Schizophrenia. Halle, Germany, Carl Marhold, 1937

Meldrum BS: Neuropathological consequences of chemically and electrically induced seizures. Ann N Y Acad Sci 462:186–193, 1986

Menken M, Safer J, Goldfarb C, et al: Multiple ECT: morphologic effects. Am J Psychiatry 136:453, 1979

Mitchell-Heggs N, Kelly D, Richardson A: Stereotactic limbic leukotomy: a follow-up at 16 months. Br J Psychiatry 128:226–240, 1976

Milstein V, Small JG, Klapper MH, et al: Uni- versus bilateral ECT in the treatment of mania. Convulsive Ther 3:1–9, 1987

Mukherjee S, Sackeim HA, Lee C: Unilateral ECT in the treatment of manic episodes. Convulsive Therapy 4:74–80, 1988

Mukherjee S, Sackeim HA, Lee C, et al: ECT in treatment resistant mania, in Biological Psychiatry. Edited by Shagass C, Josiassen RC, Bridger WH, et al. New York, Elsevier, 1986, pp 732–734,

National Institutes of Health: Electroconvulsive Therapy. National Institutes of Health Consensus Development Conference Statements, Vol 5, No 11, 1985

Nyström S: On relation between clinical factors and efficacy of ECT in depression. Acta Psychiatr Scand 181:115–118, 1964

Ottosson J-O: Experimental studies of the mode of action of electroconvulsive therapy. Acta Psychiatr Scand 145 (suppl 35):1–141, 1960

Ottosson J-O: Is unilateral nondominant ECT as efficient as bilateral ECT? a new look at the evidence. Convulsive Ther 7:190–200, 1991

Paykel ES, Klerman GL, Prusoff BA: Prognosis of depression and the endogenous-neurotic distinction. Psychol Med 4:57–64, 1974

Pippard J, Ellam L: Electroconvulsive Treatment in Great Britain, 1980. London, Gaskell, 1982

Prudic J, Sackeim HA, Devanand DP: Medication resistance and clinical response to electroconvulsive therapy. Psychiatry Res 31:287–296, 1990

Rich CL, Spiker DG, Jewell SW, et al: DSM III, RDC and ECT: depressive subtypes and immediate response. J Clin Psychiatry 45:14–18, 1984

Rifkin A: ECT versus tricyclic antidepressants in depression: a review of the evidence. J Clin Psychiatry 49:3–7, 1988

Roberts JM: Prognostic factors in the electroshock treatment of depressive states. I. clinical features from history and examination. J Ment Sci 105:693–702, 1959

Robin A, de Tissera S: A double-blind controlled comparison of the therapeutic effects of low and high energy electroconvulsive therapies. Br J Psychiatry 141:357–366, 1982

Rosenthal NE, Sack DA, Carpenter CJ, et al: Antidepressant effects of light in seasonal affective disorder. Am J Psychiatry 142:163–170, 1985

Rosenthal NE, Sack DA, Gillin JC, et al: Seasonal affective disorder: a description of the syndrome and preliminary findings with light therapy. Arch Gen Psychiatry 41:72–80, 1984

Royal College of Psychiatrists (eds): The Royal College of Psychiatrists memorandum on the use of electroconvulsive therapy. Br J Psychiatry 131:261–272, 1977

Sackheim HA, Decina P, Malitz S, et al: Postictal excitement following bilateral and right-unilateral ECT. Am J Psychiatry 140:1367–1368, 1983

Sackeim HA, Decina P, Prohovnik I, et al: Dosage, seizure threshold, and the antidepressant efficacy of electroconvulsive therapy, in Electroconvulsive Therapy. Edited by Malitz S, Sackeim HA. Ann N Y Acad Sci 398–410, 1986

Sackeim HA, Decina P, Kanzler M, et al: Effects of electrode placement on the efficacy of titrated, low-dose ECT. Am J Psychiatry 144:1449–1455, 1987

Sackeim HA, Prudic J, Devanand DP, et al: The impact of medication resistance and continuation pharmacotherapy on relapse following response to electroconvulsive therapy in major depression. J Clin Psychopharmacol 10:96–104, 1990a

Sackeim HA, Prudic J, Devanand DP: Treatment of medication-resistant depression with electroconvulsive therapy, in American Psychiatric Press Review of Psychiatry, Vol 9. Edited by Tasman A, Goldfinger SM, Kaufmann C. Washington, DC, American Psychiatric Press, 1990b, pp 91–115

Sackeim HA, Devanand DP, Prudic J: Stimulus intensity, seizure threshold, and seizure duration. Electroconvulsive Therapy 14:803–843, 1991

Sakel M: Neue Behandlungsmethode der Schizophrenie. Wien, Leipzig, Mortiz Perles, 1935

Salzman C: The use of ECT in the treatment of schizophrenia. Am J Psychiatry 137:1032–1041, 1980

Scott AIF, Whalley LJ, Legros J-J: Treatment outcome, seizure duration and the neurophysin response to ECT. Biol Psychiatry 25:585–597, 1989

Siesjö BK, Ingvar M, Wieloch T: Cellular and molecular events underlying epileptic brain damage. Ann N Y Acad Sci 462:207–223, 1986

Small JC: Efficacy of electroconvulsive therapy in schizophrenia, mania, and other disorders. I: schizophrenia. Convulsive Therapy 1:263–270, 1985a

Small JC: Efficacy of electroconvulsive therapy in schizophrenia, mania, and other disorders. II: mania and other disorders. Convulsive Therapy 1:271–276, 1985b

Small JG, Klapper MH, Kellams JJ, et al: ECT compared with lithium in the management of manic states. Arch Gen Psychiatry 45:727–732, 1988

Snaith RP, Price DJE, Wright JF: Psychiatrists' attitudes to psychosurgery: proposals for the organization of a psychosurgical service in Yorkshire. Br J Psychiatr 144:293–297, 1984

Sørensen PS, Hammer M, Bolwig TG: Vasopressin release during electroconvulsive therapy. Psychoneuroendocrinology 7:303–308, 1982

Spitzer RL, Endicott J, Robins E: Research Diagnostic Criteria: rationale and reliability. Arch Gen Psychiatry 35:773–782, 1978

Squire LR: Memory functions as affected by electroconvulsive therapy. Ann N Y Acad Sci 462:307–314, 1986

Squire LR, Chace PM: Memory functions six to nine months after electroconvulsive therapy. Arch Gen Psychiatry 32:1557–1564, 1975

Squire LR, Slater PC: Electroconvulsive therapy and complaints of memory dysfunction: a prospective three-year follow-up study. Br J Psychiatry 142:1–8, 1983

Squire LR, Slater PC, Miller PL: Retrograde amnesia and bilateral electrocon-·vulsive therapy: long-term follow-up. Arch Gen Psychiatry 38:89–95, 1981

Strömgren LS: Unilateral versus bilateral electroconvulsive therapy. investigations into the therapeutic effect in endogenous depression. Acta Psychiatr Scand 240:8–65, 1973

Taylor P, Fleminger JJ: ECT for schizophrenia. Lancet 1:1380–1382, 1980

Terman M: On the question of mechanism in phototherapy: considerations of clinical efficacy and epidemiology. J Biol Rhythms 3:155–172, 1988

Terman M, Quitkin FM, Terman JS, et al: The timing of phototherapy: effects on clinical response and the melatonin cycle. Psychopharmacol Bull 23:354–357, 1987

Thomas J, Reddy B: The treatment of mania. J Affective Disord 4:85–92, 1982

Tooth GC, Newton MP: Leukotomy in England and Wales 1942–1954. Reports on Public Health and Mental Subjects No 104. Ministry of Health, London, Her Majesty Stationery Office, 1961

Tsuang MT, Dempsey GM, Fleming JA: Can ECT prevent premature death and suicide in "schizoaffective" patients? J Affective Disord 1:167–171, 1979

Ungerleider JT: Acute myocardial infarction and electroconvulsive therapy. Dis Nerv Syst 21:149–153, 1960

Valentine M, Keddie KMG, Dunne D: A comparison of techniques in electroconvulsive therapy. Br J Psychiatry 114:989–996, 1968

Visotsky HM: Impressions of Soviet psychiatry: the treatment system. Am J Psychiatry 125:650–655, 1968

Weaver LA Jr, Williams RW: The electroconvulsive therapy stimulus, in Electroconvulsive Therapy: Biological Foundations and Clinical Applications. Edited by Abrams R, Esman WB. New York, Spectrum, 1982, pp 129–156

Weaver L, Ravaris C, Rush S, et al: Stimulus parameters in electroconvulsive shock. J Psychiatr Res 10:271–281, 1974

Wehr TA, Rosenthal NE: Seasonality and affective illness. Am J Psychiatry 146:829–839, 1989

Weinberger DR, Torrey EF, Neophytides AN, et al: Lateral cerebral ventricular enlargement in chronic schizophrenia. Arch Gen Psychiatry 36:735–739, 1979

Weiner RD: Does ECT cause brain damage? Behav Brain Sci 7:1–54, 1984

West ED: Electrical convulsion therapy in depression: a double-blind controlled trial. Br Med J 282:355–357, 1981

Wing JK, Cooper JE, Sartorius N: The Measurement and Classification of Psychiatric Symptoms. New York, Cambridge University Press, 1974

Young RC, Alexopoulos GS, Shamoian CA: Dissociation of motor response from mood and cognition in a Parkinsonian patient treated with ECT. Biol Psychiatry 20:566–569, 1985

Section III

Psychological Treatments

Introduction to Section III

Fifteen years ago, a book on psychiatric treatment would have focused on the treatment advances in psychopharmacology. This field now appears to have stabilized, the available information is well known, and critical questions are appropriate. Fifteen years ago there were little empirical data on psychological treatments, but the picture has now changed. Hence this section has four chapters: one—by Nishizono, Docherty, and Butler—to represent the traditional psychodynamic view, two—one by Perris and Herlofson and one by Cottraux—to review the advances in cognitive-behavior therapy, and one—by Andrews—to compare the benefits likely to be obtained from such therapies. The field is moving rapidly and the new point of view appears to be stabilizing. Presentations such as those in this book will help the available evidence to become known and accepted. Then chapters that ask critical questions, such as the pharmacotherapy chapter in the preceding section, will be in order. Two critical types of questions are asked in the concluding section of the book: questions about the need to identify the essential psychological treatments without which no health service is complete, and questions about the need for regulation and quality assurance of psychological treatments used in health care. The chapters in this section provide some of the data needed for these decisions.

CHAPTER 5

Evaluation of Psychodynamic Psychotherapy

Masahisa Nishizono, M.D.
John P. Docherty, M.D.
Stephen F. Butler, Ph.D.

Introduction

The birth of modern psychotherapy is commonly traced to Josef Breuer's famous patient Anna O. who gained relief from her hysterical difficulties by means of the *talking cure*. Sigmund Freud, Breuer's young colleague, built on Breuer's early insights. His subsequent discoveries of psychological dynamics ushered in a revolution that continues to have profound effects on contemporary clinical thinking and practice. The method and theory of therapy pioneered by Freud and Breuer, and then later developed by Freud into psychoanalysis, branched into a variety of approaches, subsumed under the rubric of psychodynamic or psychoanalytic psychotherapy.

Earlier in this century, most mental health professionals underwent extensive training in psychodynamic theory and therapy. Over the last 20 to 30 years, however, many nonpsychodynamic treatments have emerged. For example, pharmacotherapy, other somatic therapies, social skills training, recreation therapy, and occupational therapy and rehabilitation have all been demonstrated to be important, effective remedial procedures for various mental disorders. In addition, other psychotherapy approaches, such as cognitive therapy, have been developed as alternatives to psychodynamic psychotherapy.

These treatment developments and the current climate of concern about the cost-effectiveness of mental health treatments have raised the question of the role of psychodynamic theory and treatment in modern psychiatry. In this chapter, we examine the fundamentals of psychodynamic psychotherapy, review the relevant research literature on effectiveness, and discuss future research and clinical considerations.

Definition of Psychodynamic Psychotherapy

Psychodynamic psychotherapy, as discussed here, refers to psychological treatment based on methods that were developed and refined by Freud, including those approaches that have evolved from Freud's seminal ideas. In general, psychodynamic theory assumes that symptoms and maladaptive patterns of relating reflect underlying conflicts that have their origin in conflicted relationships with significant others in the past, usually the parents. By ascertaining the nature of these conflicts, the meaning of heretofore inexplicable behaviors and symptoms can be understood. This understanding, when imparted to the patient in a deep, experiential manner, usually involving a corrective experience in the relationship with the therapist, promotes growth and maturation of personality in the individual. The individual becomes more capable of controlling anxiety, anger, and depression and achieves a deepening sense of personal capability in managing problematic interpersonal relationships. The resulting improvement in life satisfaction and more rewarding relationships presumably lessens the debilitating symptoms associated with the mental disorders.

To facilitate the therapist's understanding, the various schools of psychodynamic psychotherapy provide perspectives on personality development that essentially are maps for guiding the therapist's formulation of a patient's diagnosis (i.e., a conception of what is "wrong") and for guiding interventions. All dynamic therapies follow the same basic outline for conceptualizing the therapeutic endeavor. As Freud observed, despite the patient's conscious endorsement of the therapeutic aim of release from symptoms, the therapist meets with "a violent and tenacious resistance, which persists throughout the whole length of treatment"

(Freud 1920, p. 286). These resistances reflect the maladaptive patterns of behaving that sustain the symptoms and prevent change. Transference occurs when these maladaptive patterns incongruently become manifested in the relationship with the therapist. Analysis of this reaction to the therapist—that is, analysis of the transference—is the sine qua non of dynamic therapy. All dynamic therapies assume that, in some manner or another, the patient repeats attitudes and emotional reactions from earlier relationships with the therapist. It is thought that this repetition within the therapeutic relationship of earlier relationship problems permits the therapist to facilitate changes in emotional problems that originated in the past.

Essentials of the
Psychotherapeutic Process

The most important elements in the process of therapy may be summarized as follows:

1. The first and foremost therapeutic element involves the formation of a therapeutic relationship (often referred to as the therapeutic alliance, working alliance, or helping alliance). Achievement of such an alliance requires empathy and empathetic listening by the therapist (Marmor 1968, 1971) and the development in the patient of trust in the therapist and the feeling of being cared for and understood.
2. As the therapist works to develop the alliance, he or she encourages free expression by the patient. The therapist listens carefully to the statements of the patient, attempting to understand what the patient is communicating. During this process it is necessary to clarify ambiguous comments and cryptic explanations and to help the patient confront accounts of significant events that are contradictory.
3. Eventually the patient's conflicts are brought to light in the therapist-patient relationship (i.e., the transference). Conflictual themes common to the patient's relationship-experience in earlier life, the present therapeutic relationship, and extratherapeutic relationships in daily life point to the patient's core areas of conflict (e.g., see Luborsky 1984; Strupp and Binder 1984).

4. As these conflicts emerge in the therapeutic relationship, the therapist draws the patient's attention to them through the use of interpretations. These interpretations usually link patterns of relating to significant others across the various relationship domains (past, present, and the therapeutic relationship).
5. During the therapeutic process, the therapist strives to minimize responding to the patient's transference in a countertherapeutic manner (that is, acting out the countertransference) and, thus, reinforcing the conflictual mode of interaction.
6. Thus therapeutic change is hypothesized to occur via two primary mechanisms. One is as a result of the therapist's pointing out (interpreting), rather than acting out (countertransference), the patient's conflicts. This fosters the patient's awareness of hitherto unconscious or automatic maladaptive modes of relating. The second is the therapist's affording the patient the experience of new, more mature and satisfying modes of relating within the therapeutic relationship itself. This fosters the development and expression of such modes of relating in daily life.

Long-Term and Short-Term Psychodynamic Psychotherapy

The first analyses of patients by Breuer and Freud were only a few months long; a few were as short as a single session of several hours duration (i.e., the cases of Katharina [Breuer and Freud 1895] and Gustav Mahler [Jones 1955]). Rapidly, however, psychoanalysis became virtually defined by its frequency (four or five times per week), its duration (5 to 7 years), and use of the couch. Efforts to extend psychotherapy to more patients and more disturbed patients led to variations in the standard, psychoanalytic technique. Currently, psychodynamic psychotherapy typically involves one or two meetings per week with the therapist and patient facing each other. These weekly sessions may continue for several years.

Time-limited psychotherapy was developed as a further attempt to make psychotherapy more accessible. In contrast to 300 to 500 hours typical of a course of psychoanalysis, time-limited dynamic psychotherapy generally means about 12 to 40 weekly sessions. This type of brief psychotherapy is also termed *focal psychotherapy,* because the effort is to shorten the work by limiting the content of the therapy to a single, central dynamic focus (Balint et al. 1972; Malan 1963; Mann 1973; Sifneos 1979). More recent versions of brief dynamic therapy (e.g., see Luborsky 1984; Strupp and Binder 1984) outline specific procedures for developing a dynamic focus, typically in interpersonal rather than intrapsychic terms. The therapist avoids digression away from the defined focus and relates the focal pattern to the state of the patient-therapist relationship and the presenting symptoms. Given the dramatically shrinking funding resources for mental health care in general, it seems likely that the future of psychodynamic psychotherapy will increasingly take the form of these brief, dynamic psychotherapies.

Research

General Considerations

In 1952, Hans Eysenck challenged the psychiatric field, which at that time was dominated by psychoanalysis, when he purported to show that response rates to psychotherapy were no greater than would be expected with the passage of time (i.e., the *spontaneous remission* concept). Nearly 35 years later, Lambert et al. (1986), in their comprehensive and rigorous review of the psychotherapy research literature, were able to draw the following conclusion:

> Psychotherapy outcome research shows that some control patients improve with the passage of time, that a variety of placebo control procedures produce gains that exceed those in no-treatment controls, and that psychotherapies produce gains that exceed those obtained through the use of placebo controls. Psychotherapists are more than "placebologists" (Lambert et al. 1986, p. 163).

In addition, these authors also documented that the gains made in psychotherapy tend to be lasting. However, despite these optimistic conclusions, psychotherapy research has failed to identify any theory or set of techniques as clearly superior, in general, to any other (e.g., see DiLoreto 1971; Elkin et al. 1989; Klein et al. 1983; Miller and Berman 1983; Pilkonis et al. 1984; Sloane et al. 1975; Smith et al. 1980; Strupp and Hadley 1979). Luborsky et al. (1975) evoked the *Alice in Wonderland* quality of this predicament by quoting the dodo bird's ruling, "Everybody has won and all must have prizes." Recent work with highly selected patients presenting with specific diagnoses, such as obsessive-compulsive disorder or panic disorder (e.g., Barlow et al. 1989), appears to establish some superiority of one treatment over others. Such highly specialized treatments notwithstanding, the general finding with psychiatric patients remains "no difference" between treatments.

Long-Term Versus Short-Term Therapy

Investigations of the effectiveness of long-term psychotherapy and its relative effectiveness vis-à-vis short-term or less intensive dynamic psychotherapy have yielded equally equivocal findings (e.g., Kernberg et al. 1972; Nishizono 1975; Weber et al. 1985). On the other hand, Howard et al. (1986) plotted improvement rates for a large number of studies as a function of time and concluded that 50% of patients show significant improvement by the eighth session and 75% by the 26th session (consistent with the 25-session limit of many brief dynamic therapies).

Evaluation of such findings must consider the inherent limitations (see section on external validity, below) of research with long-term psychotherapies. For pragmatic reasons, research on long-term therapies usually involves observation of therapies in naturalistic studies, resulting in loss of experimental control possible in studies of shorter duration. Because more severely disturbed patients often end up in longer term or more intensive treatment, naturalistic studies may be biased and random assignment to long- or short-term treatment can be hard to implement. Furthermore, patients continuing in longer term therapy are presumably working on issues not directly reflected in symptom checklists (MacKenzie 1988) so the effects of such treatment are not detected by standard measures. While the position that these are additional benefits of long-term treatment needs to be supported by research, it is certainly premature to accept the alternative conclusion, namely that long-term treatment is without value.

Research on Short-Term Therapy

Because of the practical difficulties of research on long-term treatment, the main body of dynamic research to date involves the brief dynamic therapies. Two recent reviews of the literature on the effectiveness of brief dynamic psychotherapy demonstrated the difficulties of achieving a clear consensus from these data. The first is a meta-analysis by Svartberg and Stiles (1991), which reported "a small but significant superiority" (p. 710) of brief dynamic psychotherapy to waiting list patients at posttreatment, a small-sized inferiority to other treatments at posttreatment, and a large-sized inferiority to other treatments at 1-year follow-up. These authors continued by noting that brief dynamic psychotherapy performed as well as other therapies with mixed neurotic patients "unless the patients were young or therapists are clinically experienced" (Svartberg and Stiles 1991, p. 710).

Crits-Christoph (1992), on the other hand, conducted a meta-analysis and arrived at quite different conclusions. He included only state-of-the-art psychotherapy studies that used a treatment manual, involved bona fide patient groups, and used therapists trained in brief treatment. He found that brief dynamic psychotherapy demonstrated large effects relative to waiting list controls, slight superiority to nonpsychiatric treatments (e.g., placebo, clinical management, self-help groups, low contact control), and equal effects to other psychotherapies and medications.

As with any single study, the conclusions of meta-analyses may be limited by such factors as sample size, quality of the studies included, and so forth. Both meta-analyses discussed here examined very small numbers of studies (19 in the Svartberg and Stiles study, 11 in the Crits-Christoph study). Of additional concern is the unexpected conclusions reached by Svartberg and Stiles. Whereas Crits-Christoph's conclusions are consistent with the general understanding of outcome data, Svartberg and Stiles' conclusions appear to contradict generally accepted views. Clearly, counterintuitive conclusions, such as Svartberg and Stiles' finding that experienced or trained therapists are a detrimental factor in the effectiveness of brief therapy, require close examination of a study's assumptions and methodological sophistication. Nine of the 11 studies reviewed by Crits-Christoph were published since 1987 (one 1989 study was unpublished), while 16 of the 19 studies reviewed by Svartberg and

Stiles were published before 1987. The use of older studies raises the possibility, for example, that the "experienced" therapists in the studies examined by Svartberg and Stiles may not have had specific training in brief therapy and may have been resistant to the brief format (Budman and Gurman 1988). As previously noted, Crits-Christoph included only studies using therapists specifically trained in brief therapy. Finally, the use of older, more poorly designed studies obliged Svartberg and Stiles to use various statistical transformations to make assumptions that may have affected the analyses in unknown ways.

Patient Characteristics

Patient characteristics have often been studied by focusing on static demographic variables such as age, sex, social class, education, intelligence, income, degree of psychopathology, and the like. The findings of such studies tend to find contradictory or weak relationships between such variables and outcome (Garfield 1986). More promising are studies of patients' willingness and ability to engage in verbal psychotherapies, which tend to show significantly positive association with outcome (Orlinsky and Howard 1986). In the review by MacKenzie (1988), the author identified several factors that emerge as being associated with success in brief, dynamic psychotherapy: capacity to relate, motivation, psychological mindedness, positive response to trial interpretations, higher social class, and adaptational strength. Thus, as in other areas of health services (e.g., cardiac patients), those who are healthiest respond best and most rapidly to treatments, while those with long-standing, chronic conditions and poor resources present a greater challenge.

More specifically for psychotherapy, evidence is mounting that patients who become actively involved in their therapy tend to do better than those who remain hostile or aloof (Gomes-Schwartz 1978; Orlinsky and Howard 1986). Examinations of interactions with difficult patients (Henry 1986; Henry et al. 1986; Strupp 1980a, 1980b, 1980c, 1980d) suggest that a therapist's reciprocating responses to patient's provocations (i.e., countertransference) may create a vicious cycle that culminates in early drop-out or poor outcome. Such research may eventually help to identify patients likely to present specific difficulties and foster the development of more effective strategies for dealing with them.

Research Issues, Concerns, and Promises of the Future

Research Limitations and External Validity

The methodological concerns raised in previous sections point to the critical importance of understanding the limitations of current psychotherapy research to inform public policy. Clearly a detailed knowledge of the methodology of studies and a commonsense approach to the data are required. In this context, an often overlooked issue is the external validity of psychotherapy research studies. For example, controlled research studies tend to rule out patients with difficult or complex psychiatric problems. It is not uncommon for certain conditions, such as the need for hospitalization, active suicidality or repeated suicide attempts, comorbid substance abuse, or the presence of severe personality disorder, to be exclusionary criteria in research studies. Such patients can be difficult to engage in research projects, can present data collection difficulties (e.g., follow-up), can require multiple treatments and emergency interventions, and can be generally uncooperative. While such conditions are understandably to be avoided in controlled research, the findings of these studies may not be accurately generalized to clinical settings where difficult patients cannot be turned away.

A related point involves patients who drop out or who are withdrawn from studies. Study results are typically limited to *completers* or patients who stay in the study long enough to be considered as having received treatment and for whom data exist that are amenable to traditional methods of statistical analyses. However, the questions of who these dropouts are and what has become of them have largely remained unanswered, although the incidence of patients dropping out appears to be a significant one.

For example, a study on treatment of depression (Elkin et al. 1989) reported a dropout rate of 32%, with 25% giving negative treatment-related reasons and 9% being clear symptomatic failures. This reporting is an initial step toward following *noncompleters* and determining the nature of dropouts. On the other hand, however, there is some evidence (M. Hoyt, personal communication, March 1992) that some patients quit therapy once they have achieved their goals. It is therefore important that future research should include new methods of statistical analysis that captures the full weight of these data.

Cost-Effectiveness Research

An important component of the evaluation of treatment, including psychodynamic psychotherapy, is the cost-effectiveness of the treatments offered. One important example is the meta-analysis of 58 studies by Mumford et al. (1984), who observed that patients' utilization of general medical services decreased after brief psychiatric treatment. Indeed, it has been suggested that all future psychotherapy outcome studies should include an assessment of cost-effectiveness (Krupnick and Pincus 1991). Sophisticated methodologies for assessing cost-effectiveness of various therapeutic modalities take into account not only the direct cost of delivering a particular service (e.g., the use of doctoral-level therapists versus lay counselors) but also the effect of *cost shifting* (Levin 1985). Cost shifting refers to the fact that patients given inadequate treatment often end up shifting the burden of their care to agencies and systems outside the purview of the research setting (e.g., increased use of inpatient and outpatient medical care, law enforcement, psychiatric help outside the study, increased family burden). Unless these hidden costs are systematically assessed, incorrect conclusions can be drawn about the cost-effectiveness of particular treatments (see Walsh et al. 1991 for an example how such an assessment affects research conclusions).

The Search for Curative Factors in Dynamic Psychotherapy

Luborsky et al. (in press) have proposed that future research in dynamic psychotherapy be concentrated on determining the factors responsible for the observed benefits of dynamic psychotherapy. Based largely on findings from the University of Pennsylvania Center for Psychotherapy Research (Luborsky et al. 1991), the Mt. Zion Psychotherapy Research Group (Weiss and Sampson 1986), and the Vanderbilt Psychotherapy Project (Henry et al., in press), Luborsky et al. (in press) delineated six factors that are correlated with positive outcome in dynamic therapy: psychological health, therapeutic alliance, formulation of transference, focus on transference, self-understanding, and internalization of benefits. While each factor is positively correlated with outcome, each one predicts only a small percentage of the variance in the outcome measures. Future research needs to determine if combinations of these factors might predict much more.

Reliable Measures of Psychodynamic Constructs

If dynamic psychotherapy is to make the case that its therapeutic procedures and effects are valuable, useful methods for operationalizing its constructs are essential. Some gains have been made in this direction. For example, the Structural Analysis of Social Behavior (SASB) method developed by Benjamin (1974, 1982) permits interpersonal conflicts to be operationally defined along with other dynamic concepts, such as introjection. Other powerful examples include efforts to operationalize the dynamic focus. Two prominent examples are the Core Conflictual Relationship Theme (CCRT) method (Luborsky and Crits-Christoph 1990) and the Cyclical Maladaptive Pattern method (Butler and Binder 1987; Schacht et al. 1984).

Psychodynamic Treatment Manuals and Measures of Adherence

In the last decade, the psychotherapy research field has witnessed a small revolution in research and practice—manuals have been written for each of the main forms of psychotherapy and for the main types of dynamic psychotherapy. The general manuals for dynamic psychotherapies are those written by Luborsky (1984) and Strupp and Binder (1984), and a specific one for borderline patients by Kernberg and colleagues (Clarkin and Kernberg, in press; Kernberg et al. 1989). To ensure their best use, each research group developed an adherence measure for their manual (Butler and Strupp, in press). Interestingly, research on adherence has led to a heightened awareness of the necessity of understanding therapist skill (Butler et al., in press).

Examination of Therapist Differences

There are studies that show significant differences among therapists in their success with their patients (e.g., Luborsky et al. 1985, 1986;

McLellan et al. 1988). A recent meta-analysis of therapist effects on outcome revealed a medium-sized effect (Crits-Christoph et al. 1991). These findings serve as a reminder that in psychotherapy research the person of the therapist is more critical in understanding the treatment than in evaluating the effect of medications (e.g., see Butler and Strupp 1986). A future task of psychotherapy research will be to delineate the nature of therapist differences and examine how these differences affect therapy process and outcome for different patients.

Psychotherapies for Specific Types of Patients

Because it appears that no form of psychotherapy, including psychodynamic, shows special benefits for certain types of patients, the next step will be to devote efforts to developing specific therapies for specific types of patients. While other therapies (e.g., cognitive and behavioral therapies) have well-developed treatments designed specifically for particular disorders, such as depression (Beck et al. 1979) and panic disorders (Barlow et al. 1989), dynamic therapies tend to be conceptualized as applicable to psychiatric patients in general. Greater efficacy, however, may be obtained by tailoring dynamic approaches to the conflicts and interpersonal problems commonly encountered in particular patient groups. Recent attempts to develop specialized dynamic treatment approaches to specific populations are Clarkin and Kernberg's (in press) treatment for borderline personality disorder and Mark et al.'s supportive-expressive therapy for cocaine addiction (D. Mark and L. Luborsky, unpublished manuscript, April 1992). The efficacy of these specific approaches is currently being tested.

Combined Treatments

Psychotherapy outcome research has largely been concerned with contrasting the various approaches against each other to determine the single "treatment of choice." However, a case can be made for combining different approaches. To date, investigations of combined treatments typically involved psychotherapies combined with medication treatments. For some disorders these combined treatments tend to produce more benefits than single treatments. For example, combining psychotherapy and antidepressant medication for depressed patients has been shown to produce the best outcome at 1-year follow-up when compared to either treatment alone (Weissman et al. 1981). These conclusions were supported by a later review of combined treatments for depression (Conte et al. 1986). Although much work remains to be done in this area, Karasu (1992) recently proposed that, for depression, optimal treatment appears to be combination treatment. As he stated, "Drugs have their major effects on symptom formation and affective distress, whereas psychotherapy more directly influences interpersonal relations and social adjustment" (p. 5).

Conclusions

This is a time of change in the way mental health services are provided; the changes will affect how psychotherapists think about and use psychodynamic psychotherapy. In the introduction we posed the question, What is the role of psychodynamic theory and treatment in modern psychiatry? In essence, it will retain its traditional role, albeit in a new form. It still represents the major effort to understand or modify maladaptive patterns of interpersonal relatedness. Clearly there will be increased use of the briefer versions of dynamic treatment, increased efforts to target dynamic approaches to specific kinds of patients, and increased use of combined treatments (dynamic therapy with medication and possibly with cognitive and behavioral interventions as well). Thus, although the longer term, unfocused, intrapsychic psychoanalysis may become less frequently practiced, in this new form the utility of a dynamic, interpersonal understanding of psychopathology and the rich body of clinical observation it embodies will endure.

The clinical challenge is to understand and improve treatments for those patients who do not easily respond to the available treatments. This includes not only those who fail to respond to the treatments, but also those plagued by repeated relapses. The chronic and intractable nature of the problems endured by these individuals is not well understood. It is likely, however, that many of these people are unable to make use of standard treatments due to pervasive mistrust, immaturity, and hostility. In other words, these are patients usually described as having personality disorders. Personality disorders, in turn, are typically conceptualized as involving chronic interpersonal maladaptations. Dynamic psychotherapy directly addresses such interpersonal problems and any approach to these kinds of problems will, of necessity, make use of the understanding that dynamic theory and therapy provide of chronic interpersonal problems. The greatest strides in the science and art of psychotherapy are yet to come, and we expect that dynamic psychotherapy will continue to occupy a prominent place in the future of psychological treatments.

References

Balint M, Ornstein P, Balint E: Focal Psychotherapy. London, Tavistock Publications, 1972

Barlow DH, Craske MG, Cerny JA, et al: Behavioral treatment of panic disorders. Behavior Therapy 20:261–282, 1989

Beck AT, Rush AJ, Shaw BF, et al: Cognitive Therapy for Depression. New York, Guilford, 1979

Benjamin LS: Structural analysis of social behavior. Psychological Rev 81:392–425, 1974

Benjamin LS: Use of structural analysis of social behavior (SASB) to guide intervention in psychotherapy, in Handbook of Interpersonal Psychotherapy. Edited by Anchin JC, Kieslerpp DJ. New York, Pergamon Press, 1982, pp 190–212

Breuer J, Freud SL: Studies on hysteria (1895), in The Standard Edition of the Complete Psychological Works of Sigmund Freud, Vol 12. Translated and edited by Strachey J. London, Hogarth Press, 1955, pp 125–134

Budman SH, Gurman AS: Theory and Practice of Brief Psychotherapy. New York, Guilford Press, 1988

Butler SF, Binder JL: Cyclical psychodynamics and the triangle of insight: an integration. Psychiatry 50:218–231, 1987

Butler SF, Strupp HH: "Specific" and "nonspecific" factors in psychotherapy: a problematic paradigm for psychotherapy research. Psychotherapy 23:30–40, 1986

Butler SF, Strupp HH: The effects of training psychoanalytically oriented therapists to use a manual, in Handbook of Dynamic Psychotherapy Research and Practice. Edited by Miller NE, Luborsky L, Barber JP, et al. New York, Basic Books (in press)

Butler SF, Henry WP, Strupp HH, et al: Measuring adherence and skill, in Time-Limited Dynamic Psychotherapy (in press)

Clarkin JF, Kernberg OF: Development of a disorder specific manual: the treatment of borderline personality disorder, in Handbook of Dynamic Psychotherapy Research and Practice. Edited by Miller NE, Luborsky L, Barber JP, et al. New York, Basic Books (in press)

Conte HR, Plutchik R, Wild KV, et al: Combined psychotherapy and pharmacotherapy of depression: a systematic analysis of the evidence. Arch Gen Psychiatry 46:471–479, 1986

Crits-Christoph P: The efficacy of brief dynamic psychotherapy: a meta-analysis. Am J Psychiatry 149:2:151–158, 1992

Crits-Christoph P, Baranackie K, Kurcias JS, et al: Meta-analysis of therapist effects in psychotherapy outcome studies. Psychotherapy Research 1:81–91, 1991

DiLoreto AO: Comparative Psychotherapy: An Experimental Analysis. Chicago, Aldine-Atherton, 1971

Eysenck HJ: The effects of psychotherapy: an evaluation. J Consult Clin Psychol 16:319–324, 1952

Elkin I, Shea T, Watkins JT: National Institute of Mental Health treatment of depression collaborative research program: general effectiveness of treatments. Arch Gen Psychiatry 46:971–982, 1989

Freud S: Resistance and repression, in Introductory Lectures on Psychoanalysis. Edited by Strachey J. New York, Norton, 1966 (1920), pp 286–302

Garfield SL: Research on client variables in psychotherapy, in Handbook of Psychotherapy and Behavior Change, Vol 3. Edited by Garfield SL, Bergin AE. New York, John Wiley, 1986, pp 213–256

Gomes-Schwartz B: Effective ingredients in psychotherapy: predictions of outcome from process variables. J Consult Clin Psychol 46:1023–1035, 1978

Henry WP: Interpersonal Process in Psychotherapy. PhD thesis, Vanderbilt University, 1986

Henry WP, Schacht TE, Strupp HH: Structural analysis of social behavior: application to a study of interpersonal process of differential therapeutic outcome. J Consult Clin Psychol 54:27–31, 1986

Henry WP, Bulter SF, Schacht TE, et al: The effects of training in time-limited dynamic psychotherapy: changes in therapists' behavior. J Consult Clin Psychol (in press)

Howard KI, Kopta SM, Krause MS, et al: The dose effect relationship in psychotherapy. Am Psychol 41:159–164, 1986

Jones D: The Life and Work of Sigmund Freud, Vol 2. New York, Jason Aronson, 1955

Karasu TB: The worst of times, the best of times: psychotherapy in the 1990s. Journal of Psychotherapy Practice and Research 1:2–15, 1992

Kernberg OF, Bernstein ED, Coyne L, et al: Psychotherapy and psychoanalysis: final report of the Menninger Foundation's psychotherapy research project. Bull Menninger Clin 36:1–276, 1972

Kernberg O, Selzer M, Koenigsberg H, et al: Psychodynamic psychotherapy of borderline patients. New York, Basic Books, 1989

Klein DF, Zitrin CM, Woerner MG, et al: Treatment of phobias: II. behavior therapy and supportive psychotherapy: are there any specific ingredients? Arch Gen Psychiatry 40:139–145, 1983

Krupnick J, Pincus HA: Cost-effectiveness of psychotherapy discussion paper. Draft report of the Task Force on the Cost-Effectiveness of Psychotherapy. Washington, DC, American Psychiatric Association, 1991

Lambert MJ, Shapiro DA, Bergin AE: The effectiveness of psychotherapy, in Handbook of Psychotherapy and Behavior Change, Vol 3. Edited by Garfield SL, Bergin AE. New York, John Wiley, 1986, pp 157–211

Levin HM: Cost-effectiveness: a primer. Beverly Hills, CA, Sage Publications, 1985

Luborsky L: Principles of psychoanalytic psychotherapy: a manual for supportive-expressive treatment. New York, Basic Books, 1984

Luborsky L, Crits-Christoph P: Understanding Transference: The Core Conflictual Relationship Theme Method. New York, Basic Books, 1990

Luborsky L, Singer B, Luborsky L: Comparative studies of psychotherapy. Arch Gen Psychiatry 32:995–1008, 1975

Luborsky L, McLellan AT, Woody GE, et al: Therapist success and its determinants. Arch Gen Psychiatry 42:602–611, 1985

Luborsky L, Crits-Christoph P, McLellan T, et al: Do therapists vary much in their success: findings from four outcome studies. Am J Orthopsychiatry 56:501–512, 1986

Luborsky L, Crits-Christoph P, Barber J: The Penn Psychotherapy Research Projects, in Psychotherapy Research—An International Review of Programmatic Studies. Edited by Beutler L, Crago M. Washington, DC, American Psychological Association, 1991

Luborsky L, Miller N, Barber J, et al: What has been learned and what's next?, in Handbook of Dynamic Psychotherapy Research and Practice. Edited by Miller NE, Luborsky L, Barber JP, et al. New York, Basic Books (in press)

MacKenzie KR: Recent developments in brief psychotherapy. Hosp Community Psychiatry 39:742–752, 1988

Malan DH: A Study of Brief Psychotherapy. London, Tavistock Publications, 1963

Mann J: Time-Limited Psychotherapy. Cambridge, MA, Harvard University Press, 1973

Marmor J (ed): Modern Psychoanalysis: New Directions and Perspectives. New York, Basic Books, 1968

Marmor J: Dynamic psychotherapy and behavior therapy. Arch Gen Psychiatry 24:22, 1971

McLellan AT, Woody G, Luborsky L, et al: Is the counsellor an "active ingredient" in methadone treatment? an examination of treatment success among four counsellors. J Nerv Ment Dis 176:423–430, 1988

Miller RC, Berman JS: The efficacy of cognitive behavior therapies: a quantitative review of the research evidence. Psychol Bull 94:39–53, 1983

Mumford E, Schlesinger HJ, Glass GV, et al: A new look at evidence about reduced cost of medical utilization following mental health treatment. Am J Psychiatry 141:1145–1158, 1984

Nishizono M: Differences of healing picture between different techniques of psychotherapy, in Theory and Practice of Psychoanalysis, Vol 1 (in Japanese). Kongo, Tokyo, 1975

Orlinsky DE, Howard KI: Process and outcome in psychotherapy, in Handbook of Psychotherapy and Behavior Change, Vol 3. Edited by Garfield SL, Bergin AE. New York, John Wiley, 1986, pp 311–381

Pilkonis PA, Imber SD, Lewis P, et al: A comparative outcome study of individual, group, and conjoint psychotherapy. Arch Gen Psychiatry 41:431–437, 1984

Schacht TE, Binder JL, Strupp HH: The dynamic focus, in Psychotherapy in a New Key. A Guide to Time-Limited Dynamic Psychotherapy. Edited by Strupp HH, Binder JL. New York, Basic Books, 1984, pp 65–109

Sloane RB, Staples FR, Cristol AH, et al: Psychotherapy Versus Behavior Therapy. Cambridge, MA, Harvard University Press, 1975

Sifneos PE: Short-Term Dynamic Psychotherapy—Evaluation and Technique. New York, Plenum, 1979

Smith ML, Glass GV, Miller TI: The Benefits of Psychotherapy. Baltimore, MD, Johns Hopkins University Press, 1980

Strupp HH: Success and failure in time-limited psychotherapy: a systematic comparison of two cases. Arch Gen Psychiatry 37:595–603, 1980a

Strupp HH: Success and failure in time-limited psychotherapy: a systematic comparison of two cases. Arch Gen Psychiatry 37:708–716, 1980b

Strupp HH: Success and failure in time-limited psychotherapy: a systematic comparison of two cases. Arch Gen Psychiatry 37:831–841, 1980c

Strupp HH: Success and failure in time-limited psychotherapy: a systematic comparison of two cases. Arch Gen Psychiatry 37:947–954, 1980d

Strupp HH, Binder JL (eds): Psychotherapy in a New Key: A Guide to Time-Limited Dynamic Psychotherapy. New York, Basic Books, 1984

Strupp HH, Hadley SW: Specific versus nonspecific factors in psychotherapy: a controlled study of outcome. Arch Gen Psychiatry 36:1125–1136, 1979

Svartberg M, Stiles TC: Comparative effects of short-term psychodynamic psychotherapy: a meta-analysis. J Consult Clin Psychol 39:704–714, 1991

Walsh DC, Hingson RW, Merrigan DM, et al: A randomized trial of treatment options for alcohol-abusing workers. New Engl J Med 325:775–782, 1991

Weber JJ, et al: Factors associated with the outcome of psychoanalysis: report on the Columbia Psychoanalytic Center Research Project. International Review of Psychoanalysis 12:251–262, 1985

Weiss J, Sampson H: The Psychoanalytic Process. New York, Guilford, 1986

Weissman MM, Klerman GL, Prusoff BA, et al: Depressed outpatients: results one year after treatment with drugs and/or interpersonal psychotherapy. Arch Gen Psychiatry 38:51–55, 1981

CHAPTER 6

Cognitive Therapy

Carlo Perris, M.D.
Jörgen Herlofson, M.D.

The Growing of a New Approach in the Conceptualization of Psychotherapeutic Interventions

It would be beyond the scope of this chapter to discuss the ever increasing emphasis on cognitive processes in the conceptualization of mental disorders and their treatment that has occurred during the last few decades. A critical discussion of this multifaceted issue is available elsewhere (e.g., Mahoney 1988; Perris 1988), hence a repetition here would be superfluous. At this juncture, instead, it may suffice to mention the impact that a more explicit acknowledgment of the importance of cognitive processes has on the theory and practice of psychotherapies of different orientation, without even touching on the issue of how this impact is related to a changing conception of man. The reader interested in the historical and philosophical underpinnings of the present-day focus on cognitions is referred to the works mentioned above.

Whereas traditional behaviorism has consistently avoided taking into account private events or cognitive mechanisms that mediate behavior, a shift has occurred with the more recent development of social-learning theory. This latter theoretical model is more comprehensive in its scope because it acknowledges both the role of classical and operant conditioning processes and the importance of cognitive mediational processes. Two concepts, both introduced by Bandura (1978), have added further important cognitive features to social learning theory. The first concept, *self-efficacy,* emphasizes that all procedures for changing behavior work by changing expectations of self-efficacy. The second, *reciprocal deter-*

minism, acknowledges that humans not only are determined by their environment but also greatly contribute to determining it. Hence, a gradient is evident from the traditional environment-deterministic conception of man, proper of behaviorism, to an interactionistic and constructivistic conception, proper of cognitive therapy.

Attention to cognitive processes is paid, more often implicitly than explicitly, in most of the insight-oriented psychotherapies that have been developed ever since Freud's introduction of psychoanalysis. A few psychoanalysts have emphasized the role of cognitions in the occurrence of mental disorders both in their theoretical formulations and in their therapeutic practice, even though their main concern has been with emotions. Eventually, a psychoanalytical orientation with an emphasis on cognitive processes has become well established (e.g., Arieti 1974) and apparently is growing (e.g., Basch 1981; Horowitz et al. 1984; Peterfreund 1971), but its followers clearly remain within the realm of psychoanalysis.

Cognitive therapy and cognitive-behavior therapy (CBT) have contributed to the changed orientation occurring in the other two major psychotherapy systems (i.e., behavior therapy and psychoanalysis) rather than being a direct consequence of those changes. It has been developed mainly during the last 25 years and has rapidly expanded into becoming one of the most well-established methods of treatment for a great variety of mental disorders. Its underlying theoretical assumptions, including the view of humans endorsed by cognitive therapists, clearly differ from those of both psychoanalysis and traditional behavior therapies (Liotti and Reda 1981; Mahoney 1988; Perris 1988). Accordingly, it would be unjustified, for example, to lump together the cognitive therapies with behavior therapy in an evaluation of efficacy.

The main scope of the present review will be an evaluation of empirical studies that support the efficacy of cognitive therapy when used with patients with various mental disorders. Further, some recent areas in which the use of a cognitive-behavioral treatment approach seems to be highly promising, even if controlled studies are not yet available, will be pointed out. Finally, a few conclusive remarks regarding the feasibility of this treatment procedure at various levels in the health care system, and a few concerning training, will be made. Because some variants of CBT are so closely related to the more traditional behavior therapies that a clear-cut distinction is difficult, those relationships will also be considered, and those studies in which a more cognitive and a more behavioral treatment approach have been compared will be emphasized.

Origins and Development of the Cognitive-Behavior Therapies (CBTs)

Comprehensive reviews of the philosophical foundations and the development of CBT are available in the literature, the most recent by Mahoney (1988), Perris (1988), and Ellis (1989). Hence, only some key features of this development will be mentioned at this juncture. In particular, as the term *cognitive-behavior therapy* is a comprehensive label covering similar approaches that are based on different theoretical conceptions, (for a recent review, see Mahoney 1988), it is necessary to examine the original relationship to psychoanalysis on the one side and to behaviorism on the other to account for similarities and differences among the various clinical usages.

Cognitive Therapy and Rational-Emotive Therapy

Very likely, one of the first authors to explicitly use the term cognitive therapy was the Freudian analyst Hans Lungwitz (1881–1967), who used it as the title of an article published in 1926. In a monumental, 10-volume textbook, *Lehrbuch der Psychobiologie,* first published in the 1930s, Lungwitz (1955) expanded his theory, devoting one whole volume (number 7) to the description of a short-term type of cognitive therapy that he had developed. Lungwitz's cognitive therapy is deeply rooted in biological concepts, has a manifest educative orientation, and emphasizes the active work of the patient (including homework assignments) in correcting misconceptions through active learning. However, Lungwitz's work, which was never translated into English, has had a relatively modest impact on the theory and practice of psychotherapy, despite its striking similarities with the therapeutic approach advocated by more recent proponents of cognitive therapy. In particular, Lungwitz's work seems to have been completely unknown to the Americans Albert Ellis and Aaron Beck, who are regarded as the founders of modern cognitive therapy. Unfortunately, only anecdotal reports have been published by Lungwitz's followers and no controlled studies have yet been reported in which Lungwitz's original conceptions have been applied in practice.

Ellis, a Horneyan analyst, began to develop his rational psychotherapy (rational-emotive therapy [RET])in the mid-1950s whereas Beck, a Freudian analyst, developed his theoretical formulation of cognitive therapy in the early 1960s, both doing so because of dissatisfaction with classical psychoanalytical conceptions. Their respective approaches share important characteristics and represent the mainstream of CBT from which further developments are still occurring.

Common to both Ellis's and Beck's theorizing is an almost exclusive emphasis on cognitions in the complex dysfunctional pattern of interactions among cognitions, emotions, and behavior that characterize most mental disorders. This emphasis on cognitions obviously does not imply that emotions are neglected. Both in RET and cognitive therapy, the primary concern is with the identification of dysfunctional cognitions (irrational beliefs in Ellis's terminology, faulty thinking and basic dysfunctional assumptions in Beck's) assumed to underlie various mental disorders, and with an active and directive orientation toward challenging and eventually correcting such dysfunctional cognitions. RET and cognitive therapy do not put any particular emphasis on the development and resolution of transference, as in psychoanalysis and analytically oriented psychotherapies, even though they both emphasize the relationship between therapist and patient and pay due attention to the occurrence of transference and countertransference reactions. The therapist-patient working relationship is mainly conceptualized in cognitive therapy and RET as being similar to the one that develops between two research workers actively working together to solve a research problem, putting forward various hypotheses and testing their validity.

In both therapies, the Socratic method of dialogue is actively used to help the patients become aware of the relationship occurring between dysfunctional cognitions, painful emotions, and maladaptive behaviors. Both RET and cognitive therapy incorporate a large number of behavioral and other techniques (cognitive, behavioral, emotive-expressive, and so on). These technical procedures, however, serve as a mean for eliciting and pinpointing dysfunctional cognitions in the patient and as a tool to guide the patient in correcting them, rather than for the direct training of more adaptive behavioral responses.

Because of the almost consistent use of various behavioral techniques, both RET and cognitive therapy clearly qualify for the more comprehensive label *cognitive-behavior therapy*. However, the theoretical and epistemological foundations of RET and cognitive therapy are clearly different from those underlying other types of CBT, which are more related to behavior therapy (see Table 6–1). One illustrative example of a fundamental difference between a more behavioral and a more cognitive approach is the modification of maladaptive self-instructions as used by therapists of a different orientation. In behavior therapy, the direct training of alternative and more adaptive self-instructions is literally used. In cognitive therapy, the validity of negative self-instructions (often conceptualized in terms of negative automatic thoughts) is challenged and the patient is stimulated to search for alternatives.

An important distinguishing characteristic of RET and cognitive therapy, that is also shared by behavior therapy, has been the formulation of their underlying theoretical conceptions in a way that is amenable to empirical verification. Hence, from the very beginning, concern has been shown for the development and the use of assessment instruments to measure dysfunctional cognitions and to assess their change as a consequence of the treatment. Even more important has been a concern with the implementation of empirical studies to document the therapeutic efficacy. Furthermore, a large number of treatment manuals have been developed for use with patients of various ages (i.e., children, adults, and elderly people) or with patients presenting with a variety of mental disorders (e.g., depression, anxiety disorders, alcohol- and drug-abuse, anorexia, disorder of impulse control).

Table 6–1. A selection of main cognitive-behavior therapy approaches

More "cognitive"	More "behavioral"
Rational-emotive therapy	Self-instructional training
Cognitive therapy	Problem-solving training
Cognitive appraisal therapy	Self-control therapy
Cognitive-experiential therapy	Rational-behavior therapy
Structural cognitive therapy	Systematic rational restructuring
	Social skills training

Other CBTs

A large group of therapeutic approaches, subsumed under the comprehensive heading *cognitive-behavior therapy* (for example, cognitive-behavioral modification, cognitive restructuring, systematic rational restructuring, self-instructional training, a modern reformulation of social skills training that takes into account cognitions), were born within the context of what has been called the *cognitive revolution*, which took place in psychology in the late 1960s and early 1970s (see Mahoney 1988 for a thorough discussion of this particular development of cognitive therapy). The essence of this revolution, as concerns the development of CBTs, is the acknowledgment of the scientific legitimacy of examining the client's thoughts and the shift in the interpretation of the learning process as one involving cognitive mechanisms rather than only conditioning (Perris 1988). However, not all leading behavior therapists have fully endorsed these views. Accordingly, the same therapeutic procedure (i.e., systematic desensitization) is conceptualized differently by traditional behavior therapists, who refer to *counterconditioning* or *reciprocal inhibition* to explain the dissolution of symptoms, and by cognitive therapists who emphasize the modification of conceptual systems.

Besides those mentioned above, there are other therapeutic approaches that are currently understood as belonging to the group of CBTs (e.g., multimodal therapy [Lazarus 1971], rational behavior training [Maultsby 1984], lay epistemic therapy [Kruglanski 1981], problem-solving therapies [D'Zurilla and Goldfried 1971; Spivack and Shure 1974], cognitive-experiential therapy [Weiner 1985], self-management therapies [Rehm and Kokke 1988]). Particular mention has to be made of Kelly's (1955) fixed-role therapy (derived from his personal construct theory), which is unequivocally cognitive in its conception. However, Kelly's impact has been greater on the theoretical and research level than through the therapy method that he proposed. Further therapies that qualify for an inclusion under the comprehensive heading *cognitive-behavior therapy* are logotherapy (Frankl 1985), developmental therapy (Ivey 1986), strategic therapy (Haley 1963), and the Japanese psychotherapy developed by Morita (Reynolds 1976), which has a strong resemblance to logotherapy, especially as concerns conceptions of neurosis and cure (Marks 1969). Morita's psychotherapy uses both cognitive (with a particular focus on attentional processes) and behavioral techniques (e.g., the use of diaries, the training of assertive responses, and the behavioral application of Moritist principles to daily life). One major target in Morita therapy is a reorientation of self-focused attention (or *torraware* as it is labeled in Moritist terminology). However, it would be a serious mistake to interpret similarities in techniques between the Japanese therapy and Western-style CBTs with a similarity in the underlying theoretical conceptions. Unfortunately, outcome studies of Morita psychotherapy are almost inaccessible in Europe. Hence, no further mention of this therapy method will be made in this chapter. (Table 6–2 shows a survey of various therapies that are often included in a broad conception of CBT.)

Empirical Evidence of the Efficacy of Cognitive Therapies

The increase in the number of different psychotherapies that have occurred during the last 20 years makes it important to document their effectiveness. However, psychotherapy research is still a young and growing discipline that only recently has begun to approach the level of methodological sophistication that has been reached, for example, in studies of psychopharmacotherapy. Hence, in spite of a number of high-level outcome studies concerning the use of the various psychotherapeutic approaches taken into account in this review, many more of the small-scale studies suffer from shortcomings.

Overall, research carried out with students or with groups of volunteers (amounting to thousands of articles that can hardly be discussed

Table 6–2. Other therapies that belong to the broad cognitive-behavior therapy domain

Logotherapy	Lay espitemic therapy
Fixed-role therapy	Developmental therapy
Strategic psychotherapy	Morita therapy
Multimodal therapy	Cognitive-behavior hypnotherapy

here) is, for obvious reasons, of a higher methodological standard than studies carried out with psychiatric patients in unnaturalistic settings. The results from a sizable number of these studies support the assumption that cognitive-behavioral treatments have effects that are clearly superior to no treatment for a large array of behavioral problems, at the same time as they contribute to elucidating process issues. However, favorable results obtained in nonclinical subjects cannot be generalized to patient populations as subjects who volunteer for experiments and patients who seek treatment clearly differ in several ways (Marks 1978).

Quantitative Reviews of the Research Evidence

One means of comparing the efficacy of various psychotherapies across a large body of studies is through using the technique of meta-analysis (Glass 1976). However, the unavoidable contamination of important variables in the studies, a factor that is taken into account, greatly limits the degree to which one can make clear statements about the effects of particular treatments for particular types of patients. With this warning in mind, let us consider a few recently published quantitative reviews of the efficacy of CBTs. In this context it must be emphasized, however, that at the time when these reviews were published, CBT was still in its beginning stages and subject to refinements, whereas the other psychotherapies used for comparison had been well established for a longer time.

In an early study, Smith and Glass (1977) analyzed 375 studies of psychotherapy outcome in which investigations of RET, systematic desensitization, implosion, and behavior modification (apparently not the cognitive variant) were included. An additional group, labeled *eclectic therapies* also included verbal, cognitive, nonbehavioral treatments. Other therapies taken into account were psychodynamic, Adlerian, transactional analysis, Gestalt, and client-centered. In this study, systematic desensitization showed the largest average effect size (.9 sigma) and RET the second largest (.8 sigma), almost equal to behavior modification. Implosive therapy showed a mean effect size of .6, about equal to that of Rogerian and psychodynamic therapies and transactional analysis.

Smith et al. (1980) reported a further quantitative evaluation of the effectiveness of 17 types of therapy based on the analysis of 475 studies. The average outcome score for all treated groups was .85 SD more improved than the mean of all control groups. The effect size of cognitive therapies was considerably higher than any of the other types.

Shapiro and Shapiro (1982) reported a meta-analysis of comparative therapy outcome studies, which was prompted by criticisms against meta-analytic studies of psychotherapy reported in the literature. In their investigation, the authors surveyed 143 studies that had been published from 1974 to 1979. Among the therapy methods examined, a large proportion consisted of behavior therapy variants, such as self-control and monitoring, rehearsal, biofeedback, systematic desensitization, flooding, and covert behavioral. Included also were studies of cognitive therapy, dynamic/humanistic psychotherapies (e.g., psychodynamic, client-centered) and mixed or unclassified methods (mainly behavioral). Consistent with previous studies, the mean effect size obtained from the 414 treated groups approached one SD unit. The comparison of treatment methods showed a significant superiority of mixed ($P < .01$) and cognitive ($P < .001$) methods whereas negative scores indicated inferior results for dynamic and humanistic therapies and unclassified methods. Covert behavioral, rehearsal/self-control, systematic desensitization, social skills training, and unclassified treatments were significantly superior to minimal or placebo treatments. Cognitive therapy and mixed methods were superior to systematic desensitization. By and large, comparisons among the behavioral methods suggested that these have rather similar effects. In their conclusion, they emphasized that the results of their analysis showed "a modest but undeniable superiority of behavioral and cognitive methods and a corresponding relative inferiority of dynamic and humanistic methods" (Shapiro and Shapiro 1982, p. 595).

R.C. Miller and Berman (1983) assessed the efficacy of cognitive behavior therapies in an analysis of 48 studies. In line with the studies previously quoted, they too found a mean effect size of .83 for CBTs in comparison with no treatment. However, they did not find that these therapies were superior to other psychotherapies, independently of whether or not cognitive therapies gave more or less emphasis to behavioral procedures and of whether they were administered individually or in a group. In Miller and Berman's review, a large proportion of the studies concerned student or community volunteers and only a small number (six or seven) of studies with outpatients. In studies of outpatients, treatment effects were larger than in either group of volunteers.

In their analysis, Latimer and Sweet (1984) specifically addressed the issue of cognitive versus behavioral procedures in CBTs. Their review comprised 12 studies that involved a variety of clinical problems (phobias, obsessive-compulsive disorder, tension headache, unassertive behavior, social anxiety, social skills deficits, depression). A number of the studies reviewed demonstrated a superiority of behavioral methods, and only 1 the superiority of cognitive therapy. It should be noted, however, that in 8 of the 12 studies reviewed, patients had been recruited by means of advertisements in community newspapers.

Berman et al. (1985) re-addressed the findings reported by Shapiro and Shapiro (1982), which suggested a superiority of cognitive therapy in comparison with systematic desensitization. Berman et al. considered three forms of psychotherapy: cognitive therapy, systematic desensitization, and treatments that combined both cognitive and desensitization techniques. They analyzed 25 studies in which cognitive and desensitization therapies were compared either with each other or with a mixed treatment that combined both techniques. A majority (76%) of the studies used volunteers: 64% with student volunteers and 12% with volunteers from the community. In 60% of the studies the patients were treated for some form of anxiety problem and in 28% for phobias. Both cognitive therapy and desensitization showed similar mean effect sizes. Therapies combining both cognitive and desensitization treatments did not appear to be more effective than either treatment alone.

In summary, the results of the reviews reported so far are consistent in showing that treatment with cognitive and behavioral therapies gives effect sizes that are significantly superior to no treatment or minimal treatment. Both cognitive and behavioral treatments appear to be at least slightly superior to psychodynamic therapies. The evaluation of the superiority of more cognitive versus more behavioral therapies has yielded inconsistent results. However, the overall trend indicates an equivalence of cognitive and behavioral therapies with a possibly slight superiority for the former.

Efficacy of CBTs for Defined Disorders

In the following sections, evidence of efficacy will be considered for defined morbid conditions. However, the use of CBT for a large amount of minor behavioral problems will be subsumed under a common heading and only cursorily surveyed.

Depressive Disorders

Undoubtedly, outcome studies of depressive disorders, comprising a large number of controlled investigations, represent the most solid piece of evidence for the therapeutic efficacy of CBT. Such an emphasis on depression stems from the fact that Beck's cognitive therapy was originally conceived in the context of the treatment of depressive illnesses (Beck 1966). Particularly important is the fact that several controlled studies of CBT for depression have contrasted this method of treatment to drug treatment. For no other morbid condition, and for no other psychotherapy method as well, has such a comprehensive documentation been made available.

Several detailed reviews of the cognitive treatment of depression have been published (Albersnagel and Rouwendal 1984; Beckham and Watkins 1989; Blackburn 1988; Blaney 1981; DeRubeis and Beck 1988; Hollon 1981; Jansson and Öst 1984; Steinbrueck et al. 1983). Hence, no detailed report of each study will be made at this juncture. Instead, only the major findings will be emphasized.

It seems appropriate to begin this section by quoting the results of a meta-analysis of psychotherapy and drug therapy in the treatment of adult unipolar depressed patients published by Steinbrueck et al. (1983). Those authors analyzed 56 outcome studies comprising five types of psychotherapy (behavioral; social-learning interpersonal; cognitive; a combination of cognitive, social-learning, and behavioral therapy; and marital therapy) and 35 types of drug therapy, the most common consisting of the use of tricyclic antidepressants. Effect sizes of all treatment with control comparisons were significantly ($P < .001$) higher for the psychotherapies (mean effect size 1.2) than for drug-therapy (mean effect size .6). Even when the comparison was restricted to psychotherapy versus tricyclic antidepressants the results did not change: the average effect size for tricyclic antidepressants was .67 and the difference versus psychotherapy was still highly significant ($P < .001$). This finding is consistent with the results of a quantitative analysis reported by Albersnagel and Rouwendal (1984); in that study, however, meta-analysis techniques were not used.

In Tables 6–3 and 6–4, we summarize the main results of the outcome studies of CBT used with clinical populations that were based on a
controlled design. Table 6–3 comprises studies of individual therapy and
Table 6–4 comprises group therapy. Studies concerning college students
or community volunteers who did not fulfill operationalized criteria of
currently acknowledged diagnostic systems have not been included in
the tables. Also not included are findings reported in single-case studies
and experimental investigations whose primary aim was not the treatment of sick people. (Most of these studies have been reviewed by
Blaney [1981] and by Rush and Giles [1982].)

Two of the studies of individual CBT (Gallagher and Thompson
1982; Jarvik et al. 1982) and two of the studies of group CBT (Beutler et
al. 1987; Steuer et al. 1984) concerned depressed, nondemented elderly
patients. No studies of children and adolescent patient populations are
included in the tables. There are, so far, no controlled studies in which
the cognitive-behavioral treatment of depression in childhood has been

Table 6–3. Survey of the results of outcome studies *(discussed in text)* of
individual cognitive-behavior therapies (CBTs) versus other
treatment modalities for depression

		Outcome of patients receiving individual CBT compared with those receiving alternative treatments					
		Posttreatment			Follow-up		
Alternative treatments	*n* studies	Better	Same	Worse	Better	Same	Worse
Control conditions							
Waiting list	9	9			1		
Attention placebo	1	1					
Other treatments							
TCAs	8		8		4		
TCAs and CBT	4		4		3		
Behavior therapy	8		7	1	1		
Psychodynamic	3	2	1				
Client-centered	1		1				
Nonspecified standard	2	2					

Note. TCAs = tricyclic antidepressants.

specifically addressed. However, single case reports with a long follow-up (e.g., Asarnow and Carlson 1988) suggest the feasibility of cognitive therapy with depressed children. Regarding adolescents, a few anecdotal reports claiming the feasibility of cognitive therapy and one controlled study (Reynolds and Coasts 1986) in which CBT was found superior to relaxation training are presently available. However, further research in these areas is in progress.

As concerns CBT administered in the individual format, at least 10 studies included a nontreatment control condition. In all of them, the active treatment was significantly superior to the control condition. Comparisons with other types of treatment have been reported in at least 26 studies (note, however, that comparisons with different treatments may have been carried out in the same study). In evaluating the results of the comparisons in which different findings concerning different ratings were evidenced, more stress was placed on the proportion of patients

Table 6–4. Survey of the results of outcome studies *(discussed in text)* of group cognitive-behavior therapies (CBTs) versus other treatment modalities for depression

Alternative treatments	*n* studies	Outcome of patients receiving individual CBT compared with those receiving alternative treatments					
		Posttreatment			Follow-up		
		Better	Same	Worse	Better	Same	Worse
Control condition							
Waiting list	7	5	2		1		
Other treatments							
Individual CBT	2		1	1			
Behavior therapy	3		2			3	
Insight-oriented group therapy	5	4	1		1		
Individual CBT and TCAs	2		1	1			
Interpersonal group therapy	1	1					
Nonspecified standard	1	1					

Note. TCAs = tricyclic antidepressants.

who had globally improved than on differences in the rating scores.
The largest number of studies (12) compared CBT and treatment
with tricyclic antidepressants or a combination of both treatments (Beck
et al. 1979, 1985a; Blackburn et al. 1981, 1986; Dunn 1979; Hollon et al.
1983; I.W. Miller et al. 1989; Murphy et al. 1984; Rötzer-Zimmer et al.
1985; Rush and Watkins 1981; Rush et al. 1977; Teasdale et al. 1984).
The type of CBT used in these studies, almost consistently, was Beck's
cognitive therapy for which a detailed treatment manual is available
(Beck et al. 1979). In all those studies, CBT, alone or in combination
with tricyclic antidepressants, proved to be as effective and produced results equal to treatment with tricyclic antidepressants alone.

Eight studies compared CBT with other types of behavior therapy
(Comas-Diaz 1981; de Jong et al. 1981; Fleming and Thornton 1980;
Gallagher and Thompson 1982; McNamara and Horan 1986; P.H. Wilson et al. 1983; Zeiss et al. 1979), with equal results. Of the remaining
studies, three concerned psychodynamic psychotherapy, one used client-
centered therapy, two a "non-specified standard treatment," nine a waiting list control condition, and one placebo. In all, CBT proved to be
significantly superior to the no-treatment or placebo condition.

Five of the CBT alone versus tricyclic antidepressant treatment studies included a follow-up evaluation 1 to 2 years after the end of treatment. In all instances, patients treated with CBT showed a significantly
better outcome. A similar result applies to follow-up evaluations in comparison with other methods of treatment. It is important to note that patients treated with CBT alone have consistently shown a better long-term
outcome at follow-up than patients treated with a combination of CBT
plus tricyclic antidepressants. Furthermore, patients treated with cognitive therapy have consistently shown a significantly lower rate of attrition than patients treated with tricyclic antidepressants.

In Table 6–4 the results of 14 outcome studies in which CBT in a
group format was compared with a control condition (almost exclusively
a waiting list) or another active treatment are summarized (Covi and Lipman 1987; Jarvik et al. 1982; LaPointe 1977; LaPointe and Rimm 1980;
Magers 1978; Neimeyer et al. 1985; Ross and Scott 1985; Rush and
Watkins 1981; Shaw 1977; Steuer et al. 1984; Wierzbicki and Bartlett
1987; also see discussion by Besyner, cited in Blaney 1981, and discussion by Kelly, cited in Haaga and Davison 1989).

A waiting list control condition was included in seven studies. In all of them CBT proved to be significantly superior. Comparisons with other active treatments included insight-oriented (psychodynamic) group therapy (five studies), behavioral group therapy (three studies), interpersonal therapy (one study), and nonspecific group therapy (one study). In five studies CBT in a group format was compared with individual CBT (three studies) and individual CBT plus tricyclic antidepressant treatment (two studies). In four of the five studies of CBT versus psychodynamic group therapy, the former proved to be more effective. The difference between individual CBT and group CBT appears to be inconsistent. Of the three studies comparing CBT with behavioral group therapy, two yielded similar results whereas in one CBT was superior. In their controlled study, Neimeyer et al. (1985) included a comparison of cognitive therapy with homework (CTH) and cognitive therapy without homework (CTN), against interpersonal therapy (IPT) and a waiting list control condition. CTH generally outperformed CTN in the magnitude and universality of treatment gains. Overall results were roughly equal between CTH, CTN, and IPT. Yet, both cognitive therapy conditions did significantly better on cognitive measures. CTN had the lowest rate of attrition (3%) over the 10 weeks of therapy (CTH, 16%; IPT, 12%).

Besides the general survey shown in Tables 6–3 and 6–4, there are some other relevant studies. Two of them concern the treatment of severe and chronic drug-refractory patients (de Jong et al. 1986; Harpin et al. 1982). Harpin et al. assigned 12 chronically depressed outpatients either to CBT or to a waiting list control condition for 10 weeks. By the end of treatment, the treated group but not the control group had improved significantly both on clinical measures of depression and anxiety and on two indexes of social skills. This significant difference persisted at a follow-up evaluation 6 months after completed treatment. de Jong et al. admitted 33 chronically depressed inpatients to a study with treatment options comprising 1) cognitive restructuring (CR), based on Beck's cognitive therapy but with the total exclusion of the use of behavior modification techniques and activity scheduling; 2) a package consisting of CR plus cognitive-behavioral modification techniques and activity scheduling (COMB); and 3) a waiting list control condition (WL). The results of this study differed depending upon the source of data. Clinical observers rated changes following CR and COMB equally favorably and considered both more effective than WL. According to self-report measures, COMB patients experienced more improvement than CR-treated patients. The degree of improvement assessed at the end of treatment was still present at a follow-up 6 months later.

A further study of severely depressed inpatients has been reported by I.W. Miller et al. (1989). The authors randomly assigned 47 inpatients to one of three treatment conditions: 1) standard treatment (pharmacotherapy according to a semi-structured medication protocol and management sessions), 2) cognitive therapy plus standard treatment, and 3) social skills training plus standard treatment. All those treatments were continued for a period of 20 weeks after discharge. All treatment groups showed significant improvement of depressive symptoms at discharge and at the end of outpatient treatment. At discharge there were no significant differences between the treatment groups except that patients who had participated in cognitive therapy and in social skills training manifested lower levels of symptoms than did the standard treatment patients.

Larcombe and Wilson (1984) addressed the issue of secondary depression in patients with multiple sclerosis. Twenty depressed multiple sclerotic patients were assigned either to CBT or to a waiting list control condition. At the end of treatment, and at a 4-week follow-up, CBT-treated patients in comparison to controls showed a clinically and statistically significant improvement on most measures of depression. Turner and Wehl (1984) found that CBT was significantly superior to standard (nonspecified) inpatient treatment in treating depression in alcoholics.

There are only two anecdotal reports of the use of cognitive therapy in patients with a bipolar affective disorder (Chor et al. 1988; Kingdon et al. 1986), although bipolar patients have not been explicitly mentioned in any of the studies listed in Tables 6–3 or 6–4. Hence, no conclusions can be drawn from the present evidence about the feasibility of CBT with bipolar patients. However, studies concerning this particular patient population are now in progress. The case report by Kingdon et al. concerned a patient who developed a hypomanic episode between 4 and 6 weeks of treatment with cognitive therapy. The case history reported by Chor et al. was that of a bipolar patient who had frequent relapses, who had refused lithium treatment and who apparently benefited from cognitive therapy, having no relapses during a follow-up period of 4 years. Cochran (1984), however, reported the results of a controlled study, comprising 28 patients, that showed that treatment compliance can be improved in bipolar depressive patients by adding cognitive therapy to lithium treatment.

Hautzinger (1988) described an interesting trial carried out in mildly depressed patients. Five patients watched 12 videotaped sessions of cognitive therapy three times a week over two 2-week periods separated by a 2-week break. At the end of each session patients received a homework assignment identical to that for the patient in the tape. All patients participating in the study improved, and only one asked for further treatment.

Suicidal behavior. Related to the issue of depression is that of the efficacy of CBT in suicide-prone patients. Rush et al. (1982) addressed this issue by investigating the effect of cognitive therapy in comparison to treatment with imipramine on measures of hopelessness and self-concept, which are significantly related to suicidal behavior (Beck et al. 1985b; Minkoff et al. 1973). Thirty-five unipolar patients participated in the study, which lasted 11 weeks. Compared with imipramine, cognitive therapy resulted in significantly greater improvements in hopelessness and more generalized gains in self-concept. A single case report by Nidiffer (1980) of a suicidal depressive adult treated with cognitive therapy and followed-up over 42 months, supported the assumption that cognitive therapy may be of value in the prevention of suicidal behavior in depressed patients.

In summary, even though some of the studies reviewed in this section could be criticized because they do not fulfill all the requirements for high standard psychotherapy research, the evidence supporting the efficacy of cognitive therapy in the treatment of depressive disorders appears to be fairly strong both in terms of magnitude and stability. Such a conclusion applies not only to mild depressive disorders but also to moderately and severely depressed patients, independent of whether or not they are labeled "endogenous" (Gallagher and Thompson 1983). Also severe chronically depressed patients, refractory to previous (pharmacological and psychological) treatments, appear to significantly improve when treated with cognitive therapy. There is a consistency across different settings and in different ethnic groups.

In none of the studies in which cognitive therapy was compared with treatment with tricyclic antidepressants was there any significant difference between the outcomes at the end of treatment. Nor was there any difference in immediate outcome in patients treated with cognitive therapy alone compared to patients treated with cognitive therapy and tricyclic antidepressants. Cognitive therapy in the studies reviewed did not appear to be superior to behavior therapies on assessments made at the end of treatment. On the other hand, cognitive therapy was reported to be superior in those studies that included a long-term follow-up.

Anxiety Disorders

The largest number of studies carried out on nonclinical populations concern test anxiety and speech anxiety; these studies are mentioned in this chapter even though they do not concern psychiatric patients because these disorders may be severely incapacitating for selected populations. In the treatment of this type of minor disorder, CBT (in particular as conceptualized by Ellis, Beck, and Meichenbaum) frequently yielded favorable results (Barabasz and Barabasz 1981; Fremouw and Gross 1983; Fremouw and Zitter 1978; Goldfried et al. 1978; Karst and Trexler 1970; Meichenbaum 1972; Moleski and Tosi 1976; Trexler and Karst 1972). Only results of controlled outcome studies carried out in clinical populations will be emphasized. This implies that neither single-case studies, nor studies of college students and of community volunteers besides those mentioned above, will be scrutinized. An exception will be made for studies in which it was explicitly stated that participants fulfilled recognized diagnostic criteria for an anxiety disorder.

Evidence of efficacy based on quantitative analyses. Andrews and Harvey (1981) reanalyzed data that had been reported by Smith et al. (1980), cited above. The reason for such a reanalysis was to limit the investigation to 81 studies of patients who had neuroses or emotional-somatic disorders. Eighty-eight percent of the patients had neuroses or true phobias, and 12% had emotional-somatic complaints. No studies focused only on depressed patients. The authors divided the therapies into 1) verbal (subdivided into dynamic, cognitive, and developmental), 2) behavioral (comprising traditional behavioral and cognitive behavioral methods), and 3) developmental (consisting of client-centered counseling, personal development, vocational, or undifferentiated counseling). The mean effect size across all treatments was .72, with the behavioral (.97) and the verbal (.74) having the largest effect size. The developmental therapies had an average effect size of .35, which was smaller than that for placebo treatment (.55). Among the subtypes in each class, cognitive and Gestalt therapies had the largest mean effect size (1.21); next largest were traditional behavioral (.99) and cognitive-behavioral (.74).

Dushe et al. (1983) examined 69 studies in a review focused on self-statement modification (SSM) techniques and found a mean effect size of .74 in comparison to no-treatment controls, in contrast to an effect size of .49 among the 42 non-SSM studies. Larger effect sizes were found in studies comprising more intensive cognitive treatments, and efficacy consistently increased with the addition of those techniques. Complex phobias yielded an average effect size of 1.26. Similar findings were reported by Barrios and Shigatomi (1980) who analyzed 22 studies of SSM. SSM was consistently found to be superior to attention-placebo controls. In comparison with other treatment methods, SSM was found to be superior in 37% of the comparisons and equal in 45%. It should be noted that Barrios and Shigatomi included RET under the heading SSM.

Lyons and Woods (1991) compiled a quantitative review of the efficacy of RET by means of meta-analysis. Seventy studies of RET were included and 236 comparisons of RET to baseline, control conditions, cognitive behavior modification, behavior therapy, and other psychotherapies were analyzed. The average effect size for RET for comparisons against no treatment was .91. This translated to a 72% improvement rate for RET compared to a 28% improvement rate for the nontreatment conditions. Comparisons with other treatments did not yield significant differences, nor did differences emerge when individual RET was compared to group RET.

A critical analysis of 17 studies of cognitive-behavioral treatment of social phobia was reported by Heimberg (1989). Seven of those studies did not include any control condition, and only five included a nontreatment (waiting list) control. Heimberg pointed out that the large number of interventions (including several cognitive restructuring techniques) used in this small number of studies limits the conclusions that may be drawn. In his review, Heimberg stated that there might be reason for cautious optimism concerning the efficacy of the cognitive and behavioral treatment of social phobia, but that more refinements are necessary before definite statements can be made. In a separate analysis of the techniques most frequently applied, Heimberg, on the one hand, emphasized the many shortcomings in their use and, on the other, stressed the particular importance of the integration of cognitive techniques in other treatment procedures.

Tyrer et al. (1988) reported overall outcome data of a comprehensive study comprising 210 psychiatric outpatients with neurotic disorders (71 with generalized anxiety disorder [GAD], 74 with panic attacks, and 65 with dysthymic disorder). The patients were allocated by constrained randomization to one of five treatments: 28 to diazepam, 28 to dothiepin, 28 to placebo, 84 to cognitive and behavior therapy, and 42 to a self-help treatment program. In this large study, diazepam appeared to be less effective than dothiepin, cognitive and behavior therapy, or self-help, the latter three treatments being of similar efficacy. Patients in the placebo group required significantly more psychotropic drugs, while patients in the cognitive and behavioral group required the least.

Evidence of efficacy based on controlled studies. A few studies particularly emphasized the use of a cognitive approach to the treatment of anxiety disorders, and important research work in this field is now in progress in many quarters. However, before moving into an analysis of those studies, a few general remarks on the use of cognitive techniques and on the assessment of their usefulness are appropriate.

We will begin our review with a comment on a much publicized finding by Emmelkamp and his group that apparently indicated that the addition of cognitive interventions (self-instructional training or an approach derived from Ellis RET) did not enhance the gains obtainable with exposure in the treatment of agoraphobics (Emmelkamp and Mersh 1982; Emmelkamp et al. 1978). The inferences drawn from the studies by Emmelkamp and colleagues were criticized by Michelson (1987). At least two serious shortcomings were emphasized. On the one hand, cognitive therapies were used for too short a time in all studies (3 weeks at most) to give a fair opportunity for the subjects to learn and incorporate coping strategies based on the cognitive approach. On the other hand, in almost all studies students of psychology served as therapists. Hence, even though they had access to treatment manuals and to clinical supervision, there was no objective analysis of treatment fidelity or therapist competency. Both conditions are known to relate negatively to outcome.

Further, Emmelkamp and Mersh (1982) reported that evaluations at follow-up showed that patients in the cognitive group continued to improve whereas the subjects treated with exposure alone experienced mild relapse. A similar result was reported by Mavissakalian et al. (1983). Consistent with those results is a similar finding reported by Durham and Turvey (1987) who compared behavior therapy (relaxation, distraction, and graded exposure) with Beck's cognitive therapy in the treatment of 51 patients with GAD. Whereas there were no differences between the two methods in the amount of improvement at the end of treatment, by the 6-month follow-up, cognitive therapy treated patients maintained their gains or improved further while behavior therapy patients tended to revert toward their pretreatment scores.

A sizable number of studies, besides those already mentioned, have been concerned with a comparison of cognitive therapies (mostly Beck's cognitive therapy, Ellis's RET, or procedures explicitly derived from those two approaches) and other therapies or a no-treatment control condition in the treatment of a variety of anxiety disorders, including agoraphobia (e.g., Marchione et al. 1987), social phobia (e.g., Heimberg et al. 1990), GAD (e.g., Barlow et al. 1984; Blowers et al. 1987; Lindsay et al. 1987; Lipsky et al. 1980; Woodward and Jones 1980), panic disorder (e.g., Barlow et al. 1989; Beck 1988), obsessive-compulsive disorder (e.g., Emmelkamp et al. 1988), posttraumatic stress disorder (PTSD) (e.g., Barlow et al. 1984), or mixed or unspecified conditions (e.g., anxiety and depression, Shaffer et al. 1981, 1982). The treatment of combat-related PTSD with CBT has to our knowledge been reported in only a single-case study by investigators who used a combination of systematic desensitization and RET, with a favorable outcome at 2-year follow-up.

In all studies that included a no-treatment control condition, the active treatment proved to be superior. In comparison with other treatments, the results appeared to be inconsistent, possibly with the exception of the consistent superiority of supportive psychotherapy, which had been one of the treatments modalities in four studies (Beck 1988; Blowers et al. 1987; Borkovec et al. 1987; Heimberg et al. 1990). Two studies included a benzodiazepine derivative as a treatment modality. In one of the studies (Klosko et al. 1988) CBT was as effective as a benzodiazepine and in the other study (Lindsay et al. 1987) CBT was superior to a benzodiazepine.

Abuse of Benzodiazepines

The issue of the abuse of anxiolytics has become a matter of concern (Borg et al. 1986; Lader 1978), and some reports, including one controlled study, have suggested that CBT treatment may be a satisfactory treatment for benzodiazepine dependence (Crouch et al. 1988; Sanchez-Craig et al. 1986; Skinner 1984; Tyrer et al. 1985). Our own unpublished findings (C. Perris, J. Herlofson, April 1992) were consistent with this suggestion. Hamlin (1988) recently presented a detailed, integrated treatment program for tranquilizer withdrawal. The program combines elements of Beck's cognitive therapy with elements of transactional analysis and was designed to be carried out in a group format. Preliminary results from this project revealed that the short-term group program (8 sessions) was effective in helping clients to reduce and withdraw from tranquilizers, with the results being maintained at a 6-month follow-up. Crouch et al. (1988) treated 12 patients who had entered a withdrawal program. Three patients did not complete the treatment. At the end of the treatment, which lasted for 5 weeks with boosters at 2 and 4 weeks after completion, 4 patients had stopped taking tranquilizers, 3 were taking less than 25% of their initial dose, and 2 were still taking between 25% and 50% of the initial dose. At 3-month follow-up, 6 patients were evaluated. All of them had stopped taking their tranquilizers.

In summary, CBTs appear to have a promising place in the treatment of patients with anxiety disorders. There is evidence that CBTs are superior to no-treatment and to placebo, and that they may have some advantage compared with other types of psychotherapy. Even though further studies are needed to justify a definite statement, there seems to be a trend in the literature suggesting that behavioral therapy may be equally effective or even more powerful in the short term than the CBT therapies that have been tested. Cognitive-behavioral treatments, on the other hand, may have a clear advantage in the long term. As CBT is further developed, with more emphasis on interventions directed to promote schematic changes rather than on molecular interventions, we consider (and others agree with us, e.g., Biran 1988) that the potential efficacy of CBT will become even more evident in the future.

In view of the concern with the rapid expansion of the use and abuse of benzodiazepines and of the possible dangers that this entails, the suggestion that CBT may be effective in the treatment of this condition should be particularly welcome and should be followed up by more comprehensive investigations.

Eating Disorders

Anorexia. Despite the fact that detailed guidelines for the CBT treatment of anorexia have been made available (Garner and Bemis 1985), and the rationale for the use of CBT has been emphasized in the literature (Garner and Bemis 1985; Guidano and Liotti 1983; Sasson Edgett and Prout 1989), comprehensive and controlled outcome studies of CBT in the treatment of anorexia are still lacking. A majority of the treatment packages used with anorexic inpatients include both behavioral and cognitive components (e.g., Garfinkel et al. 1985; Powers and Powers 1984). Levendusky et al. (1983) emphasized the importance of cognitive-behavioral strategies in structuring the inpatients' milieu in the treatment of anorexic patients. Preliminary results from this project have indicated the usefulness of this treatment.

Guidano and Liotti (1983) report on a large series ($N = 38$) of patients with eating disorders (12 with anorexia, 15 with obesity, and 11 with bulimia nervosa. Those patients were part of a much larger series of patients (comprising 115 agoraphobic patients, 21 obsessive-compulsive patients, and 24 depressed patients) who had been treated by the authors and their co-workers during an 8-year period. Thus it is difficult to deduce to what extent the favorable outcome reported by the authors (success in 70% of the whole series) applied to the eating disorders group.

The results of a preliminary, uncontrolled study of CBT for anorexic patients was reported by Cooper and Fairburn (1984). Five patients in this study received a treatment approach similar to that used by Fairburn in the treatment of bulimia (see below). The results were mixed, both at the end of treatment and at 1-year follow-up, with the patients who also had episodes of bulimia responding best.

Bulimia. In contrast to anorexia, the evidence of efficacy of CBT in the treatment of bulimia seems to be more satisfactory. Recent qualitative reviews of outcome studies have been reported by Rosen (1987) and by Cox and Merkel (1989).

Cox and Merkel analyzed 32 individual and group therapy studies of the psychosocial treatment of bulimia, published between 1976 and 1986. Twelve of the group therapy studies concerned either behavior therapy (5 studies) or CBT (7 studies). All but 1 in the individual treatment series ($n = 17$) concerned behavior therapy and CBT. However, only 2 studies (both CBT) included a controlled condition. Furthermore, 8 of the studies reviewed were single case reports, and 5 used two to six patients. It is unfortunate that several controlled studies that appeared within the time limits supposedly covered by this analysis were not included. Out of the 12 group therapy studies dealing with behavior therapy or CBT, 7 included a control group and were judged as being of high or medium quality, according to stipulated evaluation criteria. Overall, patients in the treatment condition improved more than patients in the control condition. The results, however, varied among the studies with a proportion of abstinent patients at the end of treatment ranging from 0% to 80%. On the other hand, at follow-up (range 6 weeks to 2 years), the proportion of abstinent patients was rather similar across the studies (range 16% to 20%). A study reported by Kirkley et al. (1985) is noteworthy as it included a nondirective group treatment for comparison: the CBT-treated group had fewer dropouts and yielded a significantly greater decrease in bingeing and vomiting than the nondirective condition group. At 3-month follow-up, the difference had become greater.

Besides the studies reviewed by Cox and Merkel, there are five additional controlled studies of individual treatment (Freeman et al. 1985, 1988; Lee and Rush 1986; Leitenberg et al. 1988; Ordman and Kirschenbaum 1985) and one of group therapy (Agras et al. 1989), all of which were of high quality according to the criteria adopted by Cox and Merkel. In all those studies, a waiting list control condition was included. In addition, both the studies carried out by Freeman and his co-workers and the studies reported by Leitenberg et al. and Agras et al. included other treatments for comparison. Patients treated with CBT consistently showed a better outcome than patients in the waiting list condition. In the four studies that included other types of treatment, CBT appeared to be equally effective in two and superior in the other two.

Obesity. Behavioral interventions are claimed to be particularly effective in the treatment of mild obesity. However, the most favorable immediate posttreatment results are clearly transient and the long-term success of behavior therapy is unequivocally modest. This statement is supported by the results of some 200 controlled studies that have been reviewed by G.T. Wilson and Brownell (1980) and Brownell and Wadden (1986). Recently, Kramer and Stalker (1989) published guidelines for a CBT program in the treatment of obesity, the cognitive component being inspired by Beck. However, no experimental data are yet available. Results of uncontrolled cognitive therapy interventions in obese or mildly obese patients reported by Guidano and Liotti (1983) have been mentioned above.

Collins et al. (1986) investigated the comparative efficacy of cognitive and behavioral approaches to the treatment of obesity. Sixty obese females were recruited in the study, and assigned to one of four treatments: 1) cognitive therapy, 2) behavior therapy, 3) cognitive therapy plus behavior therapy, and 4) a nutrition-exercise group as a minimal treatment control condition. At posttreatment, behavior therapy subjects had lost more weight than the other groups. At 7-month follow-up, the cognitive therapy group was the only group that showed a continuing decrease in weight.

Only one controlled study of RET in a group format in the treatment of obesity was located in our search of the literature (Block 1980). Bloch allocated 40 overweight clients to three treatments: 1) RET, 2) relaxation training with discussion of weight problems, and 3) no treatment as a control condition. RET was significantly more effective than the relaxation and discussion treatment and the nontreatment condition. RET patients were an average of some 25 pounds overweight before treatment, 16 after treatment, and 6 pounds at 18-week follow-up. Patients in the other two groups were on average some 20 pounds overweight before treatment and maintained this weight throughout the follow-up period.

In summary, evidence for the efficacy of CBT in the treatment of anorexia is still lacking. The preliminary results of uncontrolled studies do not allow any definitive statement. Evidence of the efficacy of CBT in the treatment of bulimia is much more promising. It is based on findings obtained in good quality controlled studies, and additional investigations are in progress. The evidence of the efficacy of CBT in the treatment of obesity is presently very limited and does not allow for any statement. The only controlled study of RET has shown favorable results but the finding has not yet been replicated. Such replications are badly needed, especially in view of the cognitive orientation of obesity emphasized in many quarters (Kreitler and Chemerinski 1988).

Alcohol and Substance Abuse

The issue of alcoholism and substance abuse was an early concern in cognitive therapy, and a special treatment manual for the treatment of patients with those conditions was made available at the Cognitive Therapy Center of the University of Pennsylvania in Philadelphia. However, documentation of the efficacy of cognitive therapy in the treatment of those conditions remains anecdotal, except for a few well-designed, controlled studies.

Woody et al. (1986) reported one of the most thorough studies of CBT for substance-abusing patients (methadone-maintained opiate addicts). The authors enrolled 150 patients in the study and assigned them to one of three treatments: 1) supportive-expressive psychotherapy plus drug counseling, 2) CBT plus drug counseling, and 3) drug counseling alone. Each treatment was described in a manual and these manuals were used for training and ongoing supervision. The CBT treatment was Beck's while the supportive-expressive psychotherapy was an analytically oriented, focal psychotherapy. Complete 7-month data were available for 110 patients (out of 121 who completed the trial). Average effect sizes for the active treatment groups were greater and patients in those groups showed more gains than those receiving drug counseling alone, without any significant difference in the comparison of the two types of psychotherapy. Furthermore, the patients treated with either psychotherapy showed less use of prescribed and self-administered medications. The authors cautiously concluded that professional psychotherapy can be helpful with this particular patient population.

Oei and Jackson (1982) enrolled 32 problem drinking inpatients in a comparative study and assigned them to one of four treatments: 1) social skills training, 2) cognitive restructuring, 3) a combination of social skills training and cognitive restructuring, and 4) traditional supportive therapy. At 3, 6, and 12 months after discharge, the patients participated in an additional booster group session and were evaluated. (It should be mentioned that the social skills training as practiced in this study incorporated cognitive-behavioral procedures.) The findings of this study showed that cognitive restructuring, social skills training, and cognitive restructuring plus social skills training were superior on all measures (including amount of alcohol intake) to supportive therapy. In their conclusion, the authors emphasized that "long-term persistence and, in fact continuing improvement in social skills, were produced by the cognitive restructuring method compared with social skills training" (Oei and Jackson 1982, p. 544).

Other studies have been concerned with a CBT program for problem drinkers assigned to abstinence and controlled drinking (Sanchez-Craig et al. 1984) and with a pilot investigation of cognitive group therapy for wives of alcoholics (Farid et al. 1986). The results of those investigations are promising.

An important, multimodal approach to relapse prevention, including cognitive treatment and a social skills training component, has been developed by Marlatt and Gordon (1984). Overall, their relapse prevention approach would appear to contribute substantially in a variety of conditions characterized by abuse.

Rosenberg and Brian (1986) combined RET with the model proposed by Marlatt to devise a treatment for multiple driving-under-the-influence offenders. The new model was comprised of RET, coping skills training, and unstructured therapy. No significant differences in outcome were found among the groups except for assertiveness. On this measure, RET and the coping skills treatment proved to be equally superior to the control condition.

Botvin et al. (1984) described a particular cognitive-behavioral approach to substance abuse prevention in a population of 1,311 seventh grade students from 11 suburban New York junior high schools. The approach consisted of 20 sessions. The program was implemented either by older students (condition A), or by regular classroom teachers (condition B). A third group (condition C) consisted of pretest/multiple posttest control. Four schools participated in the experimental conditions while two were assigned to the control condition. Training sessions were organized and a special manual containing detailed lesson plans for each session was provided. No significant differences were found between treatment conditions B and C. Students participating in treatment condition A showed a significantly lower proportion of smokers, a significantly lower proportion of marijuana users, and a significantly lower frequency of drunkenness than students in the other two treatment conditions, a very interesting finding.

In summary, on the basis of the findings reported above, any definitive claim about the efficacy of CBT in the treatment and prevention of alcohol and substance abuse could not be justified. However, both the studies carried out in abusers of tranquilizers reported earlier (see section on abuse of benzodiazepines, above) and the few studies in this section, together with the studies reviewed in Marlatt and Gordon (1984), have yielded promising findings. The approach by Botvin et al. aimed at a large-scale preventive application of cognitive-behavioral procedures is particularly important.

Schizophrenia

Therapeutic interventions with patients who have been given a diagnosis of schizophrenia create a number of conceptual issues that are difficult to disentangle. On the top of the many problems, there is the very definition of the disorder due to its polymorphous manifestations, and to the relative unpredictability of the long-term course in the single patient (Perris 1989). However, there is a consensus that the complex clinical picture mostly frequently observed in patients with a schizophrenic disorder is in part the product of the morbid process. Premorbid social handicaps and negative environmental influences (including the effects of hospitalization and prolonged medication) greatly contribute to the total picture. Hence, it is not always possible to identify the target of the therapeutic interventions. There is a growing consensus that the treatment of most patients with a schizophrenic disorder has to be multimodal and should encompass pharmacological, environmental, psychotherapeutic, and family interventions if it is to be effective. It is against this background that the use of CBT is considered.

Findings in isolated case reports and small-scale uncontrolled studies have suggested that CBT can modify important aspects of delusional and hallucinatory experiences in chronic schizophrenic patients (Adams et al. 1981; Alford et al. 1982; Hole et al. 1979; Watts et al. 1973), hence promoting clinical improvement. In a small controlled study of confrontation versus belief modification in persistently deluded patients, with 16 subjects randomly allocated to either treatment, Milton et al. (1978) found that belief modification was superior to confrontation in producing changes on a measure of delusion, on a rating of psychiatric status, and on a measure of social anxiety assessed both at the end of treatment and after 6 weeks. Favorable results concerning hallucinatory and delusional experiences were also recently reported by Fowler and Morley (1989) and by Kingdon and Turkington(1991).

On a related theme, Bishay et al. (1989) reported the results of their uncontrolled study of cognitive therapy in treating morbid jealousy. Thirteen patients were treated, and 2 patients dropped out of treatment. Among those who remained in the trial, 9 were much improved and 1 was rated as much improved at follow-up. At 6-month follow-up 10 patients still lived with their partners. In one case the relationship was terminated because of jealousy whereas in two cases the relationship was terminated for reasons other than jealousy.

An important group of studies dealing with a multistep program with a strong emphasis on cognitive treatment, was reported in the German literature (Brenner et al. 1980, 1987). Replication studies by other groups of research workers who have used the same or a slightly modified approach have also been published (Hermanutz and Gestrich 1987; Kraemer et al. 1987; Olbrich and Mussgay 1990; Peter et al. 1989). The rationale of this approach is that basic cognitive deficits greatly contribute to the global disability of the schizophrenic patient. This multistep program is related to the structured learning therapy developed by Magaro and West (1983). The studies published so far include a no-treatment control condition. Overall, the posttreatment results document the superiority of the treatment condition in the improvement of cognitive functioning as assessed by means of several outcome measures. No long-term outcome data have yet been reported.

Buchkremer and Fiedler (1987) compared a cognitive-oriented, problem-solving treatment with an action-oriented, therapeutic approach in a prospective study of relapse prevention in schizophrenic patients. Two groups of 21 patients were randomly assigned to either treatment condition whereas a further 24 patients served as a control group. During a 2-year follow-up, patients in the cognitive treatment group showed lower relapse rates and shorter hospitalizations. In addition, patients in the cognitive treatment group were rated as significantly less impaired than patients in the other two groups.

In summary, controlled trials of multimodal cognitive-behavioral treatments have yielded favorable posttreatment results that have been independently verified across several studies. The most promising approach, however, seems to be a multimodal one that also takes into account family interventions.

Cognitive therapy as conceived by Beck was used with schizophrenic patients in only a few uncontrolled studies (e.g., Fowler 1991; Greenwood 1983; Kingdon and Turkington 1991). The results suggested the feasibility of cognitive therapy with schizophrenic patients and should be regarded as a first step toward more comprehensive controlled studies.

Preliminary results of a 4-year experience of cognitive therapy with young schizophrenic patients in a community-based small center setting at Umeå in Northern Sweden (Andersson et al. 1989; Skagerlind 1991), taken together with results reported from the United Kingdom by Fowler (1989, 1991) suggest that cognitive therapy may be a particularly important part of a multicomponent treatment program (Perris 1989, in press) that aims far beyond the mere correction of social skills or the suppression of targeted psychotic behaviors.

Cognitive and Behavioral Therapies in Other Disorders

CBT has been used with patients with such a large variety of disorders as to make even a simple enumeration meaningless. In this section, an arbitrary selection of areas of application for CBT will be noted.

Impulse Control Disorders

CBT is frequently applied to the control of anger, especially as Novaco (1975, 1978) proposed a cognitive model of anger, developed appropriate treatment strategies (mostly inspired by Meichenbaum's cognitive behavior modification approach), and produced a treatment manual.

In one of his early studies, Novaco compared four treatment conditions: 1) CBT, 2) relaxation, 3) a combination of CBT and relaxation, and 4) an attention-control condition in the treatment of 34 persons who "were both self-identified and assessed as having serious anger-control problems" (Novaco 1978, p. 152). The treatment was composed of six sessions. At posttreatment all three treatments proved to be superior to the attention control condition, and CBT and relaxation were modestly superior to CBT alone and relaxation alone. No follow-up data were reported.

CBT and behavior therapy treatments of disorders of impulse control have been used, most frequently, with populations of delinquent youngsters. A recent survey of studies in this area was made by Little and Kendall (1979). In their conclusions, the authors emphasized that a CBT approach seemed to be promising and to offer some advantages in comparison with exclusively behavioral programs (e.g., token reinforcement and contingency contracting).

More recent studies, particularly those concerning adolescents, have been reviewed by Feindler et al. (1986). These studies give cause for some optimism concerning the efficacy of cognitive and self-control interventions in the reduction of aggressive and disruptive behaviors. Feindler et al. (1986) reported a study of institutionalized psychiatric male adolescents in which 21 patients participating in a CBT treatment group were compared with patients on a waiting list and with patients on an "open ward" control group. The analysis of the results of the treatment program revealed significant differences on several measures of outcome between the CBT group and the control groups. In addition, 18 of the 21 participants in the CBT treatment could be discharged. The patients were followed for 3 years. No direct comparisons among the three groups at follow-up were reported but only 3 of the original 18 patients required further psychiatric hospitalization.

Recently, Deffenbacher et al. (1988) compared cognitive and cognitive-relaxation conditions in reducing general anger among psychology students. At 5-week follow-up no differences were found between the two treatments. Relative to controls, results in both treatment groups were equally and significantly superior as assessed by means of a battery of assessment measures.

One of the major areas of application of CBT for impulsive control (and for other behavior disorders) concerns its use with children. The reader is referred to recent reviews (Abikoff 1985; Hughes and Sullivan 1988; Urbain and Kendall 1980).

In summary, judging from the data now available, one must agree with the conclusion by Little and Kendall (1979) and Feindler et al. (1986) that CBT treatments represent a viable approach to interventions in adult patients with disorders of impulse control and merit a cautious optimism. However, the evidence of efficacy is only suggestive and much more research is required before any definitive conclusions can be reached.

Management of Pain

Traditionally, pain has been treated with drugs or by surgical means. More recently, however, a variety of CBT strategies have emerged as useful alternatives (Eimer 1989; Fordyce 1976; Holroyd and Andrasik 1982; Meichenbaum 1977; Turk and Genest 1979).

One of the most thoroughly investigated areas concerns headaches. An early study in which a direct comparison between primarily cognitive and behavioral approaches was made was carried out by Holroyd and his group in 1977 (this, and the following studies by the same group are reported, in some detail, in Holroyd and Andrasik [1982], to which the reader is referred for references). Holroyd and co-workers enrolled 31 chronic tension-headache sufferers in a study aimed at comparing cognitive therapy and biofeedback. The control condition was a waiting list. At posttreatment, about 80% of the subjects in the cognitive therapy group showed at least a 50% improvement in their symptoms, whereas 50% of the patients in the other treatment conditions showed similar results. At 2-year follow-up, subjects treated with cognitive therapy still showed substantial improvement compared with baseline levels.

In a later (1978) replication study, Holroyd and colleagues compared cognitive-behavioral treatments with coping skills (see Holroyd and Andrasik 1982). This second study showed that patients in the treatment groups responded significantly better than those in the control condition. Several other studies carried out by independent groups have verified the original findings by Holroyd and colleagues. Favorable results apply not only to the treatment of tension headache but also to migraine and mixed headache sufferers as well. Among the studies reviewed by Holroyd and Andrasik (1982), a sizable number included biofeedback, or a combination of cognitive therapy and biofeedback, for comparison; few included relaxation training. The results of those studies showed a consistent superiority for cognitive therapy (or a combination in which cognitive therapy was included) over the behavior therapy techniques alone.

Holroyd and Andrasik also reported a study by Lake et al. (1979) in which RET was used as a comparison treatment. The authors of this study noted, however, that only three 30- to 40-minute sessions were appended to biofeedback sessions. Hence, no satisfactory conclusions could be drawn concerning the efficacy of RET. A later study (Finn et al. 1991) concerned with the use of RET in comparison with progressive muscle relaxation training in the treatment of tension headache was cursorily reviewed in the otherwise comprehensive review of RET outcome studies recently published by Haaga and Davison (1989). In the study by Finn et al. (1991), RET appeared to be about as effective as muscle relaxation, achieving substantial benefits in about one-third of the subjects.

Attanasio et al. (1987) are among the few who specifically addressed the issue of efficacy and cost-effectiveness of a largely self-administered treatment format compared with a therapist-administered treatment program. This compared relaxation training alone or in combination with cognitive therapy in the treatment of headache. At 2-month follow-up patients in all treatment conditions improved in their symptoms, with a slight superiority for the cognitive treatments. On the basis of those results the authors suggested that largely self-administered treatments can result in significant improvements while substantially reducing the total amount of therapist contact.

In summary, there is a wealth of replicated controlled investigations that emphasize the efficacy of a cognitive-based treatment approach to severe headache. Long-term follow-up data (up to 2 years) suggest that therapeutic gains obtained at posttreatment are maintained for at least 2 years. A partially self-administered treatment format has been developed that would substantially reduce treatment costs for a large proportion of tension headache sufferers. Generalization of the results of these studies to the treatment of other, and perhaps more severe, pain syndromes cannot be made at this time as the available evidence only consists of anecdotal reports.

Miscellaneous Conditions

As stressed in the introduction to this section, cognitive therapies have been applied in a great array of disorders (e.g., in the management of essential hypertension, in the treatment of nausea and vomiting induced by cancer chemotherapy, in the management of stress in patients with breast cancer, in the treatment of patients after mastectomy, in the treatment of coronary patients postsurgery, in the treatment of emesis following gastrointestinal surgery, in the treatment of the Type A behavior pattern, in the treatment of psychosexual dysfunctions, and with patients suffering from writer's cramp). Most of the evidence concerning these treatments is from clinical reports or small-scale uncontrolled studies. As would be expected, the great majority of the reports express a degree of confidence in the effectiveness of the therapeutic strategy used. It is unfortunate that solid evidence based on well-designed controlled studies that have been replicated is not yet available. However, preliminary reports suggest that CBT could become an important treatment strategy for the treatment of some nonpsychiatric conditions.

General Comments and Conclusions

A summary of the efficacy of CBT for defined mental disorders has been made at the end of each pertinent section and will not be repeated here. Instead, an attempt at a more global assessment will be made.

The rise of cognitivism has added a new dimension to, and opened new venues for behavior therapy, at the same time as it has created new conceptual problems that are not easy to solve. On the other hand, the incorporation of cognitive conceptions constitutes an important step toward a convergence and rapprochement of therapies of different theoretical origins (see Goldfried 1982). This goes far beyond a superficial eclecticism. The inclusion of cognitive treatment strategies has widened the scope of behavior therapy, and the results obtained by combining more traditional strategies with techniques based on cognitive-social learning appear, in most cases, to enhance efficacy. Evidence for this statement has been presented in this review. On the other hand, a clear conceptualization of the use of cognitive strategies in otherwise strictly behavioral treatment approaches is too often lacking, and terminology is inconsistently used. For example, the term "cognitive restructuring" is used to refer to both direct training in reducing self-defeating instructions and such training coupled with an attempt at correcting "irrational" beliefs. However, the same concept, when used in cognitive therapy, primarily refers to an attempt at modifying more basic (schematic) cognitive structures. Thus, it would be impossible to understand what an author actually means if the theoretical context is unclear. The contemporaneous out of context use, of cognitive and behavioral techniques could also reduce the efficacy of traditional behavioral interventions because the patient could be distracted to pay attention to cognitive events. Clearly the necessity of a shift in theoretical stance when trying to combine treatment principles of traditional behavior therapy with treatment principles of cognitive therapy is ignored by many behavior therapists. A poor awareness of this issue cannot but lead to methodological confusion and, very likely, to poorer results.

Much of the criticism leveled above at behavior therapy, and at CBTs with a strong emphasis on behavior modification, also applies to more proper cognitive therapies. The publications dealing with the use of RET, for example, do not succeed in substantiating claims for its efficacy in various morbid conditions. Ellis himself has acknowledged that, "in comparison to some more incisive studies of Beck's cognitive therapy, RET research has been distinctly lacking" (Ellis 1989, p. 231). In those areas in which the efficacy of cognitive therapy has been subjected to empirical validation, the results have appeared to be consistent across different populations of patients and in different settings. Especially in the field of emotional disorders, cognitive therapy appears to represent a valid alternative to more traditional treatments, including pharmacotherapy. In addition, evidence is accumulating that therapeutic gains at post-treatment are not only maintained but can also increase over time.

Even though evidence in this respect is still preliminary, there are suggestions that cognitive therapy–based treatment approaches could be a viable alternative for the treatment of patients with severe personality disorders and with schizophrenia.

That CBT is feasible with patients of all ages clearly emerges from a review of the pertinent literature. Treatments comprised of cognitive therapeutic strategies have proven to be effective, both when implemented in institutions and when applied at various levels of the health system, or in the classroom, at work locations, or even at home. Large-scale, community-based programs relying on cognitive-behavioral strategies are currently underway in many places around the world and no serious obstacles have been met in implementing them.

The use of CBT in a group format, compared to individual treatment, has overall yielded similar results. The length of treatment for the average patient with an uncomplicated disorder is clearly shorter than that required by many other psychotherapeutic approaches. No side effects of any relevance have been reported in the literature for any of the therapeutic approaches under scrutiny. In none of the various types of CBT is there any commitment opposing the concomitant use of pharmacotherapy whenever such a combination is required by the particular status of the patient. In fact the issue of combining cognitive therapy and pharmacotherapy has been addressed at some length (Wright and Schrodt 1989).

A sizable number of cognitive therapy publications for home reading (bibliotherapy) are available. The use of records and videotapes has proven to be a viable alternative for promoting clinically relevant changes in patients with milder forms of mental disorders. Thus this particular method of treatment can be widely disseminated. However, it is impossible to evaluate the extent to which such approaches are of substantial help to persons troubled by everyday life problems who otherwise would become patients requiring professional attention.

The issue of efficacy in relation to costs has only had preliminary examination. The cost of a treatment can be assessed in several ways: for example, by taking into account the cost of professional training required to apply a given treatment, or by considering which individuals can be trained. Patient costs are the actual monetary costs and the emotional ones that relate to how taxing a certain treatment is to the patient. The concept of "acceptability" is pertinent in this context. In many of the quantitative analyses reported above, a significant correlation has been found between the therapist's level of competence and the outcome. Training programs in cognitive therapy require a shorter time span than training for other therapies. Also, those programs can easily be designed to suit the needs of particular categories of mental health workers (Bowers 1989; Perris 1989, in press). In principle, it is possible to train nurses and other mental health workers operating in the field to perform meaningful interventions. This can be done in a much shorter time than would be required to train the same people in other types of psychotherapy.

There is no direct information about the acceptability of CBT to patients of various categories. However, judging from the low attrition rates emphasized in most reports, CBT appears to be acceptable to a sizable number of patients at all levels of the health system.

In conclusion, there is strong evidence for the efficacy of CBT in various morbid conditions, and especially in the treatment of emotional disorders. In patients with disorders of this type, CBT appears to be not only an equally effective alternative to other treatments, but also a type of treatment where therapeutic gains are maintained and increased over time. CBT is, apparently, easily accepted by a sizeable number of patients. Low attrition rates have been consistently reported in studies of outcome. No noxious side effects have been noted. The length of treatment is relatively short for the treatment of the average patient (12–15 sessions), and is shorter than that required for a number of other treatments. CBT can be applied at various levels of the health system by professionals, as well as by trained nonprofessionals, especially trained nurses. CBT can be widely disseminated in various formats.

References

Abikoff H: Efficacy of cognitive training interventions in hyperactive children: a critical review. Clinical Psychology Review 5:479–512, 1985

Adams HE, Brantley PJ, Malatesta V, et al: Modification of cognitive processes: a case study of schizophrenia. J Consult Clin Psychol 49:460–464, 1981

Agras WS, Schneider JA, Arnow B, et al: Cognitive-behavioral and response-prevention treatments for bulimia nervosa. J Consult Clin Psychol 57:215–221, 1989

Albersnagel F, Rouwendal J: Cognitive gedragstherapie van depressie: overzicht en evaluatie van gecontroleerd outcome-onderzoek. Gedragstherapie 17:27–44, 1984

Alford GS, Fleece L, Rothblum E: Hallucinatory-delusional verbalizations: modification in a chronic schizophrenic by self-control and cognitive restructuring. Behav Modif 6:421–435, 1982

Andersson BO, Thoresson P, Skagerlind L, et al: Preliminary results of an intensive cognitive-behavioral treatment program for patients with schizophrenic syndromes. Paper presented at the World Congress of Cognitive Therapy, Oxford, England, June 28–July 2, 1989.

Andrews G, Harvey R: Does psychotherapy benefit neurotic patients? Arch Gen Psychiatry 38:1203–1212, 1981

Arieti S: The cognitive-volitional school, in American Handbook of Psychiatry, 2nd Edition, Vol 1. Edited by Arieti S. New York, Basic Books, 1974, pp 877–903

Asarnow JR, Carlson GA: Childhood depression: five-year outcome following combined cognitive-behavior therapy and pharmacotherapy. Am J Psychother 42:456–464, 1988

Attanasio V, Andrasik F, Blanchard EB: Cognitive therapy and relaxation training in muscle contraction headache: efficacy and cost-effectiveness. Headache 27:254–260, 1987

Bandura A: The self system in reciprocal determinism. Am Psychol 33:344–358, 1978

Barabasz AE, Barabasz M: Effects of rational-emotive therapy on psychophysiological and reported measures of test anxiety arousal. J Clin Psychol 37:511–514, 1981

Barlow DH, Cohen AS, Waddell MT, et al: Panic and generalized anxiety disorders: nature and treatment. Behavior Therapy 15:431–449, 1984

Barlow DH, Craske MG, Cerny JA, et al: Behavioral treatment of panic disorder. Behavior Therapy 20:261–282, 1989

Barrios BA, Shigatomi C: Coping skills training for the management of anxiety: a critical review. Behavior Therapy 10:491–522, 1980

Basch MF: Psychoanalytic interpretation and cognitive transformation. Int J Psychoanal 62:151–175, 1981

Beck AT: Depression. Philadelphia, University of Pennsylvania Press, 1966

Beck AT: Cognitive approaches to panic disorder: theory and therapy, in Panic: Psychological Perspectives. Edited by Rachman S, Maser J. Hillsdale, NJ, Lawrence Erlbaum, 1988, pp 91–109

Beck AT, Rush AJ, Shaw BF, et al: Cognitive Therapy of Depression. New York, Guilford, 1979

Beck AT, Hollon SD, Young JE, et al: Treatment of depression with cognitive therapy and amitriptyline. Arch Gen Psychiatry 42:335–344, 1985a

Beck AT, Steer RA, Kovacs M, et al: Hopelessness and eventual suicide: a 10-year prospective study of patients hospitalized with suicidal ideation. Am J Psychiatry 142:559–563, 1985b

Beckham EE, Watkins JT: Process and outcome in cognitive therapy, in Comprehensive Handbook of Cognitive Therapy. Edited by Freeman A, Simon KM, Beutler LE, et al. New York, Plenum, 1989

Berman JS, Miller RC, Massman PJ: Cognitive therapy versus systematic desensitization: is one treatment superior? Psychol Bull 97:451–461, 1985

Beutler LE, Scogin F, Kirkish P, et al: Group cognitive therapy and alprazolam in the treatment of depression in older adults. J Consult Clin Psychol 55:550–556, 1987

Biran M: Cognitive and exposure treatment for agoraphobia: reexamination of the outcome research. Journal of Cognitive Psychotherapy 2:165–178, 1988

Bishay NR, Petersen N, Tarrier N: An uncontrolled study of cognitive therapy for morbid jealousy. Br J Psychiatry 154:386–389, 1989

Blackburn IM: An appraisal of comparative trials of cognitive therapy, in Cognitive Psychotherapy: Theory and Practice. Edited by Perris C, Blackburn IM, Perrisberg H. Heidelberg, Springer, 1988, pp 160–179

Blackburn IM, Bishop S, Glen AIM, et al: The efficacy of cognitive therapy in depression: a treatment trial using cognitive therapy and pharmacotherapy, each alone and in combination. Br J Psychiatry 139:181–189, 1981

Blackburn IM, Eunson KM, Bishop S: A two-year naturalistic follow-up of depressed patients treated with cognitive therapy, pharmacotherapy and a combination of both. J Affective Disord 10:67–75, 1986

Blaney PH: The effectiveness of cognitive and behavioral therapies, in Behavior Therapy for Depression. Edited by Rehm LP. New York, Academic Press, 1981, pp 1–32

Block J: Effects of rational-emotive therapy on overweight adults. Psychotherapy, Theory, Research and Practice 17:277–280, 1980

Blowers C, Cobb J, Mathews A: Generalized anxiety: a controlled treatment study. Behav Res Ther 25:493–502, 1987

Borg S, Blennow G, Sandberg P, et al: Bensodiazepinberoende och andra långtidsbiverkningar—en översikt. Läkartidningen 83:321–326, 1986

Borkovec TD, Mathews AM, Chambers A, et al: The effects of relaxation training with cognitive or nondirective therapy and the role of relaxation-induced anxiety on the treatment of generalized anxiety. J Consult Clin Psychol 55:883–888, 1987

Botvin GJ, Baker E, Renick NL, et al: A cognitive-behavioral approach to substance abuse prevention. Addict Behav 9:137–147, 1984

Bowers WA: Cognitive therapy with inpatients, in Comprehensive Handbook of Cognitive Therapy. Edited by Freeman A, Simon KM, Beutler LE, et al. New York, Plenum, 1989, pp 583–596

Brenner HD, Stramke WG, Mewes J, et al: Erfahrungen mit einem spezifischen Therapieprogramm zum Training kognitiver und kommunikativer Fähigkeiten in der Rehabilitation chronisch schizophrener Patienten. Nervenarzt 51:106–112, 1980

Brenner HD, Hodel B, Kube G, et al: Kognitive therapie bei schizophrenen: problemanalyse und empirische Ergebnisse. Nervenarzt 58:72–83, 1987

Brownell KD, Wadden TA: Behavior therapy for obesity: Modern approaches and better results, in Handbook of Eating Disorders. Edited by Brownell KD, Foreyt JP. New York, Basic Books, 1986, pp 180–197

Buchkremer G, Fiedler P: Kognitive versus handlungsorientierte Therapie. Vergleich zweier psychotherapeutischer Methoden zur Rezidivprophylaxe bei schizophrenen Patienten. Nervenarzt 58:481–488, 1987

Chor PN, Mercier MA, Halper IS: Use of cognitive therapy for treatment of a patient suffering from a bipolar affective disorder. Journal of Cognitive Psychotherapy 2:51–58, 1988

Cochran SD: Preventing medical noncompliance in the outpatient treatment of bipolar affective disorders. J Consult Clin Psychol 52:873–878, 1984

Collins RL, Rothblum ED, Wilson GT: The comparative efficacy of cognitive and behavioral approaches to the treatment of obesity. Cognitive Therapy and Research 10:299–318, 1986

Comas-Diaz L: Effects of cognitive and behavioral group treatment on the depressive symptomatology of Puerto Rican women. J Consult Clin Psychol 49:627–632, 1981

Cooper PJ, Fairburn G: Cognitive behavior therapy for anorexia nervosa: some preliminary findings. J Psychosom Res 28:493–499, 1984

Covi L, Lipman RS: Cognitive behavioral group psychotherapy combined with imipramine in major depression. Psychopharmacol Bull 23:173–176, 1987

Cox GL, Merkel WT: A qualitative review of psychosocial treatments for bulimia. J Nerv Ment Dis 177:77–84, 1989

Crouch G, Robson M, Hallström C: Benzodiazepine dependent patients and their psychological treatment. Prog Neuropsychopharmacol Biol Psychiatry 12:503–510, 1988

Deffenbacher JL, Story DA, Brandon AD, et al: Cognitive and cognitive-relaxation treatments of anger. Cognitive Therapy and Research 12:167–184, 1988

de Jong R, Henrich G, Ferstl R: A behavioral treatment program for neurotic depression. Behavior Analysis and Modification 4:275–287, 1981

de Jong R, Treiber R, Henrich G: Effectiveness of two psychological treatments for inpatients with severe and chronic depressions. Cognitive Therapy and Research 10:645–663, 1986

DeRubeis RJ, Beck AT: Cognitive therapy, in Handbook of Cognitive-Behavioral Therapies. Edited by Dobson KS. New York, Guilford, 1988, pp 273–306

Dunn RJ: Cognitive modification with depression-prone psychiatric patients. Cognitive Therapy and Research 3:307–317, 1979

Durham RC, Turvey AA: Cognitive therapy versus behavior therapy in the treatment of chronic general anxiety. Behav Res Ther 25:229–234, 1987

Dushe DM, Hurt ML, Schroeder H: Self-statement modification with adults: a meta-analysis. Psychol Bull 94:408–442, 1983

D'Zurilla TJ, Goldfried MR: Problem-solving and behavior modification. J Abnorm Psychol 78:107–126, 1971

Eimer BN: Psychotherapy for chronic pain: a cognitive approach, in Comprehensive Handbook of Cognitive Therapy. Edited by Freeman A, Simon KM, Beutler LE, et al. New York, Plenum, 1989, pp 449–466

Ellis A: Comments on my critics, in Inside Rational-Emotive Therapy. Edited by Bernard ME, DiGiuseppe R. New York, Academic Press, 1989, pp 199–260

Emmelkamp PMG, Mersch PP: Cognition and exposure in vivo in the treatment of agoraphobia: short-term and delayed effects. Cognitive Therapy and Research 6:77–88, 1982

Emmelkamp PMG, Kuipers A, Eggeraat J: Cognitive modification versus prolonged exposure in vivo: a comparison with agoraphobics. Behav Res Ther 16:33–41, 1978

Emmelkamp PMG, Visser S, Hoekstra RJ: Cognitive therapy versus exposure in vivo in the treatment of obsessive-compulsives. Cognitive Therapy and Research 12:103–114, 1988

Farid B, El Sherbini M, Raistrick: Cognitive group therapy for wives of alcoholics—a pilot study. Drug Alcohol Depend 17:349–358, 1986

Feindler EL, Ecton RB, Kingsley D, et al: Group anger-control training for institutionalized psychiatric male adolescents. Behavior Therapy 17:109–123, 1986

Finn T, DiGiuseppe R, Culver C: The effectiveness of rational-emotive therapy in the reduction of muscle contraction headache. Journal of Cognitive Psychotherapy Int Q 5:93–103, 1991

Fleming BM, Thornton DW: Coping skills training as a component in the short-term treatment of depression. J Consult Clin Psychol 48:652–654, 1980

Fordyce WE: Behavioral methods for chronic pain and illness. St Louis, MO, Mosby, 1976

Fowler DG: Cognitive-behavioral interventions with schizophrenic patients at high risk of relapse. Paper read at the World Congress of Cognitive Therapy, Oxford, United Kingdom, June 28–July 2, 1989

Fowler DG: The cognitive-behavioral management of patients with schizophrenia. Paper read at the Tenth International Symposium for the Psychotherapy of Schizophrenia, Stockholm, Sweden, Aug 11–15, 1991

Fowler D, Morley S: The cognitive-behavioral treatment of hallucinations and delusions: a preliminary study. Behavioral Psychotherapy 17:267–282, 1989

Frankl VE: Logos, paradox, and the search for meaning, in Cognition and Psychotherapy. Edited by Mahoney MJ, Freeman A. New York, Plenum, 1985, pp 259–277

Freeman C, Sinclair F, Turnbull J, et al: Psychotherapy for bulimia: a controlled study. J Psychiatr Res 19:473–478, 1985

Freeman CPL, Barry F, Dunkeld-Turnbull J, et al: Controlled trial of psychotherapy for bulimia nervosa. BMJ 296:521–525, 1988

Fremouw WJ, Gross R: Issues in cognitive-behavioral treatment of performance anxiety. Advances in Cognitive-Behavioral Research and Therapy 2:279–306, 1983

Fremouw WJ, Zitter RE: A comparison of skills training and cognitive restructuring-relaxation for the treatment of speech anxiety. Behavior Therapy 9:248–259, 1978

Gallagher DE, Thompson LW: Treatment of major depressive disorder in older adult outpatients with brief psychotherapies. Psychotherapy: Theory, Research and Practice 19:482–490, 1982

Gallagher DE, Thompson LW: Effectiveness of psychotherapy for both endogenous and nonendogenous depression in older adult outpatients. J Gerontol 38:707–712, 1983

Garfinkel PE, Garner DM, Kennedy S: Special problems of inpatient management, in Handbook of Psychotherapy for Anorexia Nervosa and Bulimia. Edited by Garner DM, Garfinkel PE. New York, Guilford, 1985, pp 344–359

Garner DM, Bemis KM: Cognitive therapy for anorexia nervosa, in Handbook of Eating Disorders. Edited by Garner DM, Garfinkel PE. New York, Guilford, 1985, pp 107–146

Glass GV: Primary, secondary, and meta-analysis of research. The Educational Researcher 10:3–8, 1976

Goldfried M (ed): Converging Themes in Psychotherapy. New York, Springer, 1982

Goldfried MR, Linehan MM, Smith JL: Reduction of text anxiety through cognitive restructuring. J Consult Clin Psychol 46:32–39, 1978

Greenwood VB: Cognitive therapy with the young adult chronic patient, in Cognitive Therapy With Couples and Groups. Edited by Freeman A. New York, Plenum, 1983, pp 183–198

Guidano V, Liotti G: Cognitive Processes and the Emotional Disorders. New York, Guilford, 1983

Haaga DAF, Davison GC: Outcome studies of rational-emotive therapy, in Inside Rational-Emotive Therapy. A Critical Appraisal of the Theory and Therapy of Albert Ellis. Edited by Bernard ME, DiGiuseppe R. New York, Academic Press, 1989, pp 155–197

Haley J: Strategies of Psychotherapy. New York, Grune & Stratton, 1963

Hamlin M: An integrated cognitive-behavioral approach to withdrawal from tranquilizers, in Developments in Cognitive Psychotherapy. Edited by Dryden W, Trower P. London, Sage, 1988, pp 153–176.

Harpin RE, Liberman RP, Marks I, et al: Cognitive-behavior therapy for chronically depressed patients: a controlled pilot study. J Nerv Ment Dis 170:295–301, 1982

Hautzinger M: Cognitive therapy with depressed outpatients: a summary of four outcome and process related studies, in Cognitive Psychotherapy. An Update. Edited by Perris C, Eisemann M. Umeå, DOPUU Press, 1988, pp 63–66

Heimberg R: Cognitive and behavioral treatments of social phobia: a critical analysis. Clinical Psychology Review 9:107–128, 1989

Heimberg RG, Dodge CS, Hope DA, et al: Cognitive behavioral group treatment for social phobia: comparison with a credible placebo control. Cognitive Therapy and Research 14:1–23, 1990

Hermanutz M, Gestrich J: Kognitives Training mit Schizophrenen. Beschreibung des Trainings und Ergebnisse einer kontrollierten Therapiestudie. Nervenarzt 58:91–96, 1987

Hole RW, Rush AJ, Beck AT: A cognitive investigation of schizophrenic delusions. Psychiatry 42:312–318, 1979

Hollon SD: Comparisons and combinations with alternative approaches, in Behavior Therapy for Depression. Edited by Rehm LP. New York, Academic Press, 1981, pp 32–71

Hollon SD, Tuason VB, Wiemer MJ, et al: Combined cognitive-pharmacotherapy versus cognitive therapy alone and pharmacotherapy alone in the treatment of depressed outpatients. Paper read at the meeting of the Association for the Advancement of Behavior Therapy, Washington, DC, December 10, 1983

Holroyd KA, Andrasik F: A cognitive–behavioral approach to recurrent tension and migraine headache. Advance in Cognitive-Behavioral Research and Therapy 1:275–320, 1982

Horowitz M, Marmar C, Krupnick J, et al: Personality Styles and Brief Psychotherapy. New York, Basic Books, 1984

Hughes JN, Sullivan KA: Outcome assessment in social skills training with children. J School Psychol 26:167–183, 1988

Ivey AE: Developmental Therapy. San Francisco, Jossey Bass, 1986

Jansson L, Öst L-G: Psykologisk behandling av klinisk depression: en evaluerande översikt. Nordisk Psykiatrisk Tidsskrift 21:467–480, 1984

Jarvik LF, Mintz J, Steuer J, et al: Treating geriatric depression: a 26-week interim analysis. J Am Geriatr Soc 30:713–717, 1982

Karst TO, Trexler LD: Initial study using fixed-role and rational-emotive therapy in treating public-speaking anxiety. J Consult Clin Psychol 34:360–366, 1970

Kelly G: The Psychology of Personal Constructs. New York, Norton, 1955

Kingdon DG, Turkington D: The use of cognitive behavior therapy with a normalizing rationale in schizophrenia. J Nerv Ment Dis 179:207–211, 1991

Kingdon D, Farr P, Murphy S, et al: Hypomania following cognitive therapy. Br J Psychiatry 148:103–104, 1986

Kirkley, BG, Schneider JA, Agras WS, et al: Comparison of two group treatments for bulimia. J Consult Clin Psychol 53:43–48, 1985

Klosko JS, Barlow DH, Tassinari RB, et al: Comparison of alprazolam and cognitive behavior therapy in the treatment of panic disorder: a preliminary report, in Panic and Phobias, Vol 2. Edited by Hand I, Wittchen H-U. Berlin, Springer, 1988, pp 54–65

Kraemer S, Sulz KHD, Schmid R, et al: Kognitive Therapie bei standardversorgten schizophrenen Patienten. Nervenarzt 58:84–90, 1987

Kramer FM, Stalker LA: Treatment of obesity, in Comprehensive Handbook of Cognitive Therapy. Edited by Freeman A, Simon KM, Beutler LE, et al. New York, Plenum, 1989, pp 385–401

Kreitler S, Chemerinski A: The cognitive orientation of obesity. Int J Obes 12:403–415, 1988

Kruglanski AW: The epistemic approach in cognitive therapy. International Journal of Psychology 16:275–297, 1981

Lader M: Benzodiazepines—the opium of the masses? Neuroscience 3:159–165, 1978

Lake A, Rainey J, Papsdorf JD: Biofeedback and rational-emotive therapy in the management of migraine headache. J Appl Behav Anal 12:127–140, 1979

LaPointe KA: Cognitive therapy versus assertive training in the treatment of depression, in Dissertation Abstracts International, No 37,4689B, 1977

LaPointe KA, Rimm DC: Cognitive, assertive, and insight-oriented group therapies in the treatment of reactive depression in women. Psychotherapy: Theory, Research and Practice 17:312–321, 1980

Larcombe NA, Wilson PH: An evaluation of cognitive-behavior therapy for depression in patients with multiple sclerosis. Br J Psychiatry 145:366–371, 1984

Latimer PR, Sweet AA: Cognitive versus behavioral procedures in cognitive-behavior therapy: a critical review of the evidence. J Behav Ther Exp Psychiatry 15:9–22, 1984

Lazarus AA: Behavior Therapy and Beyond. New York, McGraw-Hill, 1971

Lee NL, Rush AJ: Cognitive-behavioral group therapy for bulimia. International Journal of Eating Disorders 5:599–615, 1986

Leitenberg H, Rosen JC, Gross J, et al: Exposure plus response-prevention treatment of bulimia nervosa. J Consult Clin Psychol 56:535–541, 1988

Levendusky PG, Berglas S, Dooley CP, et al: Therapeutic contract program: preliminary report on a behavioral alternative to token economy. Behav Res Ther 21:137–142, 1983

Lindsay WR, Gamsu CV, McLaughlin E, et al: A controlled trial of treatments for generalized anxiety. Br J Clin Psychol 26:3–15, 1987

Liotti G, Reda MA: Some epistemological remarks on cognitive therapy, behavior therapy, and psychoanalysis. Cognitive Therapy and Research 5:231–236, 1981

Lipsky MJ, Cassinove H, Miller NJ: Effects of rational-emotive therapy, rational role reversal, and rational-emotive imagery on the emotional adjustment of community mental health center patients. J Consult Clin Psychol 48:366–374, 1980

Little VL, Kendall PC: Cognitive-behavioral interventions with delinquents: problem solving, role-taking, and self-control, in Cognitive-Behavioral Interventions: Theory, Research, and Procedures. Edited by Kendall PC, Hollon SD. New York, Academic Press, 1979, pp 81–116

Lungwitz H: Zeitschrift für des gesamte. Neurologie und Psychiatrie 100:4–5, 1926

Lungwitz H: Die Psychobiologie der Krankheit. 7 Band: Die Neuronlehre. Die Erkenntnistherapie. Berlin, W De Gruyter, 1955

Lyons LC, Woods PJ: The efficacy of rational-emotive therapy: a quantitative review of the outcome research. Clinical Psychology Review 11:357–369, 1991

Magaro PA, West AN: Structured learning therapy: a study with chronic psychiatric patients and level of pathology. Behav Modif 7:29–40, 1983

Magers BD: Cognitive-behavioral short-term group therapy with depressed women, in Dissertation Abstracts International, no 38, 2816B, 1978

Mahoney MJ: The cognitive sciences and psychotherapy: patterns in a developing relationship, in Handbook of Cognitive-Behavioral Therapies. Edited by Dobson KS. New York, Guilford, 1988, pp 357–386

Marchione KE, Michelson L, Greenwald M, et al: Cognitive behavioral treatment of agoraphobia. Behav Res Ther 25:319–328, 1987

Marks IM: Fears and Phobias. London, Heinemann, 1969

Marks IM: Exposure treatments: clinical applications, in Behavior Modification: Principles and Clinical Applications, 2nd Edition. Edited by Agras WS. Boston, Little, Brown, 1978

Marlatt GA, Gordon JR: Relapse Prevention: Maintenance Strategies in Addictive Behavior. New York, Guilford, 1984

Maultsby MC: Rational Behavior Therapy. Englewood-Cliffs, NJ, Prentice-Hall, 1984

Mavissakalian M, Michelson L, Greenwald D, et al: Cognitive-behavioral treatment of agoraphobia: paradoxical intention versus self-statement training. Behav Res Ther 21:75–86, 1983

McNamara K, Horan JJ: Experimental construct validity in the evaluation of cognitive and behavioral treatments for depression. Journal of Counseling Psychology 33:23–30, 1986

Meichenbaum D: Cognitive modification of test-anxious college students. J Consult Clin Psychol 39:370–380, 1972

Meichenbaum D: Cognitive-Behavior Modification. New York, Plenum, 1977

Michelson L: Cognitive-behavioral assessment and treatment of agoraphobia, in Anxiety and Stress Disorders. Edited by Michelson L, Ascher LM. New York, Guilford, 1987, pp 213–279

Miller IW, Norman WH, Keitner GI, et al: Cognitive-behavioral treatment of depressed inpatients. Behavior Therapy 20:25–47, 1989

Miller RC, Berman JS: The efficacy of cognitive behavior therapies: a quantitative review of the research evidence. Psychol Bull 94:39–53, 1983

Milton F, Patwa VK, Hafner RJ: Confrontation versus belief modification in persistently deluded patients. Br J Med Psychol 51:127–130, 1978

Minkoff K, Bergman E, Beck AT, et al: Hopelessness, depression and attempted suicide. Am J Psychiatry 130:455–459, 1973

Moleski R, Tosi DJ: Comparative psychotherapy: rational-emotive therapy versus systematic desensitization in the treatment of stuttering. J Consult Clin Psychol 44:309–311, 1976

Murphy GE, Simons AD, Wetzel RD, et al: Cognitive therapy and pharmaco-therapy. singly and together in the treatment of depression. Arch Gen Psychiatry 41:33–41, 1984

Neimeyer RA, Twentyman CT, Prezant D: Cognitive and interpersonal group therapies for depression: a progress report. The Cognitive Behaviorist 7:21–22, 1985

Nidiffer FD: Combining cognitive and behavioral approaches to suicidal depression: a 42-month follow-up. Psychol Rep 47:539–542, 1980

Novaco RW: Anger Control: The Development of an Experimental Treatment. Lexington, MA, DC Heath, Lexington Books, 1975

Novaco RW: Anger and coping with stress: cognitive behavioral interventions, in Cognitive Behavior Therapy. Edited by Foreyt JP, Rathjen DP. New York, Plenum, 1978 pp 135–173

Oei TPS, Jackson PR: Social skills and cognitive behavioral approaches to the treatment of problem drinking. J Stud Alcohol 43:532–547, 1982

Olbrich R, Mussgay L: Reduction of schizophrenic deficits by cognitive training: an evaluative study. European Archives of Psychiatry and Neurological Sciences 239:366–369, 1990

Ordman AM, Kirschenbaum DS: Cognitive-behavioral therapy for bulimia: an initial outcome study. J Consult Clin Psychol 53:305–313, 1985

Perris C: The foundations of cognitive psychotherapy and its standing in relation to other psychotherapies, in Cognitive Psychotherapy. Theory and Practice. Edited by Perris C, Blackburn IM, Perris H. Heidelberg, Springer, 1988, pp 1–43

Perris C: Cognitive therapy with schizophrenic patients. New York, Guilford Press, 1989

Perris C: An integrating cognitive-behavioral treatment program for patients with a schizophrenic disorder, in Innovations in Psychiatric Rehabilitation. New Directions in Mental Health Services (Special Issue). Edited by Liberman RP. San Francisco, CA, Jossey-Bass, (in press)

Peter K, Glaser A, Kühne G-E: Erste Erfahrungen mit der kognitiven Therapie Schizophrener. Psychiat Neurol med Psychol 41:485–491, 1989

Peterfreund E: Information, Systems, and Psychoanalysis. New York, Academic Press, 1971

Powers PS, Powers HP: Inpatient treatment of anorexia nervosa. Psychosomatics 25:512–527, 1984

Rehm LP, Kokke P: Self-management therapies, in Handbook of Cognitive Behavioral Therapies. Edited by Dobson KS. New York, Guilford, 1988, pp 136–166

Reynolds DK: Orita Psychotherapy. Berkeley, CA, University of California Press, 1976

Reynolds WM, Coasts KI: A comparison of cognitive behavioral therapy and relaxation training for the treatment of depression in adolescents. J Consult Clin Psychol 54:653–660, 1986

Rosen JC: A review of behavioral treatments for bulimia nervosa. Behav Modif 11:464–486, 1987

Rosenberg H, Brian T: Cognitive-behavioral group therapy for multiple-DUI offenders. Alcoholism-Treatment Quarterly 3:47–65, 1986

Ross M, Scott M: An evaluation of the effectiveness of individual and group cognitive therapy in the treatment of depressed patients in an inner city health center. Journal of the Royal College of General Practitioners 35:239–242, 1985

Rötzer-Zimmer FT, Axmann D, Koch H, et al: One year follow-up of cognitive behavior therapy for depressed patients: a comparison of cognitive behavioral therapy alone, in combination with pharmacotherapy and pharmacotherapy alone. Paper presented at the 15th annual meeting of the European Association for Behavior Therapy, Munich, August 29–September 1, 1985

Rush AJ, Watkins JT: Group versus individual cognitive therapy: a pilot study. Cognitive Therapy and Research 5:95–103, 1981

Rush AJ, Giles DE: Cognitive therapy: theory and research, in Short-Term Psychotherapies for Depression. Edited by Rush AF. Chichester, John Wiley, 1982, pp 143–181

Rush AJ, Beck AT, Kovacs M, et al: Comparative efficacy of cognitive therapy and pharmacotherapy in the treatment of depressed outpatients. Cognitive Therapy and Research 1:17–37, 1977

Rush AJ, Beck AT, Kovacs M, et al: A comparison of the effects of cognitive therapy and pharmacotherapy on hopelessness and self-concept. Am J Psychiatry 139:862–866, 1982

Sanchez-Craig M, Annis HM, Bornet AR, et al: Random assignment to abstinence and controlled drinking: evaluation of a cognitive-behavioral program for problem drinkers. J Consult Clin Psychol 52:390–403, 1984

Sanchez-Craig M, Kay G, Busto U, et al: Cognitive-behavioral treatment for benzodiazepine dependence. Lancet 1:388, 1986

Sasson Edgett J, Prout MF: Cognitive and behavioral approaches to the treatment of anorexia nervosa, in Comprehensive Handbook of Cognitive Therapy. Edited by Freeman A, Simon KM, Beutler LE, et al. New York, Plenum, 1989, pp 367–384

Shaffer CS, Shapiro J, Sank LI, et al: Positive changes in depression, anxiety, and assertion following individual and group cognitive behavior therapy intervention. Cognitive Therapy and Research 5:149–157, 1981

Shaffer CS, Sank LI, Shapiro J, et al: Cognitive behavior therapy follow-up: maintenance of treatment effects at six months. Journal of Group Psychotherapy, Psychodrama and Sociometry 35:57–64, 1982

Shapiro DA, Shapiro D: Meta-analysis of comparative therapy outcome studies: a replication and refinement. Psychol Bull 92:581–604, 1982

Shaw BF: Comparison of cognitive therapy and behavior therapy in the treatment of depression. J Consult Clin Psychol 45:543–551, 1977

Skagerlind L: Behandlingserfarenhet från de kognitive behandlingscentra i Umeå. Paper read at the spring meeting of the Swedish Psychiatric Association, Linköping, Sweden, May 1991

Skinner PT: Skills not pills: learning to cope with anxiety. Journal of the Royal College of General Practitioners 34:258–260, 1984

Smith ML, Glass GV: Meta-analysis of psychotherapy outcome studies. Am Psychol 32:752–760, 1977

Smith ML, Glass GV, Miller TI: The Benefits of Psychotherapy. Baltimore, MD, John Hopkins University Press, 1980

Spivack G, Shure M: Social Adjustment of Young Children: A Cognitive Approach to Solving Real-Life Problems. San Francisco, Jossey-Bass, 1974

Steinbrueck SM, Maxwell SE, Howard GS: A meta-analysis of psychotherapy and drug therapy in the treatment of unipolar depression with adults. J Consult Clin Psychol 51:856–863, 1983

Steuer JL, Mintz J, Hammen CL, et al: Cognitive-behavioral and psychodynamic group psychotherapy in treatment of geriatric depression. J Consult Clin Psychol 42:180–189, 1984

Teasdale JD, Fennell MJ, Hibbert GA, et al: Cognitive therapy for major depressive disorder in primary care. Br J Psychiatry 144:400–406, 1984

Trexler LD, Karst TO: Rational-emotive therapy, placebo, and no-treatment effects on public-speaking anxiety. J Abnorm Psychol 79:60–67, 1972

Turk DC, Genest M: Regulation of pain: the application of cognitive and behavioral techniques for prevention and remediation, in Cognitive-Behavioral Interventions. Theory, Research and Procedures. Edited by Kendall PC, Hollon SD. New York, Academic Press, 1979, pp 287–318

Turner RW, Wehl CK: Treatment of unipolar depression in problem drinkers. Advances in Behav Res Ther 6:115–125, 1984

Tyrer P, Murphy S, Oates G, et al: Psychological treatment for benzodiazepine dependence. Lancet 1:1042–1043, 1985

Tyrer P, Murphy S, Kingdon D, et al: The Nottingham study of neurotic disorder: comparison of drug and psychological treatments. Lancet 30:235–240, 1988

Urbain ES, Kendall PC: Review of social-cognitive problem-solving interventions with children. Psychol Bull 88:109–143, 1980

Watts FN, Powell GE, Austin SV: The modification of abnormal beliefs. Br J Med Psychol 46:359–363, 1973

Weiner ML: Cognitive-Experiential Therapy. New York, Brunner/Mazel, 1985

Wierzbicki M, Bartlett TS: The efficacy of group and individual cognitive therapy for mild depression. Cognitive Therapy and Research 11:337–342, 1987

Wilson GT, Brownell KD: Behavior therapy for obesity: an evaluation of treatment outcome. Advances in Behav Res Ther 3:49–86, 1980

Wilson PH, Goldin JC, Charbonneau-Powis M: Comparative efficacy of behavioral and cognitive treatments of depression. Cognitive Therapy and Research 7:111–124, 1983

Woodward R, Jones RB: Cognitive restructuring treatment: a controlled trial with anxious patients. Behav Res Ther 18:401–407, 1980

Woody GE, McLellan AT, Lubursky L, et al: Psychotherapy for substance abuse. Psychiatr Clin North Am 9:547–562, 1986

Wright JH, Schrodt GR: Combined cognitive therapy and pharmacotherapy, in Comprehensive Handbook of Cognitive Therapy. Edited by Freeman A, Simon KM, Beutler LE, et al. New York, Plenum, 1989, pp 267–281

Zeiss RD, Lewinsohn PM, Munoz RF: Nonspecific improvement effects in depression using interpersonal skills training, pleasant activity schedules, or cognitive training. J Consult Clin Psychol 47:427–439, 1979

CHAPTER 7

Behavior Therapy

Jean Cottraux, M.D., Ph.D.

General Overview

Behavior therapy (BT) could be defined as the application of scientifically based psychological principles to the solution of clinical problems. Antecedents of the behavioral approach are to be found in the works of the French psychologist Pierre Janet (1920). The traditional Japanese Morita therapy represents an attempt to treat phobic, obsessive, and depressive problems through a process of social isolation and mental and physical relaxation followed by a *life training period,* which is similar to graded exposure (Murase and Johnson 1974). BT started in the mid-1950s with narrow applications (i.e., specific phobias) and has become a well-established psychotherapy school with techniques that represent treatments of choice for phobias, panic attacks, obsession-compulsions, and sexual problems and for the rehabilitation of people with chronic mental diseases. Other major applications have been in the field of depression and in the prevention and psychological management of some physical diseases. Child psychiatry and psychology, education, and psychogeriatrics have also benefited from principles or techniques derived from BT research.

Behavior or Cognitive-Behavior Therapy

In the last 10 years BT has become more and more cognitive, and it would be more realistic today to speak of *cognitive-behavioral therapy.* But this label is not accepted by all the BT practitioners. Some think that adding cognitive theory and therapeutic principles to the classical BT, rooted in the conditioning model, represents a methodologically wrong step. Others contend that there is no longer any justification, at the theoretical, practical, or research level, for distinguishing cognitive therapy and BT. Results obtained with classical behavioral methods can be better explained in cognitive terms than in conditioning ones. Even though BT acts to modify behaviors and emotions, its final action is on cognitions. The patient becomes more confident, less demoralized, and more able to cope with stressful or distressing situations that were previously avoided (Bandura 1977). This cognitive change has been variously labeled as self-efficacy enhancement, internalization of the locus of control, or modification of danger or failure self-schemas.

The limits of BT can be expanded with cognitive methods, as shown by research on depression, panic attacks, or bulimia. The information processing model now dominates the fields of neuroscience, computer science, neuropsychology, and psychology. Since the early 1970s it has been extended to the treatment of depression and anxiety disorders by Beck and his followers (Beck et al. 1979). Moreover, surveys of clinical practice have indicated that most members of BT associations define their practice as both cognitive and behavioral.

In general terms, the criteria that define BT are as follows:

1. The therapy is structured and an agenda is set for each session. Patients and therapists interact on the basis of an empirical collaboration to solve psychological problems.
2. The therapy is centered on current problems. Therapist and patient agree on the selection of target behaviors and on the goals of the treatment.
3. Functional analysis (or behavioral analysis) is carried out with the patient. It consists of isolating target problems to analyze their current antecedents and consequences. Mediating cognitive variables (images, thoughts, emotions, and beliefs) are related to ongoing emotions and behaviors. While the main focus is on those factors that maintain current behavior, the patient's history is also noted if it has some relevance to "here and now" problems.
4. Continuing measurement of target problem behaviors occurs before, during, and after therapy, and at follow-up (usually 6–12 months after the end of the treatment). Other measures, especially cognitive

or personality measures, should be used to complement the measurement of target behaviors.

5. A written treatment program (usually 10 to 25 sessions) is defined with the patient. Its rationale and techniques are explained to the patient. The term of the therapy is fixed in advance. Sessions are given once or twice a week.

6. The therapy aims to develop the patient's control over personal problem behaviors.

7. The therapy has a structured format. Each session starts with an agenda, and at the end of each session real-life homework is agreed on with the patient, which is evaluated at the next session. Ongoing functional analysis is carried out to understand new or unexpected problems. At the last session patient and therapist agree on a maintenance program. Booster sessions are scheduled if needed. The patient is followed up 6–12 months after the end of the treatment to ensure the quality of the outcomes and assess the durability of the treatment.

8. The techniques are designed to teach the patient new coping skills or improve old ones that are failing. Three basic techniques are used: a) modification of emotional and psychophysiological responses (e.g., through relaxation); b) behavior modification (e.g., prolonged exposure to anxiety-provoking situations in imagination, in vivo, until anxiety and avoidance subsides); and c) cognitive modification (e.g., questioning and challenging irrational depressive thoughts or implementing problem-solving strategies to cope with a difficult social encounter).

9. Techniques have been empirically tested in single-case experimental designs and later in controlled trials. They are based on learning principles (classical and operant conditioning, social learning theory) and on cognitive principles related to an information processing model.

BT and Other Psychotherapeutic Schools

A positive therapeutic relationship (therapeutic alliance) is a necessary but not sufficient condition for a successful treatment. Transference with insight into deep unconscious structures and meanings related to psychodynamic theories is not central to BT practice. Behavior therapists give as many explanations to patients as do psychoanalysts (Sloane et al. 1975); these explanations refer to learning and cognitive principles and also to the biological bases of learning. Past history of learning is not neglected, especially by cognitive therapists who conceptualize depression as the result of negative self-schemas that are deep seated in long-term memory and related to early learning. Behavior therapists give advice and support as *supportive therapists* do; but in addition they use specific learning-based or cognitive techniques that have been tested in controlled trials. Accordingly, the therapeutic relationship and the search for meaning are not banished from BT settings: they are used in another way and with reference to a theoretical model other than psychoanalysis.

Scope of the Chapter

The main aim of this chapter is to review the most important controlled trials aimed at assessing the effectiveness of BT. More general meta-analyses comparing the effectiveness of different psychotherapies are discussed in this book. This review is limited to adult psychopathological problems; interested readers can find a general overview of BT as applied to child pathology in Ollendick (1986). The cognitive therapy of depression is discussed by Perris and Herlofson in this book (see Chapter 6), while the contribution of BT to rehabilitation of psychotic states is discussed by Burti and Yastrebov (see Chapter 10). Thus in this chapter I will focus on anxiety disorders, sexual and marital problems, and the applications of BT to medical problems (behavioral medicine).

Agoraphobia and Panic Attacks

Panic attacks may exist as a single disorder (panic disorder without agoraphobia), but are often the first stage of agoraphobia. Patients with panic attacks can be depressed or suicidal, have a drug or alcohol addiction, or have employment or marital problems. To my knowledge no study focusing on the prevention of agoraphobia by the treatment of panic attacks has so far been carried out, but agoraphobia and panic attacks can be treated by effective BT techniques.

Exposure Treatment

Since the pioneering work of Wolpe (1958) on systematic desensitization for phobias, in vivo exposure has been firmly established as the key factor in modifying situational anxiety and avoidance in simple phobias, social phobia, and agoraphobia with or without panic attacks. Panic attacks can also be modified by exposure treatments (Marks 1987). The rationale of such treatment is habituation to physiological responses and extinction of avoidance responses. Prolonged exposure in imagination is presented to the patient, sitting in an armchair, slightly relaxed with closed eyes. Exposure in imagination aims at ensuring subjective habituation to the phobic stimuli before real life exposure. The exposure in imagination session is stopped when the patient's subjective anxiety is decreased by 50%. At this point, the patient begins in vivo exposure. This prolonged exposure may be presented to the patient in the two following ways:

1. It may be presented through therapist-aided and -accompanied, prolonged in vivo exposure, preceded by exposure in imagination and cognitive restructuring, and followed by homework exposure assignments. Each session lasts 1–2 hours.
2. Graded exposure homework assignments are discussed with the patient and agreed on at each session. Marital and family therapy may be useful in some cases. Significant others can be enrolled as cotherapists for prolonged exposure sessions.

This self-exposure technique is the most cost-effective. Ten to 20 sessions are generally required to modify phobic behaviors. Booster sessions are often necessary in the 6 months following treatment. Prolonged in vivo exposure (2 hours) is superior to short (½ hour) in vivo exposure. Group exposure is as effective as individually conducted exposure programs (Marks 1987).

Exposure management is quickly taught to students. Indeed, Marks (1987) found that nurse-therapists trained in BT (in a 1-year course) are as effective as doctors or psychologists. Furthermore, small group treatments are feasible. Cost-effective computer-assisted treatment has been proposed by Gosh et al. (1988) who studied, in a controlled design, 71 phobic patients randomized to three groups: self in vivo exposure instructed by either a psychiatrist, a computer, or a book. The average therapist contact with each group last 3.1, 3.2, and 0 hours, respectively. All three groups improved significantly and continued improvement at 6 months follow-up. Interestingly, the therapist was perceived and rated by the patient as more tolerant, reliable, and understanding than the computer or the book.

It should be emphasized that in vivo exposure is one of the few "success stories" in the history of psychotherapy (Barlow 1984). Barlow's review showed that a significant improvement was found in 70% of the treated patients, but total symptom elimination appeared only in 18%. The drop-out rate was 12% when behavioral exposure was given alone, but reached 25%–40% if antidepressants were also given. Relapses were as high as 50%, but in general were easily treated with booster sessions. No symptom substitutions were found.

A meta-analysis of 11 studies, carried out using stringent inclusion criteria, found an average improvement rate of 58% across all data sets (Jacobson et al. 1988). Only 27% of the patients ended the therapy with little or no residual phobic behaviors. Generally the treatment gains were maintained over various follow-up periods. Jacobson et al. (1988) suggested that cognitive techniques and involvement of the spouse should be added to exposure to improve outcomes.

A review restricted to long-term follow-up studies was conducted by O'Sullivan and Marks (1990). Ten studies, ranging in duration from 1 to 9 years and conducted in England, Germany, the United States, and the Netherlands, were included (Burns et al. 1986; Emmelkamp and Kuipers 1979; Jansson and Ost 1982; Lelliot et al. 1987; McPherson et al. 1980; Munby and Johnston 1980). Out of 553 patients included in controlled studies, 474 were followed up for a mean duration of 4 years. Taking all studies together, 76% of the agoraphobic patients improved. Mean improvement from baseline was 50%. Work and social adjustment were good, but residual symptoms were the rule, and 15%–25% of the patients continued to have depressive episodes following treatment. In the longer follow-ups, up to 50% of the 553 patients had consulted doctors for their psychological problems and 25% had seen psychiatrists for depression and agoraphobia. However, the overall frequency of consultations had decreased.

Antidepressants and Exposure

Antidepressants are effective for avoidance, depression, panic, anger, hostility, rituals, and pain. According to Klein and colleagues (Klein 1964; Klein et al. 1987), antidepressants have a specific antipanic effect, which exposure does not have. Telch et al. (1985) found that imipramine and exposure had a synergistic effect, but suggested that the action of imipramine was not related to pharmacological blocking of panic. Agras (1988) suggested from the findings of a controlled study that imipramine may have antiphobic effects and exposure antipanic effects. Both treatments were synergistic.

However, the side effects caused by the drug treatment resulted in frequent noncompliance by the patients. Relapses after withdrawal of antidepressants are common (25%–100% [Noyes et al. 1986]) and the gain of combining exposure with imipramine has been shown to vanish after withdrawal of the medication (Zitrin et al. 1980). Unlike drugs, the effects of exposure are long lasting. However, antidepressants are useful in depressed agoraphobic patients (Marks 1987) and in patients who do not respond quickly enough to BT or who need a benzodiazepine withdrawal phase.

Limitations of Drug and Exposure Treatments

Clum (1989) reviewed 40 drug studies and 14 behavior or cognitive-behavioral controlled studies that compared the effectiveness of psychological intervention and drug treatments in the management of panic attacks. Three criteria were used: treatment termination, treatment success, and treatment relapse. According to this review, claims of superiority for psychological or pharmacological treatment are premature. Nonetheless, behavior therapies specifically developed to ameliorate panic attacks have the lowest relapse rate. Agoraphobics with panic attacks have, in general, higher dropout rates and lower success rates than individuals with panic disorders without avoidance, regardless of the treatment used.

In conclusion, despite the clearly demonstrated effectiveness of both exposure and antidepressants in these disorders, the limitations of those treatments have led to a search for new methods to treat panic disorders. From this research, cognitive therapies for panic attacks have emerged.

Rational-Emotive Therapy and
Self-Instructional Training Techniques

Rational-emotive therapy has been used for treating agoraphobia and obsessive-compulsive disorders. Typically the treatment is given in 15 1-hour individual sessions, or 6 2.5-hour group sessions. The A-B-C framework is presented in a didactic and persuasive way, with A referring to an activating event or experience, B to the person's irrational beliefs about the activating event, which is assumed to lead to the C, the irrational consequence. The therapist helps the patient to dispute his or her irrational belief system.

Self-instructional training methods have also been developed. An example is Meichenbaum's (1977) cognitive restructuring therapy, which is presented to the patient in four successive stages:

1. Preparation, which consists of explanations of anxiety management and the relations between internal dialogue and behavior
2. Covert confrontation of anxiety-provoking situations, which are rehearsed in imagination
3. Coping in imagination with phobic situations
4. Reinforcement for any progress achieved by the patient in coping with imagined situations

During each of the four stages, the patient is taught to ascertain how anxious he or she feels, to become conscious of negative self-statements, and to replace them with productive self-statements.

A general review of the results obtained with these early techniques of cognitive therapy can be found in Cottraux and Mollard (1988). The techniques were not superior to exposure, and the effectiveness of exposure was not increased when it was combined with cognitive therapy in seven studies (Barlow et al. 1984; Cullington et al. 1984; Emmelkamp and Mersch 1982; Emmelkamp et al. 1978, 1986; Mavissakalian et al. 1985; Williams and Rappoport 1983). Michelson et al. (1988) found equivalent outcomes in agoraphobia with panic attacks in a controlled study comparing three treatment groups: relaxation, paradoxical intention, and in vivo exposure. But the three groups received exposure homework, which could have been the key factor in modifying avoidance and panic attacks. In view of the unsatisfactory outcomes obtained with these intellectualistic cognitive techniques, a search for new cognitive methods became warranted.

Cognitive-Behavioral Therapy Techniques

Cognitive-behavioral therapy of phobias is a directive and didactic form of psychotherapy that aims at modifying erroneous basic assumptions concerning danger (Beck et al. 1985). Clark (1986) proposed a cognitive model to explain the interactions and the negative feedback loops between cognitions, hyperventilations, and external or internal triggering events. Therapy lasts about 15 1-hour sessions, once or twice weekly.

The therapist gives the patient an outline of general principles and basic hypotheses on cognitive therapy in panics. Functional analysis emphasizes the interactions between thoughts, emotions, and behavior. During the first sessions, Socratic dialogue, and real life self-observation, using daily recording forms, elicit inner monologues, self-verbalizations, and dysfunctional ideas concerning danger and avoidance behavior. The links between anxiety, avoidance, and some recurrent involuntary and automatic thoughts are progressively pointed out.

Emotions are elicited through exposure to internal interoceptive cues. Bodily sensations linked to anxiety that lead to catastrophic interpretations, especially the fear of becoming crazy or having a heart attack, are challenged. Inductive reasoning, Socratic dialogue, and problem-solving techniques modify the patient's logical errors.

In this way, step by step, the deeper basic schemas of danger are elicited and understood. Schemas are then progressively disputed by the therapist. The patient's catastrophic expectations are modified by reality testing, which is achieved by gradual, prolonged, and successful exposure in imagination and in vivo to feared cues (behavioral experiments).

Breathing Control Techniques

Chronic and acute hyperventilation is one of the clinical manifestations of agoraphobia and panic attacks. The treatment has two main strategies: 1) teaching patients to relabel their bodily sensations and to reattribute these sensations to hyperventilation induced by stressful stimuli, and

2) teaching patients to avoid hyperventilation by slow breathing when under stress in order to control the starting point of panic attacks.

Bonn et al. (1984) compared two groups of agoraphobic patients with panic attacks (exposure with or without respiratory control) and concluded that, although respiratory control was more effective for panic attacks and somatic symptoms, in vivo exposure was necessary to increase patients' autonomy.

Hibbert and Chan (1989) showed that respiratory training plus in vivo exposure was more effective than exposure alone in a controlled study of 40 patients with panic attacks, with or without avoidance. Respiratory control plus exposure was compared to placebo plus exposure. Observer ratings, but not self-ratings of anxiety, showed a greater improvement for the group receiving breathing training. Patients who hyperventilated did not benefit more from respiratory training than those who did not have the training.

Ost (1988) showed the superiority of an applied relaxation package, including cognitive instructions, over a classical Jacobsen's relaxation program. Barlow et al. (1989) developed a package labeled *panic control treatment*, which included hyperventilation, regulated breathing, exposure to interoceptive feared internal situations, and cognitive restructuring. This package treatment was superior to a waiting list control condition or relaxation alone, but when combined with relaxation it was significantly less effective than when used alone, at least at a 2-year follow-up (Craske et al. 1991). Relaxation seemed detrimental to panic disorders. Accordingly, the internal exposure and breathing control with cognitive restructuring emerged as the most effective technique, with about 80% of patients remaining panic free 2 years after the end of the treatment.

Other studies are in press. The Oxford study deserves mention. A preliminary report at 1-year follow-up (Salkovskis et al. 1990) has suggested that BT, with respiratory techniques, was superior (84% panic-free patients) to a waiting list control condition, to relaxation (40%), and to imipramine up to 300 mg a day (42% panic free). As all treated groups received in vivo exposure instructions, it was the cognitive treatment component that seemed the most effective for panic attacks.

A German study (Margraf et al. 1991) randomized 82 patients with panic disorder into four treatment groups: pure cognitive treatment, pure exposure treatment, combined treatment, and a waiting list control group. Over 80% of the those completing the study were panic free at 4-week follow-up in the three treated groups, versus 5% in the waiting list. Pure cognitive and pure exposure treatments alone were as effective as their combination. Specific cognitive changes in bodily sensation interpretations correlated with treatment success, while self-exposure did not. The authors' hypothesis was that specific cognitive changes could be the active therapeutic ingredient, even in pure exposure therapy.

Summary

Panic disorder with or without agoraphobia can be treated effectively with BT. The crucial component of the therapy could be the modification of catastrophic interpretation of bodily sensations. Respiratory control and cognitive restructuring in agoraphobia with panic attacks is an effective technique that adds something to in vivo exposure. Panic disorder, without agoraphobia, can be treated effectively with BT. Antidepressant medication may be useful to treat panic attacks and depression associated with agoraphobia, although it may induce a higher drop-out rate and more frequent relapse when the medication is stopped. Its benefit is short-lived and inferior to cognitive therapy. Benzodiazepines do not seem effective in controlled trials.

In terms of applicability, Barlow's panic control package, which is presented through therapist and patient manuals, seems to be the easiest to implement to date (Barlow and Craske 1988). It can be delivered by psychopharmacologically oriented clinicians (Welkowitz et al. 1991), but with a lower rate of success than usually achieved with trained behavior therapists (60% versus 85%). Barlow's panic control treatment is now being tested versus imipramine and in combination with imipramine in a large scale study ($N = 600$) being conducted by the National Institute of Mental Health. Results are expected by the end of 1994 (D. Barlow, personal communication, November 1991). The applicability of Barlow's treatment in primary care by nurses or general practitioners has yet to be tested.

The development of panic control packages that are easy to apply resulted from a project designed to treat both panic and agoraphobia (Andrews 1982). The results of the research de-emphasized the role of therapist-aided exposure, replacing it with self-managed exposure, led at a personal pace by the patient and supplemented with cognitive and respiratory techniques. As noticed by Welkowitz et al. (1991), the main problem regarding the applicability of these techniques is represented by the presence of comorbid conditions such as depression, suicide, marital problems, occupational problems, or personality disorder, all of which require an additional treatment. Flexibility and therapeutic adaptation to specific problems may therefore require an extensive training that standardized manuals cannot do.

The application of these methods according to patient personality warrants further research on predictive factors. In their study of 124 patients with panic disorder and agoraphobia, Cottraux et al. (1991) found that improvement in agoraphobia after BT was correlated with a higher Minnesota Multiphasic Personality Inventory (Hathaway and McKinley 1943) internalization ratio.

Social Phobias

Social skills training, through role-play with rehearsal, shaping, and modeling by the therapist, is effective in treating social phobias in individual or group settings. The development of social skills and assertiveness is generally used to modify social phobic behavior. The rationale of such treatment often refers to exposure principles, but social learning and cognitive theories are also invoked to explain the effects of assertiveness training, which is a cost-effective, group-treatment method. Furthermore, role-playing may be a treatment in its own right or an adjacent technique in cognitive therapy or in vivo exposure packages.

In two controlled studies (Butler et al. 1984; Marzillier et al. 1976), behavioral techniques (role-playing or systematic desensitization) proved to be better than control groups. There were no differences between the behavioral technique, systematic desensitization, or role-playing. In addition, long-term follow-up showed that gains were maintained (O'Sullivan and Marks 1990).

Psychodynamic therapies are less effective than systematic desensitization in socially anxious students. The results of psychodynamic therapies are equal to those of a waiting list control condition (Paul 1966).

There are no controlled studies comparing BT to antidepressants, which are deemed effective in this disorder (for a review see Liebowitz et al. 1985).

Good evidence exists in analogous populations to support the effectiveness of cognitive interventions for test anxiety, speech anxiety, and social anxiety (for a review see Beck et al. 1985; Liebowitz et al. 1985). Social phobias, however, represent a more enduring and stable condition marked by chronic social skills deficits. Stravinsky et al. (1982), studying socially dysfunctional patients, compared a social skills training program using role rehearsal, instructions, feedback, and homework assignments with the same program combined with a cognitive restructuring method. At 6-month follow-up, social skills training showed a significant improvement that was not enhanced by the addition of cognitive modification.

Mattick et al. (1989) compared in vivo exposure, cognitive restructuring, exposure plus cognitive restructuring, and waiting list treatments in patients with social phobias: the treated groups improved more than the control group. The two groups receiving exposure improved more than the group receiving cognitive restructuring alone on the measures of phobia at the end of the treatment. But at 3-month follow-up, the combination of the two treatments was more effective than either alone.

In a randomized design with 65 patients, Gerlentner et al. (1991) compared BT (with exposure), phenelzine plus self-exposure, alprazolam plus self-exposure, and placebo plus self-exposure. No between-group differences were found at the end of treatment, or at 2-month posttreatment follow-up. Exposure seemed to be the critical therapeutic variable in that study.

In summary, exposure treatment or social skills training are the psychological treatments of choice for social phobias. Direct comparisons with antidepressants alone are needed.

Simple Phobias

Many uncontrolled single case reports have been published on treatment of simple phobias (e.g., see Wolpe 1958). In controlled studies, simple phobias are often composed of mixed samples of phobic patients. Follow-up studies have shown a 54% improvement from baseline, which is maintained at follow-up ranging from 1 to 5 years (O'Sullivan and Marks 1990). Zitrin et al. (1978), in a controlled study, showed that imipramine was ineffective in simple phobias and may have had detrimental effects. Two controlled studies (Biran and Wilson 1981; Ladouceur 1983) reported negative outcomes of the effectiveness of cognitive therapy alone in simple phobias.

Thus, despite the paucity of controlled studies, in vivo exposure seems to be the treatment of choice for simple phobias; antidepressant medication is not effective.

Generalized Anxiety

Generalized anxiety is four times more frequent than panic disorder. However, only a handful of controlled studies have been published so far on its treatment. The inclusion of a mixed anxiety-depression category in the *International Classification of Diseases, 10th Edition* (World Health Organization 1992) and possibly in the forthcoming *Diagnostic and Statistical Manual of Mental Disorders, 4th Edition* may increase the interest in those pervasive anxiety syndromes that are commonly found in primary care. As long-term treatment with benzodiazepines is not satisfactory, there is a need for long-acting psychological treatment in such chronic and common problems.

The effectiveness of behavioral management and relaxation has been demonstrated in controlled studies using waiting list subjects as controls and using 6-month follow-ups (Blowers et al. 1987; Butler et al. 1987; Tarrier and Main 1986). Durham and Turvey (1987), in a controlled study with 51 subjects, compared two treatment groups: BT and BT according to Beck et al.'s model (1985). At 6 months BT according to Beck's model was superior to BT alone. Therefore, the dissemination of BT techniques among general practitioners may reduce the prescription of benzodiazepines and the cost to public pharmaceutical budgets.

Posttraumatic Stress Disorder

There has been a growing interest in the treatment of posttraumatic stress disorders. Only a few papers have dealt with the problem of the effectiveness of the treatment with antidepressants compared to BT (exposure in imagination). For example, exposure in imagination, when compared with a waiting list control condition, was effective for treating posttraumatic stress disorder in Vietnam war veterans (Keane et al. 1989). Self-instructional training showed clear effectiveness in the controlled study by Foa and Rothbaum (1989). Further evidence is needed to determine the treatment of choice for this disorder.

Obsessive-Compulsive Disorder

Most obsessive-compulsive patients present with both obsessions and compulsions; depression is common in about 50% of these patients. Methods have been developed to modify motor rituals and obsessive thoughts as well as depression.

In Vivo Exposure With Response Prevention

The application of this technique is now well described (Marks 1987). In vivo exposure may be presented by the therapist, who guides the patient and demonstrates, step by step, the behavior to be performed (for example, touching the ground without washing the hands for 10 minutes). Alternatively, it is just as effective, less time consuming, and less expensive to give homework assignments that are agreed upon, discussed, and re-evaluated at each session (Emmelkamp and Kraanen 1977). In general, 25 sessions are needed. If therapist-guided exposure is necessary, one to three 1-hour sessions are needed. For homework assignments alone, 30 to 45 minutes are enough. Home-based treatments are often necessary for rituals that involve cleaning the house or hoarding. Couples therapy and family contracts may be useful in some cases. In an early pilot study, Hand and Tichazky (1979) showed that group treatment of obsessive-compulsive patients with their spouses might be feasible, as well as effective.

Rituals have been successfully treated with exposure and response prevention with success rates ranging from 50% to 70% of the fully treated patients (Marks 1987). The cost-effectiveness of exposure with response prevention homework has been stressed by Marks et al. (1988).

Exposure in Imagination

In vivo exposure is the best solution for patients with washing-cleaning rituals, as these patients are similar to simple phobic patients: they avoid touching "dirty" or "contaminated" objects. Another category of patients, the "checkers," are more difficult to manage because their rituals are triggered by internal representations of catastrophes rather than by environmental cues. Prolonged exposure in imagination (Foa et al. 1980) is especially recommended for patients who fear catastrophes and who perform covert or overt checking rituals to prevent their responsibility in the events they imagine (e.g., death of significant others, car accidents).

Combined Packages

According to the results of a controlled study made by Steketee et al. (1982), the best package for treating obsessive-compulsive disorder is represented by a combination of three techniques that deal with cognitive, motor, and physiological response systems. These are

1. *Exposure in imagination.* This modifies internal checking rituals and covert rumination, which are directed toward preventing imaginary catastrophes.
2. *In vivo exposure.* This reduces anxiety through habituation.
3. *Response prevention.* This eliminates overt rituals.

Despite these results, the effectiveness of in vivo exposure treatment has been found to have some limitations. Many patients refuse treatment (25%) or drop out in the earlier phases of the therapy. Of those who remain in therapy, 25% will not be improved. Out of the 50% of improved patients, 20% will relapse within 3 months to 3 years (Salkovskis and Warwick 1988). These limitations are invoked to justify the addition of cognitive techniques or antidepressants to improve the outcomes. Long-term follow-ups of in vivo exposure have also been carried out.

O'Sullivan and Marks (1990) reviewed nine cohorts followed up after exposure in England, the United States, Greece, Australia, and Holland. Self-ratings and assessor ratings were used. Two cohorts received exposure plus either clomipramine or placebo. The overall attrition rate was 9%. Out of a total of 223 patients, 195 (87%) were followed up for 1–6 years with a mean of 3 years. In all the studies there was a significant improvement at posttreatment, which was retained at follow-up. The improvement was maintained in two studies, while there were further gains at follow-up, but two studies showed that some of the initial improvement had been lost. Improvement in obsessive-compulsive symptoms was found in 78% of the patients at follow-up, which generalized to better social adjustment, even though some residual symptoms were common. The average improvement was a 60% decrease in obsessive-compulsive symptoms compared to pretreatment. Despite this improvement in obsessions and compulsions, preexisting liability to depressive episodes continued.

Antidepressants and Exposure: Controlled Trials

Serotonergic antidepressants are effective in obsessive-compulsive disorder; their effects are independent of the level of depression (Zohar and Insel 1987). However, the effect of drugs is not long lasting, and relapses are common after drug withdrawal (Thoren et al. 1980). Side effects, especially anorgasmy, can also be a problem (Monteiro et al. 1986). The combined treatment of serotonergic drugs (clomipramine and fluvoxamine) and exposure have been assessed.

In a controlled study with 27 subjects, Solyom and Sookman (1977) compared exposure imagination, thought stopping (training the patient to eliminate his or her rumination with the word "stop"), and clomipramine. After 6 months clomipramine was equally as effective as exposure in imagination, but more effective than thought stopping in the reduction of ruminations. Clomipramine was less effective than BT in the reduction of rituals. A combination of the two treatments should be effective in treating both rituals and ruminations.

Marks and colleagues (Marks et al. 1980; Mawson et al. 1982; Stern et al. 1980) published a cross-over controlled study of 40 depressed ritualizers, treated in three different ways: relaxation, exposure, and clomipramine. Relaxation produced little change. Clomipramine had an effect on rituals, mood, and social adjustment, but only in those patients who had a depressed mood. Clomipramine had a maximum effect at weeks 10–18 and diminished thereafter. Relapses after clomipramine cessation obliged the researchers to recommence the drug treatment. At 2-year follow-up there was no drug effect but a stable exposure effect. At 6-year follow-up there was no drug effect, and better long-term outcome tended to be related to more previous exposure and better compliance with exposure. The best predictor of long-term outcome was the degree of improvement at the end of treatment. The patients who were initially the most depressed were more likely to receive psychotropic medication in the 6-year period following treatment.

In a second cross-over controlled study by Marks and colleagues, (Kasvikis et al. 1988; Marks et al. 1988; O'Sullivan and Marks 1990), 49 nondepressed ritualizers were assessed to evaluate the effectiveness of three methods: clomipramine, self-exposure (through homework assignments), and therapist-aided exposure. Of the three methods, clomipramine played a limited adjuvant role, while therapist-aided exposure had only a marginal effect. The most effective method was self-exposure, which is also a cost-effective treatment. At 2-year follow-up the improvement was retained and no difference appeared between the patients who received clomipramine and those who did not. Improvement in mood was found to be independent of improvements in rituals according to a principal components analysis of treatment effects. Taken together, these two studies showed that antidepressants were useful only in depressed obsessive-compulsive patients, while exposure and response prevention was an effective and sufficient treatment for nondepressed obsessive-compulsive patients.

In a controlled study by Cottraux et al. (1990), 60 depressed obsessive-compulsive outpatients were randomly assigned to fluvoxamine without exposure, fluvoxamine with exposure, or placebo with exposure for 24 weeks. At week 8 there was a drug between-group effect on rituals but not on depression. At week 24 there was a drug between-group effect on depression but not on rituals. The drug superiority was short-lived. At week 48 there was no between-group difference in rituals and depression. The 18-month follow-up of this study (Cottraux et al. 1990) showed that patients as a whole remained improved with no between-group differences. However, 80% of the patients receiving fluvoxamine with exposure or placebo with exposure, versus 40% of the patients receiving fluvoxamine without exposure, did not take antidepressants over a 1-year posttreatment period, and the difference was statistically significant

$(P < .05)$. The final conclusion drawn by Cottraux et al. was that, in depressed obsessive-compulsive patients, fluvoxamine helped BT in the early stages of the treatment; moreover, BT helped the patients to withdraw from antidepressants in the long-term follow-up. Accordingly, the outcomes of this study would favor commencing with a combined treatment in depressed obsessive-compulsive patients.

Cognitive-Behavior Therapy Techniques

In the last 10 years, rational-emotive therapy or self-instructional training have become the main techniques for treating obsessive-compulsive disorders. New formulations have been proposed by Salkovskis (1985). His functional analysis differentiates three levels in the obsessive thinking process: 1) intrusive thoughts, which are senseless, abnormal, immoral, and egodystonic; 2) obsessive thoughts, which are not related to a specific ideational content, but to the struggle between intrusive and normalizing thoughts (automatic neutralizing thoughts can in fact be elicited and recorded—these thoughts aim to repress intrusive thoughts); and 3) intrusive and neutralizing thoughts, which are related to danger schemas that are deep seated in the long-term memory. Schemas are made of silent assumptions, such as "I should control everything I think of; if not, scandal or catastrophes may occur."

Three main therapeutic techniques used are

1. Cognitive exposure to intrusive thoughts with prevention of neutralizing thoughts. Exposure in imagination to obsessive fantasies and exposure to tape-recorded obsessive intrusive thoughts are used. The patient is instructed that he or she should not try to neutralize or to seek reassurance. The rationale of the treatment is explained to the patient: neutralizing is a way to escape or avoid ideas that thereafter cannot habituate.
2. Questioning basic schemas. Problem solving is used to question the pros and cons of intrusive ideas, neutralizing thoughts, and basic schemas and their behavioral consequences.
3. In vivo exposure. Behavioral experiments (in vivo exposure) without neutralizations are eventually implemented to disconfirm basic schemas.

Cognitive-behavioral therapy has been tested in three controlled studies. Emmelkamp et al. (1980) did not find a superior effect of adding cognitive modification to in vivo exposure. The treatment used was self-instructional training that directed patients to modify self-statements and replace negative thoughts with positive ones. The failure of this study could be explained by the possibility that the therapeutic procedure might have been used by the patients as a neutralizing thought. Emmelkamp et al. (1988) compared cognitive therapy without exposure (self- or therapist-guided) with self-managed exposure. Six months after the end of the treatment both groups showed equivalent reduction in rituals, generalized anxiety, and social anxiety. However, only the group receiving cognitive therapy presented a positive change on depression measures. There was a clear need to replicate this study as the patients were young, well-educated, and not chronic. In a more impaired sample of 21 patients, Emmelkamp and Beens (1991) found cognitive therapy and in vivo exposure to have been equally effective at 6-month follow-up.

Summary

Exposure and response prevention seems to be the psychological treatment of choice for obsessive-compulsive disorders. No information from well-controlled studies exists on the effects of other psychotherapeutic treatments for this disorder. In vivo exposure either with or without cognitive therapy is now a recognized treatment at the cost of only 25 hours of a psychiatrist's, psychologist's, or nurse therapist's work time (Marks 1987). In the case of depression, the addition of an antidepressant drug is warranted, at least in the initial phases of the treatment. However, in the long-term, clomipramine or fluvoxamine do not enhance the effects of exposure. Cognitive therapy showed promising results (at least equal to those of in vivo exposure) in two controlled studies, and may also improve depression.

Sexual and Marital Problems

Sexual Dysfunctions

Studies examining the treatment of sexual dysfunctions have tended to use either behavior therapies or an eclectic blend of behavioral, humanistic, and psychodynamic approaches. However, it seems that no approach has reached the success reported by Masters and Johnson (1971), namely good outcomes in 80% of 510 couples with a 5% relapse rate over 5 years. These uncontrolled outcomes have been often criticized on methodological grounds, as they might be attributed to a biased selection of patients who would respond well to the study's method. Other studies with less biased samples showed 39%–98% of couples improved by treatment (Cole 1985), depending on the treated samples and some methodological difficulties. Wright et al. (1977) reached the pessimistic conclusion that nothing seemed to be demonstrated in the field of sex therapy.

In a more recent review of controlled studies on sexual dysfunctions, Cottraux (1990) found more favorable outcomes. Behavioral interventions are better than waiting list in the treatment of vaginismus and female anorgasmy. Anxiolytics were as effective as sex therapy in one study of male impotence (Ansari 1976). BT (80% success on average) is better than psychodynamic therapy, which is equal to waiting list (10% success on average) (Obler 1973). There is no difference between therapeutic interventions run by a couple of therapists or a single therapist. One important issue is the cost-effectiveness problem. The problem of the rate of "spontaneous" remission and "nonprofessional treatment" of sexual problems has never been dealt with.

Marital Problems

Behavior marital therapy applied to couples in crisis has been tested in seven controlled studies (see Gurman et al. 1986). These studies showed a superiority of behavioral interventions versus waiting list controls, but found inconsistent evidence of superiority over attention-placebo control. Compared to nonbehavior marital therapy (cognitive, strategic, insight, interactional) it seems that there is no substantial difference in terms of outcome. A meta-analysis of 17 controlled studies on behavior marital therapy (Gurman et al. 1986) suggested that the typical couple receiving this therapy improved by more than 82% compared to untreated patients or patients receiving nonspecific treatment, which represents an important finding.

Behavioral Medicine

Application of BT principles and techniques to medical illness treatment and prevention started in the mid-1970s. I will review some of the main results of the literature on the subject.

Type A Behavior and Coronary Heart Disease

Modification of the type A behavioral pattern has been proposed as a means of preventing relapses and death after coronary heart disease. One controlled study by Friedman et al. (1984) compared 270 patients who received simple medical counseling to 592 patients who received the same treatment plus type A behavior management (relaxation, cognitive therapy, life-style modification). At 3-year follow-up both coronary heart disease relapses and type A behavior were found to be significantly decreased in the group receiving the behavior modification program. The effects of the behavior modification were superior to the effects of the simple medical counseling.

Nunes et al. (1987), in a meta-analysis of 18 controlled studies, concluded that psychological interventions may have a positive effect on the prognosis of coronary heart disease. In general, more research in this area seems justified.

Chronic Pain

Pain clinics using behavior and cognitive approaches have grown rapidly in the last 10 years. Both organic and psychogenic pain states have been treated. Most of the behavior and cognitive approaches have been incorporated into multidisciplinary programs dealing with various pain problems. Chronic low back pain is one of the disorders best studied. About 70% of the patients entering an operant conditioning program for chronic low back pain demonstrated improvement after treatment, and most of these patients maintained improvement at follow-up. While problems in measuring pain limit the conclusions to be drawn, 15 controlled studies (Bono and Zasa 1988) have been conducted that tested operant techniques or some kind of relaxation. Studies on operant techniques have shown an increase in activity levels, a decrease in consumption of medication, and an improvement in mood and reported pain. Studies on relaxation have shown mixed results. The status of cognitive variables and "pure" cognitive therapies is still unclear (Bono and Zasa 1988).

Hypertension

Relaxation and blood pressure feedback have been evaluated in 13 controlled trials (Jacob et al. 1987). Their effectiveness was not confirmed in several large scale trials because of the improvement occurring in the control group. Physical exercise and restriction of sodium intake led to limited outcomes in poorly controlled studies (Jacob et al. 1987).

Headaches

Chronic headaches have been treated by BT, relaxation, cognitive therapy, and biofeedback, or a combination of these treatments. Although the physiological basis of biofeedback is not firmly established, its therapeutic applications have shown a widespread dissemination in the last 15 years. Frontal electromyographic (EMG) feedback has been proposed to treat tension headaches, and hand temperature feedback to treat migraines. The literature on headaches suggests that biofeedback, although it is not a placebo, is a technique of uncertain specificity and mode of action. Relaxation appears as effective as biofeedback for migraine. Nonspecific factors play a significant role in the therapeutic process. Self-control and self-management techniques in everyday-life should be associated with biofeedback to maintain improvement. Blanchard (1987) reviewed 10 reports with at least a 12-month follow-up and drew the following conclusions:

1. For tension headaches, the improvement obtained from cognitive therapy or relaxation is maintained for 2 and 4 years, respectively. Initial headache reduction with frontal EMG feedback alone deteriorates progressively after 2 or 3 years, but not to the pretreatment level.
2. For migraine headaches, there is a good evidence for a maintenance of improvement with frontal EMG feedback at 12 months.
3. For migraine and combined headaches (vascular and tension head-

ache), treated with relaxation and thermo-feedback, there is a progressive deterioration over 4 years.

Smoking

Sixty controlled studies, with a follow-up of at least 12 months, have been conducted in the last 10 years (see the review by Glasgow and Lichtenstein 1987). Behavioral approaches seem to be superior to control conditions, but do not differ from alternative interventions. Behavioral interventions appear to be less effective in preventing relapses among heavy than lighter smokers (i.e., less than 20 cigarettes per day). To produce long-term maintenance, an intervention must produce high rates of initial cessation. Relapse prevention strategies must be capable of reaching and involving a high percentage of recent quitters. No theory or relapse model of maintenance appears to be superior to any other.

Obesity

Effectiveness of BT for obesity has been proven in controlled studies. The improvement is generally maintained at 1-year follow-up, but beyond this there is no evidence of maintenance. Adding pharmacotherapy to BT does not enhance the effectiveness. Long-term maintenance programs may decrease the relapse rate (Wilson and Brownell 1982).

Prevention of Cardiovascular Risk Factors

Social-learning based interventions have been widely used to promote healthy life-style and reduce risk factors for cardiovascular disorders. The "five community study" (Farquhar et al. 1990) showed the effectiveness of television health advertisements, in addition to counseling, on eating behavior, obesity, plasma cholesterol levels, blood pressure, and resting pulse rate. With follow-ups ranging from 30 to 64 months, the mortality risk scores decreased by 15% and the coronary heart disease scores by 16%.

Stuttering

For treatment of stuttering, regulated breathing has been investigated in controlled studies and has shown its superiority over placebo conditions.

In general, nine 1-hour sessions are necessary, followed by a transfer-maintenance phase of 3 months. With this treatment, the reduction of the percentage of stuttered syllables was from 45% to 5% (Saint-Laurent and Ladouceur 1987).

Andrews and Craig (1988) demonstrated in several studies the objective value of a 150-hour speech retraining program using the smooth speech technique. Long-term fluency was related to the degree of speech skill mastery, normal communication attitude, and internalization of the locus of control achieved at the end of the treatment.

Alcoholism

Chemical aversion and covert sensitization are adjunct techniques with limited effectiveness in treating alcoholism. Social skills training with cognitive restructuring, which teaches the patient how to resist social pressures to drink, are especially useful in preventing relapse in socially anxious drinkers. Controlled drinking versus total abstinence has been investigated; assignment to a goal of controlled drinking does not produce a better outcome than assignment to total abstinence. Controlled drinking seems to be more successful in less severe alcoholics in terms of duration of illness, physical dependence, and psychopathology (for a review see Emmelkamp 1986).

Bulimia and Anorexia Nervosa

Bulimia and anorexia nervosa are chronic diseases with substantial morbidity and mortality. There is a non-chance crossover between the two conditions. Operant conditioning in institutional settings is restricted to a quasi-emergency treatment for anorexia nervosa, when the patient shows very significant and life-threatening weight loss. This behavioral technique has been used empirically for more than a century, and its effectiveness is well established although the long-term outcomes are not modified (for a review see Agras 1987). Nonbehavioral family therapy (following Minuchin's model) was better than individual supportive therapy at a 1-year follow-up in one study that included both bulimic and anorexic patients (Russell et al. 1987). Longer follow-ups are obviously needed to establish the effectiveness of this first positive study of family therapy in this indication.

Bulimia has been recently investigated by behavior therapists, who conceptualized bulimia as a compulsive behavior related to self-image disturbances. Cognitive restructuring associated with exposure to food and eating response prevention seemed effective in one uncontrolled and two controlled studies (Agras 1987). Another study (Pyle et al. 1990) showed the superiority of a structured, group cognitive-behavioral therapy over imipramine. Modification of body image and depression appeared crucial in two controlled trials; they showed the superiority of stress management over nutritional management (Laessle et al. 1991) and the superiority of BT over interpersonal therapy and a simplified BT program (Fairburn et al. 1991). Longer follow-ups are needed to ascertain a significant and lasting effect.

Conclusions

In the last 20 years, BT has made a significant contribution to the treatment of psychiatric problems. The benefits are better social functioning, the prevention of relapse, and simple treatment when relapse occurs.

There are few drawbacks in its application, but it is recommended that the pace of learning and unlearning in patients be respected in order to avoid depression, anxiety, or premature drop-out from therapy. Therapists should leave time for the patients and relatives to adapt to change. Some studies are showing positive changes in personality measures after BT (Cottraux et al. 1991).

BT can be accepted by sophisticated and unsophisticated patients. There is no relation between social status or intelligence level and acceptability of BT. To my knowledge, behavior therapies have been used in various cultural backgrounds in Western Europe, Eastern Europe, Australia, Africa, Asia, and South America. Their limited time and manpower costs should facilitate their use in developing countries.

BT can be used by doctors, psychiatrists, psychologists, nurses, and in some countries social workers, depending on the initial level of interpersonal and psychological understanding, skills, and training. The package presentation of most behavioral interventions tested should facilitate their teaching and use in primary care, both in developed and developing countries. Primary care treatment of mixed-anxiety depression or generalized anxiety, both common syndromes, could benefit from behavior techniques applied by general practitioners. The costs are those of 5 to 25 sessions, based on the level of expertise of the practitioner. Teaching general practitioners to prescribe less benzodiazepines in anxiety disorders and to use more behavior techniques may have a significant impact on medication budgets and quality of life measures. Prevention of relapse and improved quality of life in patients with recurrent depression should result from the use of behavior therapies. Risk factors for cardiovascular diseases can also be diminished by large-scale social-learning intervention (e.g., television advertisements, counseling).

The length of training depends on the previous level of expertise of the trainee. It also depends on the goal of training (e.g., exposure treatment for phobias requires 12 hours of seminar training in nurses working in a psychiatric team). BT for schizophrenia, depression, or personality disorders, however, may require from 1 to 3 years of training. Self-help systems and computer-based treatment in anxiety disorders (Gosh et al. 1988) and depression (Selmi et al. 1990) may decrease time and manpower costs, but need more carefully controlled evaluation.

No agreement exists at present about the training requirements. Courses are organized by universities or private nonprofit associations. Behavior therapist training lasts from 1 to 3 years in most European countries. One-year courses (120 hours with practical training and supervision of one or two cases) may be sufficient to acquire skills in exposure techniques for phobias, obsessive-compulsive disorder, and sexual problems. The optimal training however, should last 3 years (about 120 hours a year). One year should be devoted to theoretical course work and basic clinical observation; a second year to the supervision of 3–8 clinical cases and practical workshops; and a final year to the clinical supervision of clinical cases, with emphasis on clinical relationships and scientific methodology (following the standards of the "European Association of Behavior Therapy"). Medical doctors, psychiatrists, psychologists, and nurses can be trained successfully in BT with equivalent outcomes in the field of anxiety treatment (Marks 1987). Psychiatric nurses may require shorter training to implement social skills training in schizophrenic patients (Liberman 1988).

In developing countries where the function of specialists is not to treat a few selected patients but to train and supervise a large number of health workers operating at a more peripheral level, behavior psycho-therapist training could result in a concomitant shortage of resources for those in most need of short-term effective treatment (Orley 1992). More-over, depending on the country, cultural adapted techniques are neces-sary (Sobbie and Mulindi 1992). Generalization of on-site workshops given by local or foreign experts, supplemented with video and practical manuals, could therefore facilitate a transfer of cognitive-behavioral technology from developed to developing countries.

As regards research implications, it should be stressed that these therapies are the first psychotherapies in which a full description of the techniques, assessment procedures, and results, short- and long-term, are routinely available. Therefore it is feasible to plan and carry out studies aimed at evaluating the effectiveness of BT. Furthermore, the quantifica-tion of these studies allows inclusion in meta-analytical studies that com-pare drug studies and any other modality of treatment in which research is undertaken.

In conclusion, BT can be recommended for anxiety disorders as a treatment of choice either with or without medication. It can be an alter-native treatment to antidepressants in nonmelancholic depression and may prevent relapses. It has clear benefits for the community treatment of psychotic patients. It may promote physical health and treat some be-haviorally linked medical conditions. Prevention of relapse through self-management, improvement of quality of life, and the suspension of drug treatment represent its main assets. Its cost should be weighed against those of alternative treatments, especially pharmacotherapy. Dissemina-tion of such well-established techniques in developing countries requires intensive, brief on-site training workshops.

References

Agras S: Eating Disorders. Management of Obesity, Bulimia and Anorexia Nervosa. New York, Pergamon Press, 1987

Agras S: Behavior Therapy and Psychopharmacology. Untangling the Interac-tion. Paper presented at the World Congress of Behavior Therapy, Edin-burgh, September 1988

Andrews G: A treatment outline for agoraphobia: the Quality Assurance pro-ject. Aus N Z J Psychiatry 16:25–33, 1982

Andrews G, Craig A: Prediction of outcome after treatment for stuttering. Br J Psychiatry 153:235–240, 1988

Ansari J: Impotence prognosis: a controlled study. Br J Psychiatry 128:194–198, 1976

Bandura A: Social Learning Theory. Englewood Cliffs, NJ, Prentice Hall, 1977

Barlow D: The psychosocial treatment of anxiety disorders: current status future directions, in Psychotherapy Research. Edited by Williams JB, Spitzer RL. New York, Guilford Press, 1984

Barlow D, Craske M: Mastery of Your Anxiety and Panic. Graywind, Albany Center for Stress and Anxiety, Albany, NY, 1988

Barlow D, Cohen A, Wadel M, et al: Panic and generalized anxiety disorders: nature and treatment. Behavior Therapy 15:431–449, 1984

Barlow D, Craske M, Cerny J, et al: Behavioral treatment of panic disorder. Behavior Therapy 20:261–282, 1989

Beck AT, Rush AJ, Shaw BF, et al: Cognitive Therapy of Depression. New York, Guilford Press, 1979

Beck AT, Emery G, Greenberg R: Anxiety Disorders and Phobias: A Cognitive Perspective. New York, Basic Books, 1985

Biran M, Wilson GT: Treatment of phobic disorders using cognitive and exposure methods: a self-efficacy analysis. J Consult Clin Psychol 49(6):886–899, 1981

Blanchard E: Long-term effects of behavioral treatment of chronic headache. Behavior Therapy 18(4):387–400, 1987

Blowers C, Cobb J, Mathews A: Generalized anxiety: a controlled treatment study. Behav Res Ther 25(6):493–502, 1987

Bonn J, Readhead C, Timmons B: Enhanced adaptive behavioral response in agoraphobic patients pretreated with breathing retraining. Lancet 22:665–669, 1984

Bono S, Zasa M: Chronic low back pain and therapy: a critical review and overview. The Behavior Therapist 11(9):179–188, 1988

Burns L, Thorpe G, Cavallaro L: Agoraphobia 8 years after behavioral treatment: a follow-up study with interview self-report and behavioral data. Behavior Therapy 17(5):580–591, 1986

Butler G, Cullington A, Monby M: Exposure and anxiety management in the treatment of social phobias. J Clin Psychol 52:642–650, 1984

Butler G, Cullington A, Hibbert G, et al: Anxiety management for persistent generalized anxiety. Br J Psychiatry 151:535–542, 1987

Clark D: A cognitive approach to panic. Behav Res Ther 24:461–470, 1986

Clum G: Psychological interventions versus drugs in the treatment of panic. Behavior Therapy 20:429–457, 1989

Cole M: Sex therapy: a critical appraisal. Br J Psychiatry 147:337–351, 1985

Cottraux J: Les Therapies Comportementales et Cognitives. Paris, Masson, 1990

Cottraux J, Mollard E: Cognitive therapy of phobias, in The Theory and Practice of Cognitive Therapy. Edited by Perris C, Blackburn I, Perris H. Berlin, Springer Verlag, 1988

Cottraux J, Mollard E, Bouvard M, et al: A controlled study of fluvoxamine and exposure in obsessive-compulsive disorder. Int Clin Psychopharmacol 5:17–30, 1990

Cottraux J, Mollard E Bouvard M, Guerin J: Facteurs predictifs des resultats de la therapie cognitivo-comportementale dans le trouble panique avec agoraphobie. Journal de Therapie Comportementale et Cognitive 1(1):4–8, 1991

Cottraux J, Mollard E, Bouvard M, et al: One year follow-up after exposure and/or fluvoxamine in depressed obsessive-compulsive disorder. Paper presented at the meeting of the American Association for the Advancement of Behavior Therapy, New York, November 22, 1991

Craske M, Brown T, Barlow D: Behavioral treatment of panic disorder. Behavior Therapy 22:289–304, 1991

Cullington A, Butler G, Hibbert G, et al: Problem solving not a treatment for agoraphobia. Behavior Therapy 15:280–296, 1984

Durham R, Turvey A: Cognitive therapy versus behavior therapy in the treatment of chronic general anxiety. Behav Res Ther 25(3):229–234, 1987

Emmelkamp P: Behavior therapy with adults, in Handbook of Psychotherapy and Behavior Change. Edited by Garfield S, Bergin A. New York, John Wiley, 1986, pp 385–442

Emmelkamp P, Beens H: Cognitive therapy with obsessive-compulsive disorder: a comparative evaluation. Behav Res Ther 29 (3):293–300, 1991

Emmelkamp P, Kraanen J: Therapist controlled exposure versus self-controlled in vivo exposure: a comparison with obsessive-compulsive patients. Behav Res Ther 15:341–346, 1977

Emmelkamp P, Kuipers A: Agoraphobia: a follow-up study four years after treatment. Br J Psychiatry 134:352–355, 1979

Emmelkamp P, Mersch P: Cognition and in vivo exposure in the treatment of agoraphobics: short term and delayed effects. Cognitive Therapy and Research 1:77–88, 1982

Emmelkamp P, Kuipers A, Eggerraat J: Cognitive modification versus prolonged in vivo exposure: a comparison with agoraphobics as subjects. Behav Res Ther 16:34–41, 1978

Emmelkamp P, Van der Helm M, Van Zanten B, et al: Contribution of self-instructional training to the effectiveness of in vivo exposure: a comparison with obsessive-compulsive patients. Behav Res Ther 18:61–66, 1980

Emmelkamp P, Brilman E, Kuiper H, et al: The treatment of agoraphobia: a comparison of self instructional training, rational-emotive therapy, and in vivo exposure. Behav Modif 6:643–649, 1986

Emmelkamp P, Visser S, Hoekstra RJ: Cognitive therapy versus in vivo exposure in the treatment of obsessive-compulsive patients. Cognitive Therapy and Research 12(1):103–114, 1988

Fairburn C, Jones R, Peveler R, et al: Three psychological treatments in bulimia nervosa: a comparative trial. Arch Gen Psychiatry 48:463–469, 1991

Farquhar J, Fortman S, Flora J, et al: Effects of community education on cardiovascular disease risk factors: the Stanford five-city project. JAMA 264(3):359–365, 1990

Foa E, Steketee G, Turner RM, et al: Effects of imaginal exposure to feared disasters in obsessive compulsive checkers. Behav Res Ther 18:449–455, 1980

Foa E, Rothbaum B: Cognitive-behavior therapy for post-traumatic stress disorder. International Review of Psychiatry 1:219–226, 1989

Friedman M, Thoresen G, Gill J, et al: Alteration of type A behavior and reduction in cardiac recurrences in postmyocardial infarction patients. Am Heart J 108(2):237–248, 1984

Gerlentner C, Uhde T, Cimbolic P, et al: Cognitive-behavioral and pharmacological treatments of social phobia: a controlled study. Arch Gen Psychiatry 48:938–945, 1991

Glasgow R, Lichtenstein E: Long-term effects of behavioral smoking cessation interventions. Behavior Therapy 18(4):297–323, 1987

Gosh A, Marks IM, Carr AC: Therapist contact and outcome of self-exposure treatment for phobias: a controlled study. Br J Psychiatry 152:234–238, 1988

Gurman A, Kniskern D, Pinsof W: Research on the process and outcome of marital and family therapy, in Handbook of Psychotherapy and Behavior Change. Edited by Garfield SL, Bergin AE. New York, John Wiley, 1986, pp 565–624

Hand I, Tichazky M: Behavioral group therapy for obsessions and compulsions: first results of a pilot study, in Trends in Behavior Therapy. London, Academic Press, 1979

Hathaway SR, McKinley JC: Minnesota Multiphasic Personality Inventory Minneapolis, MN, University of Minnesota, 1943

Hibbert G, Chan M: Respiratory control: its contribution to the treatment of panic attacks: a controlled study. Br J Psychiatry 154:232–236, 1989

Jacob R, Wing R, Shapiro A: The behavioral treatment of hypertension: long-term effects. Behavior Therapy 18(4):325–352, 1987

Jacobson N, Wilson L, Tupper C: The clinical significance of treatment gains resulting from exposure-based intervention for agoraphobia: a reanalysis of outcome data. Behavior Therapy 19:539–554, 1988

Janet P: Les Medications Psychologiques. Paris, Alcan, 1920

Jansson L, Ost L: Behavioral treatment for agoraphobia: an evaluative review. Clinical Psychology Review 2:371–376, 1982

Kasvikis Y, Marks I: Clomipramine, self-exposure and therapist aided exposure in obsessive-compulsive ritualizers. II. two year follow-up. Journal of Anxiety Disorders 2:291–298, 1988

Keane T, Fairbank J, Cadel J, et al: Implosive (exposure in imagination) therapy reduces symptoms of PTSD in Vietnam combat veterans. Behavior Therapy 20:245–260, 1989

Klein D: Delineation of two drug responsive anxiety syndromes. Psychopharmacologia 5:397–408, 1964

Klein D, Ross D, Cohen P: Panic and avoidance in agoraphobia: application of path analysis to treatment studies. Arch Gen Psychiatry 44:377–385, 1987

Ladouceur R: Participant modeling with or without cognitive treatment for phobias. J Consult Clin Psychol 51(6):942–944, 1983

Laessle R, Beumont P, Butow P, et al: A comparison of nutritional management with stress management in the treatment of bulimia nervosa. Br J Psychiatry 159:250–261, 1991

Lelliot P, Marks I, Monteiro W, et al: Agoraphobics five years after imipramine and exposure: outcome and predictors. J Nerv Ment Dis 175(10):599–605, 1987

Liberman RP: Psychiatric Rehabilitation of Chronic Mental Patients. Washington, DC, American Psychiatric Press, 1988

Liebowitz M, Gorman J, Fyer A, et al: Social phobia: review of a neglected anxiety disorder. Arch Gen Psychiatry 42:729–736, 1985

Margraf J, Dornier C, Schneider SB: Outcome and active ingredients of cognitive-behavioral treatments for panic disorder. Paper presented at the meeting of the American Association for the Advancement of Behavior Therapy, New York, November 23, 1991

Marks I: Fears, Phobias and Rituals: Panic, Anxiety, and Their Disorders. Oxford and New York, University Press, 1987

Marks I, Stern RS, Mawson D, et al: Clomipramine and exposure for obsessive-compulsive rituals: I. Br J Psychiatry 136:1–25, 1980

Marks I, Lelliott P, Basoglu M, et al: Clomipramine, self-exposure and therapist aided exposure in obsessive-compulsive ritualizers. Br J Psychiatry 152:522–534, 1988

Marzillier J, Lambert C, Kellett J: A controlled evaluation of systematic desensitization and social skills training for socially inadequate psychiatric patients. Behavior Therapy and Research 14:225–238, 1976

Masters WH, Johnson VE: Les Mesententes Sexuelles et Leur Traitement. Paris, Laffont, 1971

Mattick R, Peters L, Clarke C: Exposure and cognitive restructuring for social phobia: a controlled study. Behavior Therapy 20:3–23, 1989

Mavissakalian M, Turner S, Michelson L: Obsessive-Compulsive Disorder. Psychological and Pharmacological Treatment. New York, Plenum Press, 1985

Mawson D, Marks I, Ramm L: Clomipramine and exposure for chronic obsessive-compulsive rituals. III. two year follow-up and further findings. Br J Psychiatry 140:11–18, 1982

McPherson F, Brougham L, McLaren S: Maintenance of improvement in agoraphobic patients treated by behavioral methods: a four year follow-up. Behav Res Ther 18:150–152, 1980

Meichenbaum D: Cognitive-Behavior Modification. New York, Plenum Press, 1977

Michelson L, Mavissakalian M, Marchione K: Cognitive, behavioral and psychophysiological treatments of agoraphobia: a comparative outcome investigation. Behavior Therapy 19:97–120, 1988

Monteiro W, Lelliott P, Marks I, et al: Anorgasmia from clomipramine, in obsessive-compulsive disorder. Br J Psychiatry 151:107–112, 1986

Munby M, Johnston D: Agoraphobia: the long-term follow-up of behavioral treatment. Br J Psychiatry 137:418–427, 1980

Murase T, Johnson F: Naikan, Morita, and western psychotherapy. Arch Gen Psychiatry 131:121–128, 1974

Noyes R, Chaudry R, Domingo D: Pharmacologic treatment of phobic disorders. J Clin Psychiatry 47(9):445–452, 1986

Nunes E, Frank K, Kornfeld D: Psychologic treatment for the type A behavior pattern and for coronary heart disease: a meta-analysis of the literature. Psychosom Med 48(2):159–173, 1987

Obler M: Systematic desensitization in sexual disorders. J Behav Ther Exp Psychiatry 4:93–101, 1973

Ollendick T: Child and adolescent behavior therapy, in Handbook of Psychotherapy and Behavior Change. Edited by Garfield S, Bergin A. New York, John Wiley, 1986, pp 525–564

Orley J: Strategy to introduce behavior therapy in a third world country. Annual Research Series in European Behavior Therapy. Proceedings of the XXth European Association of Behavior Therapy Congress, 1990. Edited by Cottraux J, L'Egeron P, Mollard E. Amsterdam, Swets, 1992, pp 115–116

Ost LG: Applied relaxation versus progressive relaxation in the treatment of panic disorder. Behav Res Ther 26(1):13–22, 1988

O'Sullivan G, Marks I: Long-term outcome of phobic, and obsessive-compulsive disorders, in Handbook of Anxiety, Vol 4. The Treatment of Anxiety. Edited by Noyes R, Roth M, Burrows GD. Amsterdam, Elsevier, 1990, pp 87–108

Paul G: Insight versus desensitization in psychotherapy. Stanford, CA, Stanford University Press, 1966

Pyle RL, Mitchell JE, Eckert ED, et al: Maintenance treatment and 6-month outcome for bulimic patients who respond to initial treatment. Am J Psychiatry 147:871–887, 1990

Russell G, Szmukler G, Dare C, et al: An evaluation of family therapy in anorexia nervosa and bulimia. Arch Gen Psychiatry 44:1047–1056, 1987

Saint-Laurent L, Ladouceur R: Massed versus distributed application of the regulated breathing method for stutterers and its long-term effects. Behavior Therapy 18:38–50, 1987

Salkovskis P: Obsessional-compulsive problems: a cognitive behavioral analysis. Behav Res Ther 23(5):571–583, 1985

Salkovskis P, Warwick H: Cognitive therapy of obsessive-compulsive disorder, in Cognitive Therapy: The Theory and Practice. Edited by Perris C, Blackburn I, Perris H. Berlin, Springer Verlag, 1988

Salkovskis P, Clark D, Hackmann A, et al: Comparative efficacy of cognitive therapy, applied relaxation and imipramine in the treatment of panic disorder. Paper presented at the XXth EABT Congress September 1990

Selmi P, Klein M, Greist J, et al: Computer administered cognitive-behavioral therapy for depression. Am J Psychiatry 147(1):51–56, 1990

Sloane RB, Staples F, Cristol AH, et al: Psychotherapy Versus Behavior Therapy. Cambridge, MA, Harvard University Press, 1975

Sobbie A, Mulindi Z: Behavior therapy in developing countries. Annual Research Series in European Behavior Therapy. Proceedings of the XXth European Association of Behavior Therapy Congress, 1990. Edited by Cottraux J, L'Egeron P, Mollard E. Amsterdam, Swets, 1992

Solyom L, Sookman D: A comparison of clomipramine hydrochloride (Anafranil) and behavior therapy in the treatment of obsessive-compulsive neurosis. J Intern Med Res 5 (suppl):49–61, 1977

Steketee G, Foa E, Grayson J: Recent advances in the treatment of obsessive-compulsive disorders. Arch Gen Psychiatry 39:1365–1370, 1982

Stern R, Marks I, Mawson D, et al: Clomipramine and exposure for compulsive rituals: II. plasma levels, side effects and outcome. Br J Psychiatry 136:161–166, 1980

Stravinsky A, Marks I, Yule W: Social skills problems in neurotic out-patients. Arch Gen Psychiatry 39:1378–1385, 1982

Tarrier N, Main C: Applied relaxation training for generalized anxiety and panic attacks. the efficacy of a learned coping strategy on subjective reports. Br J Psychiatry 149:330–336, 1986

Telch M, Agras S, Barr-Taylor C, et al: Combined pharmacological and behavioral treatment for agoraphobia. Behav Res Ther 22(3):325–335, 1985

Thoren R, Gusberg M, Cronholm B, et al: Clomipramine treatment of obsessive-compulsive disorder: a controlled study. Arch Gen Psychiatry 37:1281–1285, 1980

Welkowitz L, Laszlo A, Cloitre M, et al: Cognitive-behavior therapy for panic disorder delivered by psychopharmacologically oriented clinicians. J Nerv Ment Dis 179(8):473–477, 1991

Williams S, Rappoport A: Cognitive treatment in the natural environment for agoraphobia. Behavior Therapy 14:299–313, 1983

Wilson T, Brownell K: Behavior Therapy of obesity: an evaluation of treatment outcome. Advances in Behav Res Ther 3(2):49–86, 1982

Wolpe J: Psychotherapy by Reciprocal Inhibition. Stanford, CA, Stanford University Press, 1958

World Health Organization: International Classification of Diseases, 10th Edition. Geneva, Switzerland, World Health Organization, 1992

Wright J, Perreault R, Mathieu M: The treatment of sexual dysfunction: a review. Arch Gen Psychiatry 34:881–890, 1977

Zohar J, Insel T: Obsessive-compulsive disorder: psychobiological approaches to diagnosis, treatment and pathophysiology. Biol Psychiatry 22:667–687, 1987

Zitrin C, Klein D, Woerner M: Behavior therapy, supportive psychotherapy, imipramine and phobias. Arch Gen Psychiatry 35:307–316, 1978

Zitrin C, Klein D, Woerner M: Treatment of agoraphobia with group in vivo exposure and imipramine. Arch Gen Psychiatry 37:63–72, 1980

CHAPTER 8

The Benefits of Psychotherapy

Gavin Andrews, M.D., F.R.A.N.Z.C.P., F.R.C.Psych.

Introduction

Psychotherapy, *the talking cure*, is important to psychiatry and needs to be actively promoted and protected if it is to compete with the heavily promoted drug treatments (Andrews 1985). Ten years ago, following the original meta-analysis (Glass 1976) of psychotherapy, it seemed that the issue of efficacy was decided. In a meta-analysis of 475 controlled trials, the average treated group was better than 80% of untreated groups; that the patients had made a gain of 30 percentile ranks, or, in the language of meta-analysis, had made a gain of .85 effect size (ES) units. Smith et al. (1980) concluded that "the results show unequivocally that psychotherapy is effective." Troubled by their heavy reliance on studies involving people who would not normally enter therapy, we (Andrews and Harvey 1981) restricted a reanalysis of their data to 81 studies of patients with neurotic disorders, and compared treated groups, including placebo treatment, with waiting list controls who had also sought psychotherapy. The results were similar; the behavioral psychotherapies (average ES superiority over waiting list = .97) were significantly superior to the verbal psychotherapies (average ES = .74), and both were more effective than the counseling therapies (average ES = .35) or placebo treatments (average ES = .55 over waiting list control).

This chapter is a revised form of a paper entitled "The Evaluation of Psychotherapy," *Current Opinion in Psychiatry* 4:379–383, 1991.

Prioleau et al. (1983) conducted the third reanalysis of these data, restricting themselves to the 32 placebo-controlled trials of dynamic psychotherapy, therapy that involved "exploration and clarification of the emotional experiences of the patient within a transference relationship" and found no significant evidence of benefit in studies of psychiatric patients. The commentaries to that article, and the editorials that followed, admitted the lack of evidence, regretted that the studies analyzed were not representative of the practice of long-term psychoanalytically oriented psychotherapy, did not identify any unanalyzed trials that were representative, and called for further and more appropriate research (Bloch and Lambert 1985; Prioleau et al. 1983; "Psychotherapy" 1984; Shepherd 1984). These commentators seemed to miss the essential point. Therapies based on the work of Freud and his followers had not, in the subsequent 70 years, been shown to be of more benefit than placebo; that is, than good, nonpsychotherapeutic clinical care or even than talking to a mature and kindly advisor (Strupp and Hadley 1978).

To determine whether this is still the situation, recent evidence concerning the utility of dynamic psychotherapy for the neuroses and personality disorders will be reviewed and compared with the evidence for the effectiveness of the cognitive-behavior therapies.

Dynamic Psychotherapy

Psychoanalysis and long-term psychoanalytically oriented psychotherapy (collectively called dynamic psychotherapy) have been of great interest to psychiatry. Dominant in United States psychiatry until 20 years ago and still supported within Britain's frugal National Health Service, dynamic psychotherapy has also flourished in Australia, which has a hybrid public/private health care system with the costs of unlimited fee-for-service consultations with a private psychiatrist being reimbursed to the patient by the national health insurance system (Andrews 1989a). When surveyed, 70% of Australian psychiatrists nominated dynamic psychotherapy as the treatment they would most like to carry out, and a consensus of practitioners and experts recommended dynamic psychotherapy as the treatment of choice for neurotic depression, some anxiety disorders, and most personality disorders (Andrews et al. 1987; Hall et al. 1982;

Quality Assurance Project 1990, 1991a, 1991b). In a survey of the work of Australian psychiatrists we found that practitioners identified as specializing in dynamic psychotherapy reported that 25% of their patients had depressive neurosis and were expected to need 178 hours of therapy before "no longer needing treatment for this condition"; 12% had anxiety neuroses and were expected to need 262 hours of therapy; and 40% had personality disorders and were expected to need an average of 520 hours of therapy (Andrews et al. 1987). The cost of psychotherapy averaged $33,000 per patient, and the propriety of spending public money on a highly respected, very expensive, but still unproven treatment, became an issue.

A report by Howard et al. (1986) from the United States where fee reimbursement is not universal showed a different picture. Based on data from 15 studies of 2,431 patients in private, university, and community center clinics treated with dynamic psychotherapy, the authors concluded that the average patient with depression responded after 8 sessions and the average patient with anxiety after 13 sessions, while the average patient with a borderline disorder required 26 sessions to improve. These values were .05 those recorded by the Australian psychotherapists for patients "no longer needing treatment," a different endpoint than that used in the United States study, but the order of difficulty by diagnosis was similar. The United States group argued for peer review after 26 sessions; Andrews (1983) had earlier argued for peer review in the Australian context after 50 sessions. Intensive or long-term psychotherapy was also once dominant in the United States, but was recently noted as becoming rare in training and research programs (Altshuler 1990).

Cognitive-Behavior Therapy

Cognitive-behavior therapies have been recently developed. Loosely derived from learning theory and the notion that most learning is cognitively mediated, they have focused on ameliorating the consequences and current determinants of habit disorders, neuroses, and personality disorders. They have been largely developed by academic psychiatrists and psychologists. Their clinical use is identified with psychologists and not, as yet, with psychiatrists. In the 1986 Australian survey by Andrews and Hadzi-Pavlovic (1988), only 3% of psychiatrists' patients were recorded as receiving behavior therapy. Measuring outcome has been an integral part of these therapies, in part because of the origins in psychology, but also because of the need to show that the new techniques warranted serious consideration vis-à-vis dynamic psychotherapy. A number of therapy manuals describing how to treat each disorder are available, and their advent has been welcomed (Goldfried et al. 1990). The duration of cognitive-behavior therapy is short, usually about 20 sessions.

Strategies for Evaluating Psychotherapy

The results of placebo-controlled trials are conventionally preferred when deciding which treatments are of benefit. However, when a treatment is likely to extend over a year or more, and the outcome of interest requires a further period of observation, then keeping a group of ill people on a placebo treatment becomes difficult. I have argued elsewhere (Andrews 1989b, 1989c) that while a placebo control group receiving continuing clinical care is desirable, the criteria for evaluating such treatments may be achieved in the absence of a placebo group by comparison with another standard treatment for which placebo control data exist.

The aims of any treatment should result in the lessening of symptoms, as judged by the doctors, and complaints, as recorded by the patients. End-state functioning should show improved ability in work and personal relations, and complaints should no longer meet criteria for the original diagnosis. Ideally, risk factors, such as personality vulnerability, that could lead to relapse should also be reduced. The improvement should last after treatment has ended, and be shown to be greater than the estimated effects of three possible confounds: spontaneous remission, regression to the mean, and response to a placebo or nonspecific treatment acting over a period equivalent to the length of treatment. A waiting list or no-treatment group controls for the first two confounds, a placebo treatment for all three. The ideal placebo or control condition for a specific psychotherapy would be continuing clinical management that deliberately avoided using any specific components of the psychotherapy. Two further important indices of improvement are some evidence of a dose-response relationship and quality of life measures showing a positive change with treatment.

Benefits of Cognitive-Behavior Therapy or Dynamic Psychotherapy in Neuroses and Personality Disorders

Benefits in Outpatients

Piper et al. (1990) conducted a trial of 19 hours of dynamic psychotherapy and compared the progress of the 47 treated outpatients with the progress of a waiting list control group over the same time. All patients met criteria for a DSM-III (American Psychiatric Association 1980) Axis I or Axis II diagnosis. Therapy was described in a manual, and therapists were confirmed from session tapes to be active, interpretive, and transference oriented. Progress was measured from a battery of instruments that covered symptoms, personality, and social function. Sixteen percent of patients dropped out, and the results of those who completed the trials were shown to be stable 2 months posttherapy. Across all measures, the treated group were .52 ES units better than controls and on a broad symptom measure 56% of the treated group normalized their scores, and 36% in the waiting list group did likewise. This was a very sophisticated study; the findings were disappointing in that the degree of improvement in these outpatients over waiting list controls (ES = .52) was not greater than the superiority of placebo over waiting list control estimated in the Glass data (ES = .55), thus indicating that the therapy may not be superior to placebo but only to waiting list or no treatment.

The Piper study results are congruent with the review of short-term psychodynamic psychotherapy by Svartberg and Stiles (1991) who concluded that, while such therapy was superior to no treatment at the end of therapy, the benefit decayed within the first year, whereas the benefits of alternative psychotherapies such as cognitive-behavior therapy did not. Similarly, Crits-Christoph (1992) found that at posttreatment brief dynamic psychotherapy was significantly superior to waiting list but not to placebo-type treatments.

Bowers and Clum (1988) conducted a meta-analysis of 69 studies of behavior therapy versus placebo. When they confined their analysis to 10 studies of patients with neurotic conditions (Clum and Bowers 1990), the mean effect size compared to placebo was .86, higher than the results reported previously by Andrews and Harvey (1981) for either behavior therapy or dynamic therapy. Despite Brody's argument (1990), this is firm evidence that cognitive-behavior therapy is of benefit for neurotic conditions generally.

Benefits in Depression

The results from the National Institute of Mental Health's multicenter trial (Elkin et al. 1989) with 155 patients who had had a major depressive episode, using 16 sessions of Beck's cognitive-behavior therapy, Weissman's interpersonal psychotherapy, imipramine plus clinical management, and placebo plus clinical management, have been of major interest. As might have been expected from such an undertaking, the effects of the control condition—placebo plus clinical management— were considerable and, in terms of statistical significance, the specific treatments only barely exceeded those benefits. In clinical terms, however, 40% of patients recovered with placebo and 60% recovered with one of the specific treatments. The specific treatments were more powerful in the more severe patients. In effect size terms the superiority of cognitive-behavior therapy over placebo was .24 for the total sample and .46 for the more severe patients, while interpersonal psychotherapy was .36 and .72 respectively; with imipramine the superiority over placebo for the total sample was .50 and for the more severe patients 1.40. A major contribution of this study was defining good *clinical management* as a suitable placebo against which to compare psychotherapy. What also became clear is that for a depressed patient, it was preferable to be in one of the specific treatment categories. As Gelder (1990) noted, cognitive and interpersonal therapies are of benefit and particularly helpful for patients who cannot or do not wish to take drugs.

Dobson (1989) reported on 28 studies that compared Beck's cognitive therapy in depression with no treatment, other behavior therapy, drug treatment, or other psychotherapy. All studies used the Beck Depression Inventory (Beck 1978) as an outcome measure. Cognitive therapy was two standard deviations better than no treatment and half a standard deviation better than drug treatment, behavior therapy alone, or other psychotherapy. The use of a single outcome measure is an impressive feature of this study.

In a more wide ranging meta-analysis, Robinson et al. (1991) also found the cognitive, cognitive-behavioral, and behavioral psychotherapies to be half a standard deviation superior to general verbal psychotherapies, which did not appear to be better than placebo. This result was stable when measures were confined to formally diagnosed depressed patients and focused on classic measures of depression. There do not appear to be any recent placebo-controlled trials showing the benefits of dynamic psychotherapy in depressed patients.

Benefits in Anxiety Disorders

Since the pioneering work of Marks, it has been obvious that the behavior therapies have much to offer patients with anxiety disorders. Two recent studies of panic disorder show the power of such treatments. Both Klosko et al. (1990) and Michelson et al. (1990) used a 13–15 session cognitive-behavior therapy package and found that by the end of treatment 21 out of the 25 patients in the studies had high-end state functioning and no longer met criteria for the disorder, and 23 of 25 were free from spontaneous panic attacks. The Klosko et al. study found that patients randomly assigned to other treatments, alprazolam, placebo, or a waiting list, did significantly worse. This type of result has been seen in other centers and has been regarded as a major breakthrough (Goldfried et al. 1990).

The literature on the advantages of cognitive-behavior therapy in treating panic disorders and agoraphobia is now extensive. In addition to symptom relief, treatment produces long-term changes in personality (neuroticism, locus of control, defense style; Andrews 1991; Andrews and Moran 1988) and cognitive style (Franklin 1990) that lessen a patient's vulnerability to further neurotic difficulties. A recent and extensive meta-analytic review by Mattick et al. (1990) identified the preferred treatment programs. Franklin (1990) produced evidence from a 5-year follow-up that the cognitive learning that has occurred enables patients to deal with future difficulties more effectively than patients treated with behavior therapy alone.

Cognitive-behavior therapies appear to be the treatments of choice in generalized anxiety disorder (ES superiority over placebo = .72), social phobia (ES superiority over waiting list and placebo = 1.51), and in obsessive-compulsive disorder (ES superiority over placebo = 1.32) (Andrews 1990a). The improvement evident at the end of treatment appears to be stable (Butler et al. 1987; Foa et al. 1984; Mattick et al. 1989) and still evident months after treatment has concluded.

Benefits in Personality Disorders

Dynamic psychotherapy is regarded as the treatment of choice for patients with schizoid, borderline, histrionic, narcissistic, dependent, passive-aggressive, and avoidant personality disorders (Quality Assurance Project 1990, 1991a, 1991b). There are, however, no published placebo-controlled studies to support this contention. The evidence is confined to anecdotal case reports, supported by some naturalistic follow-up studies of treated cases. The problem with such evidence is that case selection or remission of symptoms through normal personality maturation could account for the changes reported. For example, antisocial personality disorder is deemed to be untreatable, but there is good epidemiological evidence that considerable remission occurs and that the typical patient no longer meets criteria for the disorder after his 30th birthday (Robins et al. 1990). If the other, putatively more treatable, personality disorders followed the same course, and there is some evidence that they do (Vaillant and Schnurr 1988), then the changes noted during the years of dynamic psychotherapy may only be the natural remission of these disorders that would have occurred given reasonable clinical management but no dynamic psychotherapy.

Discussion

It would not be difficult to randomly allocate patients to dynamic psychotherapy or nonspecific clinical management and compare the progress over the years. Now it probably is not ethical to continue to provide health care resources for long-term psychoanalytically oriented psychotherapy without doing such a study. Following the 1983 meta-analytical argument over the benefits of dynamic psychotherapy, many appropriate research projects were begun. We (Brodaty and Andrews 1983) conducted a study in chronic neurosis in which we found a null result; after rejection by two journals, we persuaded a third journal to publish our results. We presume that other negative studies may have been abandoned by their authors or rejected by editors. Given the 32 studies reviewed by Prioleau et al. (1983), if the file drawers are replete with negative studies, then, according to Rosenthal (1979), not one but quite a number of strong positive studies from different centers will be needed to establish that long-term psychoanalytically oriented psychotherapy is a specific treatment of benefit.

As might be expected, the cognitive-behavior therapists are exploring the treatment of personality disorder. I have already referred to evidence that personality changes, including ego defense style, can follow such therapy (Andrews 1991). Using short periods of cognitive-behavior therapy, Linehan (1987), treating borderline personality disorder, and Alden (1989), treating avoidant personality disorder, were able to significantly ameliorate key symptoms in these disorders so that end-state functioning was improved.

Psychotherapy at Differing Health Care Levels

A very real goal of psychotherapy is for patients, as a result of therapy, to be able to help themselves through future difficulties. The long-term follow-up studies of the cognitive-behavioral therapies show that this process is occurring (see Franklin 1990). There are reports (Andrews 1990b) that training in the structured problem-solving technique produces a similar effect, that is, that people who were taught the technique during a crisis continued to use the technique to resolve future difficulties. Some of the cognitive-behavioral therapies have been prepared in written form so that patients can continue to self-treat. There are now also a number of books written for laypeople to help them manage their own anxiety and depression without recourse to medical help. The book *Living With Fear* by Isaac Marks (1978) has been shown in a comparative trial to be of specific benefit. Now that we have clear directions whereby the impact of the common mental disorders of anxiety and depression could be reduced, we should take the initiative and educate the population that, for example, "if irrational fears are to be confronted they will lessen," "anxiety can be useful and facilitate decisive action," and "depressive ideas are self-defeating and should be combated by activity." Instead, many families still respond to these affects as though they are evidence of pathology quite beyond one's ability to cope.

Many professionals in primary health care are also uninformed about simple preventive mental health measures. All should be knowledgeable about the mechanisms of the more common mental disorders and all should be practiced in the structural problem-solving approach (D'Urzilla 1986) as a first line of management in many disorders. Beyond this level, the cognitive-behavioral psychotherapies require skill and patience and are best left to trained therapists. Because of the importance of these therapies, most mental health professionals should be skilled in their application, at least for the common disorders of anxiety and depression.

Conclusions

Cognitive-behavior therapy has been shown to be a powerful specific treatment in the neuroses, with some early evidence of its benefit in some personality disorders. Dynamic psychotherapy, although popular with patients and therapists (and this alone would justify the therapy if the health budget was not involved), has not been demonstrated to be superior to placebo in the neuroses or personality disorders. The reports of improvement during long-term dynamic therapy for personality disorders may be due to the combined effects of normal maturation and the nonspecific effects of continued good clinical care. It may well be that the long training in a specific psychotherapeutic model keeps clinicians interested in seeing patients repeatedly for years until natural maturation occurs, maturation potentiated by the good nonspecific clinical advice offered by the therapist. However, until sufficient controlled trials have been completed to show that dynamic psychotherapy is effective, cognitive-behavior therapy is to be preferred in terms of both specific effectiveness and cost.

References

Alden L: Short-term structured treatment for avoidant personality disorder. J Consult Clin Psychol 57:756–764, 1989

Altshuler KZ: Whatever happened to intensive psychotherapy? Am J Psychiatry 147:428–430, 1990

American Psychiatric Association: Diagnostic and Statistical Manual of Mental Disorders, 3rd Edition (DSM-III). Washington, DC, American Psychiatric Association, 1980

Andrews G: Psychotherapy and health insurance. Aust N Z J Psychiatry 17:68–72, 1983

Andrews G: On the promotion of non-drug treatments. BMJ 289:994–995, 1984

Andrews G: Private and public psychiatry: a comparison of two health care systems. Am J Psychiatry 146:881–886, 1989a

Andrews G: Which therapy is best? the role of research design, in Contemporary Themes in Psychiatry. A Tribute to Sir Martin Roth. Edited by Davison K, Kerr A. London, Gaskell, 1989b, pp 20–30, 1989b

Andrews G: Evaluating treatment effectiveness. Aust N Z J Psychiatry 23:181–186, 1989c

Andrews G: The diagnosis and management of pathological anxiety. Med J Aust 152:656–659, 1990a

Andrews G: England: an innovative community psychiatric services. Lancet 335:1087–1088, 1990b

Andrews G: Anxiety, Personality and Anxiety Disorders. International Review of Psychiatry 3:293–302, 1991

Andrews G, Hadzi-Pavlovic D: The work of Australian psychiatrists, circa 1986. Aust N Z J Psychiatry 22:153–165, 1988

Andrews G, Harvey R: Does psychotherapy benefit neurotic patients? a reanalysis of the Smith, Glass and Miller data. Arch Gen Psychiatry 38:1203–1208, 1981

Andrews G, Moran C: Exposure treatment of agoraphobia with panic attacks: are drugs essential? in Panic and Phobias II. Treatments and Variables Affecting Course and Outcome. Edited by Hand I, Wittchen H-U. Heidelberg, Springer-Verlag, 1988, pp 89–99

Andrews G, Hadzi-Pavlovic D, Christensen H, et al: Views of practicing psychiatrists on the treatment of anxiety and somatoform disorders. Am J Psychiatry 144:1331–1334, 1987

Beck AT: Depression Inventory. Philadelphia, PA, Philadelphia Center for Cognitive Therapy, 1978

Bloch S, Lambert MJ: What price psychotherapy? a rejoinder. Br J Psychiatry 146:96–98, 1985

Bowers TG, Clum GA: Relative contribution of specific and nonspecific treatment effects: meta-analysis of placebo-controlled behavior therapy research. Psychological Bulletin 103:315–323, 1988

Brodaty H, Andrews G: Brief psychotherapy in family practice: a controlled perspective intervention trial. Br J Psychiatry 143:11–19, 1983

Brody N: Behavior therapy versus placebo: comment on Bowers and Clum's meta-analysis. Psychol Bull 107:106–109, 1990

Butler G, Cullington A, Hibbert G, et al: Anxiety management for persistent generalized anxiety. Br J Psychiatry 151:535–542, 1987

Clum GA, Bowers TG: Behavior therapy better than placebo treatments: fact or artifact? Psychol Bull 107:110–113, 1990

Crits-Christoph P: The efficacy of brief dynamic psychotherapy: current status and future directions. Am J Psychiatry 149:151–158, 1992

Dobson KS: A meta-analysis of the efficacy of cognitive therapy for depression. J Consult Clin Psychol 57:414–419, 1989

D'Urzilla TJ: Problem-Solving Therapy. New York, Springer, 1986

Elkin I, Shea T, Watkins J: National Institute of Mental Health treatment of depression collaborative research program: general effectiveness of treatments. Arch Gen Psychiatry 46:971–982, 1989

Foa E, Steketee G, Grayson J, et al: Deliberate exposure and blocking of obsessive compulsive rituals. Behavioral Research Therapy 15:450–472, 1984

Franklin J: Behavioral therapy for panic disorder, in Anxiety. Edited by McNaughton N, Andrews G. Dunedin, NZ, Otago University Press, 1990, pp 84–91

Gelder MG: Psychological treatment for depressive disorder. BMJ 300:1087–1088, 1990

Glass GV: Primary, secondary and meta-analysis of research. Educational Research 10:3–8, 1976

Goldfried MR, Greenberg LS, Marmar C: Individual psychotherapy: process and outcome. Ann Rev Psychol 41:659–688, 1990

Hall W, Weekes P, Harvey R, et al: A survey of practicing psychiatrists' views on the treatment of agoraphobia. Aust N Z J Psychiatry 16:225–233, 1982

Howard KI, Kopta SM, Krause MS, et al: The dose-effect relationship in psychotherapy. Am Psychol 41:159–164, 1986

Klosko JS, Barlow DH, Tassinari R, et al: A comparison of alprazolam and behavior therapy in treatment of panic disorder. J Consult Clin Psychol 58:77–84, 1990

Linehan MM: Dialectical behavioral therapy: a cognitive behavioral approach to parasuicide. Journal of Personality Disorders 1:328–333, 1987

Marks I: Living With Fear. New York, McGraw-Hill, 1978

Mattick RP, Peters L, Clarke C: Exposure and cognitive restructuring for social phobia. Behavioral Research Therapy 20:3–23, 1989

Mattick R, Andrews G, Hadzi-Pavlovic D, et al: Treatment of panic and agoraphobia: an integrative review. J Nerv Ment Dis 178:567–576, 1990

Michelson L, Marchione K, Greenwald M, et al: Panic disorder: cognitive-behavioral treatment. Behav Res Ther 28:141–151, 1990

Piper WE, Azim HFA, McCallum M, et al: Patient suitability and outcome in short-term individual psychotherapy. J Consult Clin Psychol 58:475–481, 1990

Prioleau L, Murdock M, Brody N: An analysis of psychotherapy versus placebo studies. The Behavioral and Brain Sciences 6:275–310, 1983

Psychotherapy: effective treatment or expensive placebo? Lancet 1:83–84, 1984

Quality Assurance Project: Treatment outlines for personality disorders. Aust N Z J Psychiatry 24:339–350, 1990

Quality Assurance Project: Treatment outlines for personality disorders. Aust N Z J Psychiatry 25:392–403, 1991a

Quality Assurance Project: Treatment outlines for personality disorders. Aust N Z J Psychiatry 25:404–411, 1991b

Robins LN, Tipp J, Przybeck T: Antisocial personality, in Psychiatric Disorders in America. Edited by Robins LN, Regier DR. New York, Free Press, 1990

Robinson LA, Berman JS, Neimeyer RA: Psychotherapy for the treatment of depression: a comprehensive review of controlled outcome research. Psychol Bull 108:77–84, 1991

Rosenthal R: The "file drawer problem" and tolerance for null results. Psychol Bull 86:638–641, 1979

Shepherd M: What price psychotherapy? BMJ 288:809–810, 1984

Smith ML, Glass GV, Miller TI: The Benefits of Psychotherapy. Baltimore, Johns Hopkins University Press, 1980

Strupp HH, Hadley SW: Specific versus non-specific factors in psychotherapy: a controlled study of outcome. Arch Gen Psychiatry 36:1125–1136, 1978

Svartberg M, Styles TC: Comparative effects of short-term psychodynamic psychotherapy: a meta-analysis. J Consult Clin Psychol 59:704–714, 1991

Vaillant GW, Schnurr P: A 45 year study of psychiatric impairment within a college sample selected for mental health. Arch Gen Psychiatry 45:313–319, 1988

Section IV

Psychosocial Treatments

Introduction to Section IV

The previous chapters were concerned at length with the application of specific treatment to individual patients. The present chapters are different. In the first, concerning social interventions, Langsley, Hodes, and Grimson's discussion renews the place of family, marital, and group therapy; the function of therapeutic communities; and the role of self-help groups in reducing impairment stemming from mental disorders. In the second, which concerns rehabilitation, Burti and Yastrebov bring together a wide spectrum of information about the theory and practice of rehabilitation in general, for specific disorders, and when used to potentiate work and living skills. This chapter is a salutary reminder that good treatment is not just about reducing the key symptoms or impairment produced by the disorder, but that it should also be focused on reducing the disability and handicap that follows having been ill.

CHAPTER 9

Psychosocial Interventions

Donald G. Langsley, M.D.
Matthew Hodes, B.Sc., M.B.B.S., M.Sc., M.R.C.Psych.
Wilbur R. Grimson, M.D.

Introduction

Often psychiatry has focused attention on the individual patient and conducted its treatment on the one-to-one model of the psychiatrist-patient relationship. In many developing countries indigenous family and social therapies have been used, but until recently in most Western nations, less attention has been given to the family, marital partner, or the social setting in which the patient lives (Lin 1983). Contact with the family has been to obtain information about the patient or to enlist their aid, the "real" treatment involving the psychiatrist and patient alone. There has been a countertradition that has understood the patient in a social perspective, leading to the development of treatment approaches that are referred to as psychosocial therapies. In the psychosocial therapies, the patient is seen with other people, and the relationships between them are an important part of the treatment.

Recognition of the importance of family relationships in psychiatric disorders led to the involvement of family members in treatment; marital therapy has much in common with family therapy. Sometimes, however, it is not possible, or desirable, to treat the patient with family members, and the development of group therapy relies on the participation of the patient in a group brought together especially for the treatment of its members. Self-help groups may involve only those who meet to obtain relief from mutual distress. When group psychotherapeutic principles are applied in a residential setting, such as a hospital, it may be called a therapeutic community. These four broadly defined kinds of psychosocial interventions—family, marital, group, and therapeutic community—are discussed in this review.

There are a number of general issues that need to be addressed before these particular treatments are considered. First, the importance of nonspecific factors in all treatments, including all kinds of psychotherapies, should be borne in mind. While it is hard to quantify these nonspecific factors, they have been clearly described (Frank 1973, 1989). Psychological distress can cause demoralization that can be relieved by an emotionally charged, confiding relationship with a helping person or group. The high status of psychotherapists is reassuring to patients.

The second general issue concerns the recent rapid growth in the varieties of psychosocial interventions, and the appearance of a body of literature that describes the techniques, theory, and research of those interventions. There is considerable overlap in the theoretical bases, techniques, and applications of these treatments. What practitioners actually do is diverse, but frequently they draw on practices from different psychotherapies or offer different treatments concurrently. However, in order to discuss psychosocial interventions in a coherent way it is necessary to be highly selective.

Third, although psychosocial interventions have been described for the treatment of many psychiatric disorders, they do not all have a highly developed theoretical basis, with clearly described techniques and evidence for efficacy. In this review we summarize the theoretical rationale and techniques and emphasize research findings as a guide to informing effective treatment.

Family Therapy

Family therapy is based on ideas from general systems theory (Gorell Barnes 1985). First, it assumes that the experience and behavior of individuals is interconnected with the experience and behavior of others. Indeed the behavior of one family member is both a response to, and cause of, other family members' behavior. These processes refer to many aspects of individuals' functioning such as speech, nonverbal communication, or other behavior. The second important assumption is that in the family, as in all social systems, there is a tendency for repetition so that things stay the same. Because individuals inevitably change through aging and maturation, the family will have to change to accommodate these individual changes. However, as individuals age or die, others in the family may continue to have certain beliefs or behaviors that seemed to originate from the older relative. This relates to a third important aspect of the family therapy perspective that regards the family as an important context for human development (Stratton 1988). Communication and sharing of values—*family cultures*— are related to adults' and children's behavioral repertoires. For example, children's disobedient behavior may incur parental disapproval but in so doing gain their attention, thus possibly provoking further disobedient behavior. This sequence may have consequences for the development of aggressive and antisocial behavior (G. Patterson and Dishion 1988). It is obvious from this example that not everyone in the family has similar roles. Although the family is an open system, in that it is interconnected with other families and social groups, it can be conceptualized as consisting of separate parts. Children, parents, and grandparents occupy different subsystems, with different roles and responsibilities within the family, and yet there is a high interdependence between these roles (Minuchin 1974).

These ideas have been used in family therapy in a variety of ways. Indeed there is no single approach to family therapy. The different approaches or schools of thought and practice can be divided into four groups (Gurman and Kniskern 1981). The *psychoanalytic approach* applies psychodynamic understanding and techniques within the family. Processes of individual mental life, such as projection and splitting, are identified by the therapist who aims to produce change in the family by interpreting these processes with a view to increasing the insight of family members. This approach is related to the *intergenerational approach.* A good example is the intergenerational therapy of Bowen (1978), who described the way in which relationships between an individual and the family of origin tend to repeat through the selection of spouse and the repetition of patterns of relating. For example the overinvolved relationship between a married man and his mother will have consequences for his relationship with his wife, and this may have consequences for their joint parenting of children, so that these cross-generational alliances are repeated. Such processes are believed to be related to the development and maintenance of psychiatric disorders. As psychoanalytic and intergenerational family therapy are perhaps less practiced than the other approaches and not as well evaluated, less attention will be given to them.

The third group of family therapies are those based more directly on the *systems approach*. The structural family therapy of Minuchin and his colleagues (Minuchin 1974; Minuchin and Fishman 1981; Minuchin et al. 1967, 1978) provides a clear and readily accessible account of family function and the disturbance that occurs in the presence of psychiatric disorder. According to this approach, healthy individual functioning is a balance between closeness and distance, which requires a family to have an appropriate organization in terms of hierarchy and authority, and appropriate companionship and intimacy between those of the same generation. Psychiatric or psychosomatic disorder occurs when these boundaries are disturbed. For example, conflict between the parents may be associated with one parent forming an alliance with one of the children against the other parent. This is particularly likely to occur when the family shows a failure to accommodate to the developmental needs of its members. Therapy involves interrupting and changing aspects of communication and repeated behaviors (Minuchin and Fishman 1981).

A different approach is the Milan systems family therapy of Selvini-Palazzoli and her associates who believe that the family is organized by a belief system shared unwittingly by family members. In dysfunctional families these beliefs are related to unresolved conflict and secret coalitions across the generations. A psychiatric disorder is seen as a form of behavior that is linked to these dysfunctional beliefs and coalitions (Selvini-Palazzoli et al. 1978). Therapy involves changing the belief system of the family by making the rules explicit, in ways that resemble psychoanalytic interpretations. Another form of systems therapy is strategic family therapy. This relies on seeing family members who are involved with the problem and reframing the problem by giving it new meanings, which in turn facilitates change in the family organization (Stanton 1981).

The fourth approach to family therapy is *behavioral family therapy* (Falloon 1988a), which is derived from learning theory. Behavioral family therapists regard many psychiatric disorders and problem behaviors as maladaptive learning that can be modified by learning new behaviors. Originally, undesirable behaviors of children were reduced by the appropriate reinforcing of desired behaviors by parents. In recent years behavioral techniques have become more developed (e.g., contingency contracting in which the level of rewarding behaviors is increased by all family members). In contemporary behavioral family therapy attention can be given to speech style as well as observable behaviors; this has extended its applications dramatically.

One advantage of family therapy is that the treatments are usually short term, with less than 25 sessions offered. It is also versatile, having been applied in many settings (Berger et al. 1984), such as the general hospital, especially in pediatric wards (Lask 1987); child and adult psychiatric services (Bloch et al. 1991; Dare 1985); and primary care settings (Graham et al. 1992). It has been used to treat many problems and psychiatric disorders.

Developments of family therapy have included evaluation of its beneficial effects. Meta-analysis of a range of treatment studies (e.g., Hazelrigg et al. 1987; Markus et al. 1990) has indicated that family therapy can be favorably compared to no treatment and many alternative treatments. Increasingly, the efficacy of family therapy for particular disorders has been researched. In recent years the research has become refined enough to consider the use of family therapy with subgroups of patients (e.g., those with a particular disorder or of a particular age).

Outcome research alone in the psychosocial therapies, and also individual psychotherapies, is not enough (Gurman et al. 1986). Attention needs to be given to the process of change in order to develop more specific and effective treatments. In family therapy research, much thought has been given to the measurement of changes in family interaction. These have been studied by self-report methods, which involve family members completing questionnaires. A better way of measuring family interaction is by the use of semi-structured interviews that are then scored for certain attitudes, behaviors, or styles of problem solving. One of the most important examples of this approach is the measure of expressed emotion (EE) (Brown and Rutter 1966; Rutter and Brown 1966). Expressed emotion has a number of components: criticism, or expressions of disapproval; hostility, in which criticism is generalized to the whole person; emotional overinvolvement; and warmth and positive remarks. In EE research it is the attitudes and behaviors of relatives to psychiatric patients that are scored from recorded interviews. In this section on family therapy and in the subsequent sections on other therapies, some of the findings from EE research will be described as these inform the practice and development of the psychosocial treatments.

Family Therapy in Medical Settings

Most medical consultations take place in primary care settings. This is true for both physical and psychological disorders (Goldberg and Huxley 1980). These disorders are typically associated with distress for the whole family. Many general practitioners (primary care physicians) regard themselves as family doctors because they are aware of their responsibility to the whole family. Earlier health care experiments focusing on the whole family were not directly informed by family therapy thinking (Doherty 1985). Family therapy has been little used in primary care, although a number of reports have indicated that it is a useful way of providing help for many problems. Child behavior problems and relationship difficulties have been found to be helped in a setting that is liked by the patients (Graham et al. 1992; Neighbour 1982). Advantages of using the primary care setting are the avoidance of stigma caused by referral to psychiatric services, the familiarity of the general practitioner with the family, and the ability to obtain a quick response.

Family therapy has been used as an adjunct to the management of many physical illnesses, especially chronic illnesses. The rationale for this is an understanding of the effects of illness on family relationships and the way in which relationships may become rigidly organized around the illness. For example, the illness may lead to overprotective behaviors by parents toward their children, and fear of deterioration in the physical state may prevent the development of age-appropriate autonomy. Furthermore, the illness itself may serve a function within the pattern of family relationships. For example, the occurrence of an asthma attack may lead to reduced conflict between parents. Many of these insights came from the work of Minuchin and his colleagues (1978) and have led to the development of helpful interventions. Table 9–1 shows the range of disorders that have been treated by family therapy. A number of studies have used a controlled or comparison group to evaluate the therapy.

Family therapy also has been used extensively in the management of life-threatening illness. This is especially true for situations where children are involved, either as the member who is ill or when their parents are ill (Black 1989). It has also been used in the management of bereavement to the benefit of both parents and children. A controlled trial of six sessions involving 45 families showed beneficial effects 1 and 2 years later (Black and Urbanowicz 1987).

Family Therapy and Eating Disorders

The earliest descriptions of anorexia nervosa in the nineteenth century made an association between the disorder and a particular family constellation (Lasegue 1873). In the 1970s, with the growth of family therapy, attempts were made to clarify this association. Family therapists working from different perspectives have remarked on the high level of involvement of the parents with their anorexic child, unresolved and often covert discord between the parents, and the family's inability to change and adjust to the developmental needs of the children (Minuchin et al. 1978; Selvini-Palazzoli et al. 1978). It was remarked that the disorder itself was associated with a failure of maturation, which was seen as being interconnected with the difficulties of the families in permitting appropriate adolescent development and the failure of the family to progress to the next stage of the life cycle.

These ideas have been used to develop therapy for the disorder, mostly in adolescents and young adults. The most impressive of these

Table 9–1. Studies of family therapy in the management of physical illness

Illness	Studies
AIDS or HIV infection	Bor et al. 1988; Walker 1991
Asthma	Minuchin et al. 1978; Lask and Matthews 1979[a]; Tal et al. 1990[a]
Brain disease	Murberg et al. 1988; Lansky 1989
Diabetes mellitus	Minuchin et al. 1978
Heart disease	J. M. Patterson 1989; Bises 1990
Pain	Roy 1989
Renal disease	Altschuler et al. 1991
Systemic lupus erythematosus	Rose-Itkoff 1987

Note. AIDS = acquired immunodeficiency syndrome; HIV = human immunodeficiency virus.
[a]Study used a control or comparison group.

early studies was that carried out by Minuchin et al. (1978) who applied structural family therapy to the treatment of eating disorders. They reported on the family therapy of 53 patients with an eating disorder, whose age ranged from 9 to 21 years, with an average length of illness lasting 9 months. Their results showed that 86% made a full recovery, the condition of 4% improved, and the condition of 10% remained unchanged. This study had a number of weaknesses, such as the absence of a control group and poor outcome measures. However, these generally impressive findings provided the stimulus for a more rigorous study comparing family therapy with supportive psychotherapy for patients admitted to hospital for a weight restoration program (Dare et al. 1990; Russell et al. 1987). Family therapy was found to be superior for the younger patients, who had a short duration of illness (less than 3 years).

Further research has indicated that outpatient family therapy can be used in the absence of inpatient treatment, and that most adolescents respond well (Le Grange et al. 1992b). There is increasing empirical evidence that family therapy provides an appropriate model for outpatient treatment of anorexia nervosa in children and adolescents (Hodes et al. 1991). Even when admission is necessary, family therapy is still appropriate to prevent premature discharge and other difficulties.

A recent investigation of families in which a member has an eating disorder included measurement of EE from parents to the patient (Hodes and Le Grange 1993). The findings from this study indicated that families of patients who have bulimia nervosa have higher levels of criticism, as measured by EE, as compared to families of patients who have anorexia nervosa (Szmukler et al. 1985). This finding of a high level of discord with bulimia is in keeping with other research in this area (Strober and Humphrey 1987), and is clinically relevant in understanding certain aspects of treatment. High levels of criticism were found to be associated with a greater chance of dropping out of family treatment (Szmukler et al. 1985). Only one study reported the changing levels of EE during treatment (Le Grange et al. 1992a). It showed that during the family therapy of adolescents with anorexia nervosa, the level of criticism tended to lessen, especially in those who had a good treatment response, but there was little change in overinvolvement and warmth. This suggested that the parental achievement in ensuring that offspring ate adequately led the parents to feel less exasperated, leading to their blaming the patient less. Only one study has been carried out investigating EE and obesity (Fishman-Havstad and Marston 1984); the findings from this study showed that after a period of successful weight loss in married women, a poor response was associated with criticism by the spouse.

Family Therapy in the Management of Aggression

It has become increasingly clear that the development and persistence of aggression is closely tied to particular family interactional styles (G. Patterson 1982; G. Patterson and Dishion 1988). The family characteristics include high levels of coercive, critical, and rejecting behaviors. The children in such families tend to respond less to each command from parents as compared to children exposed to similar directives from families that have a less coercive style. There may also be increased rates of disrupted relationships, such as parental separation and parenting breakdown associated with child abuse, leading to children being cared for in alternative families or institutions (Robins 1991). In view of these findings, attempts have been made to work with the families to reduce levels of aggression shown by children and parents.

Aggressive children and adolescents who show a range of antisocial behaviors have conduct disorders and may also show delinquency. Two approaches to the involvement of the family for these problems have been tried. The first of these is more influenced by systems theory and may involve the whole family, with a view to clarifying generational differences, increasing parental authority, reducing discord between the parents, and reducing the involvement of children in parental disputes (Minuchin et al. 1967). The second kind of treatment is more influenced by social learning theory (Webster-Stratton 1991). This work often involves teaching the parents more effective skills and child control strategies. It may be augmented with individual sessions with the children, with a view to teaching them more effective social skills. The second kind of intervention has been rigorously evaluated and generally shown to produce improvement. However, many children with conduct disorder continue to have handicapping difficulties even after treatment. A comparison study (Wells and Egan 1988) of systems family therapy with more focused behavioral treatment demonstrated that the latter was more effective.

Similar work has been carried out in the treatment of delinquency. While adequately designed studies are rare, a recent review did show findings consistent with those for the treatment of conduct disorder (Tolan et al. 1986). Again, it would appear that focused and behaviorally oriented therapy is more effective than other family therapy approaches.

Aggressive behavior by parents toward their children is related to physical child abuse. Much attention has been given to the reduction of these abusive behaviors by applying family therapy techniques. Evaluation is difficult because of the need for multi-agency involvement, adequate child protection, and the high drop-out rate from treatment. Nevertheless, it would appear that family therapy can be effective in reducing the level of coercive and abusive behaviors of parents, and is superior to expressive psychotherapies (Nicol et al. 1988). Sometimes the level of aggression and risk to the child requires more intensive intervention than can be provided on an outpatient basis. Specialized programs have been developed that require all-day attendance over a period of weeks (Asen et al. 1989). Other programs involve admission of the whole family to the hospital. Such special facilities make observation of the family possible while the members carry out many everyday tasks and provide a containing environment in which parents can learn new ways of caring for their children (Brendler et al. 1991; Kennedy 1988).

Family Therapy and Substance Abuse

The family systems perspective on substance abuse views the problem behavior within the context of a pattern of relationships and a particular value system. The substance abuse is understood by the way it organizes relationships. For example, the abuser may be regarded as incompetent by others and a failure, which leads to further consumption, which in turn confirms the original view. Where abuse is shared by family members, which commonly occurs with couples, the substance becomes the "glue" that keeps the couple together but is also what prevents the development of real intimacy. Furthermore, alcoholism and drug abuse are common in the families of origin of substance abusers, and so will have had a profound effect on child development (Stanton and Todd 1982). Alcohol and drug abuse tend to be associated with high levels of conflict and disrupted relationships (Jacob et al. 1981; Stanton and Todd 1982).

There are differences in the family therapy of alcoholics and drug abusers. One difference is that alcoholics tend to enter treatment at a later age than those with drug dependency. This means they are at a different life stage and may occupy quite different family roles from those of the drug abuser. For example, the possible interventions for young substance abusers who live with their parents are quite different from the treatment of the substance abusing parent who has young dependent children. Another important difference that has appeared in the last few years is the relationship between substance abuse and the human immunodeficiency virus (HIV) and the acquired immunodeficiency syndrome (AIDS). Family therapy may have to deal with issues concerning life-threatening illness, death, and the care of children who may themselves be affected.

Evidence for the efficacy of family therapy in treating substance abuse and alcoholism comes from a range of studies, although the methodological rigor of those studies is variable (Kaufman 1985). The authors of one influential study of the treatment of heroin addiction, which included control groups (Stanton and Todd 1982), found that structural/strategic therapy was more effective than the inactive interventions. It should be borne in mind that family therapy may need to be an adjunct to inpatient management, or outpatient detoxification programs.

Family Therapy and the
Hospitalization of Psychiatric Patients

The changing attitudes toward asylum treatment of psychiatric patients, beginning in the 1950s, and the development of new patterns of community psychiatric care meant that patients were more likely to stay with their families. This provided a stimulus for the development of family therapy, which was required to support families and resolve crises. Indeed, it soon became apparent that not only was it possible to avoid hospitalization for many patients, but there were advantages of therapeutic intervention with the family.

An early study carried out in Denver, Colorado in the 1960s evaluated the effect of outpatient crisis family therapy for patients who would ordinarily have been hospitalized (Langsley et al. 1971). A group of 150 families in the experimental group were compared with another group of 150 families where the identified patient was hospitalized. Random assignment to treatment, baseline evaluation, and multiple outcome measures including independent assessment at 6-, 18-, and 30-months after discharge were used. In all 150 cases treated with family therapy, it was possible to avoid hospitalization. On measures of role functioning and symptoms, the family therapy cases did as well as the hospitalized patients, and on measures of crisis resolution and time before return to healthy functioning, the family therapy cases did better than the hospitalized cases. In another study, family therapy reduced admissions to state mental hospitals from 1200 to 30–40 per year (Langsley et al. 1978).

Family therapy has been studied as an adjunct to inpatient therapy. In a Payne-Whitney study (Glick et al. 1985; Haas et al. 1988; Spencer et al. 1988), family therapy was used to supplement standard inpatient treatment. Using a true experimental model, patients were randomly assigned to family therapy plus individual therapy or just individual therapy. The family therapy group had at least six sessions and the comparison group had an increased number of individual sessions to keep the total number of sessions the same for both groups. The final report on 186 patients included groups of 1) schizophrenic patients with good functioning for 18 months prior to hospital admission; 2) schizophrenic patients with poor prehospitalization functioning; 3) major affective disorder patients; and 4) patients with other Axis I disorders. Inpatient family intervention improved attitudes toward treatment in the families of patients with schizophrenia. There was a surprising finding for patients with affective disorders (Clarkin et al. 1990). At both 6 and 18 months after inpatient treatment, bipolar patients showed a better outcome with inpatient family intervention, while unipolar patients did better without it. Inpatient family intervention had a negative effect on males, which became evident by 18 months.

The benefits of family therapy in the management of adult psychiatric disorders are not specific to industrialized, affluent nations. One interesting study was carried out in India, where family and social organization are quite different to those of Europe and the United States. Family therapy was offered to 110 inpatients who had a variety of disorders such as hysteria, depression, and epilepsy-related psychiatric disorder. It was possible to obtain data on 55% of the patients, and it was found that two-thirds of these patients were helped by the intervention at follow-up (Prabhu et al. 1988).

Family Intervention in Schizophrenia

The relationship between the family and schizophrenia has an important place in the development of family therapy. Bateson and colleagues, working in the 1950s, were among the first to apply systems theory to the family. They observed the communication in families in which a member had schizophrenia. It was postulated that there was a particular kind of communication associated with this disorder, known as the *double bind* (Bateson et al. 1956). Other models have also related family processes to the development of schizophrenia. Later investigation of these descriptions could not confirm that these kinds of communication could be clearly identified and be shown to have an important role in schizophrenia (Dare 1985).

A different approach was adopted by a group of British investigators (Brown et al. 1958) who noticed that patients with schizophrenia who were discharged from the hospital to their relatives were more likely to relapse than those who were returned to hostels. This finding provided the stimulus for developing a measure of family life—the measure of expressed emotion (Brown and Rutter 1966; Rutter and Brown 1966). Certain components of EE—criticism and emotional overinvolvement—when scored above certain levels (high EE), were predictive of relapse in schizophrenia following discharge from the hospital (Brown et al. 1972). Many studies (see Kuipers and Bebbington 1988) carried out all over the world in different cultures and languages, such as Spanish and Hindi, have replicated this finding. The size of the effect is substantial. Vaughn and Leff (1976) showed that relapse rates at 9 months following hospital discharge was 51% among those who returned to high-EE families and 13% among those who returned to low-EE families.

There is also evidence about factors that limit the predictive effect of EE and schizophrenic relapse (Kavanagh 1992). Neuroleptic medication has been repeatedly shown to lower the rate of relapse; this effect still occurs in the presence of high-EE relatives, although the medication does not reduce relapse to a level comparable to that of low-EE environments. Another important variable is the amount of time relatives spend together. Clearly, if EE reflects communication between relatives, then high levels of contact will be associated with greater exposure to stressful interactions. A number of studies have found that when contact with relatives is less than 35 hours per week, then EE has little effect on relapse (Brown et al. 1972; Vaughn and Leff 1976; Vaughn et al. 1984).

Having shown that there is an association between EE and relapse in schizophrenia, it was then demonstrated that EE could be reduced by intervention, with an associated reduction in relapse (Leff et al. 1982). A number of subsequent studies (see Lam 1991) have replicated this finding. These studies varied in the combinations of interventions that were evaluated, although medication has become a routine part of the care. Intervention groups for relatives may receive education sessions about schizophrenia (Barrowclough and Tarrier 1987; Berkowitz et al. 1984). Other studies have evaluated the effects of relatives' groups (Leff et al. 1989) and social skills training for patients (Hogarty et al. 1986). These studies have included family treatment sessions, typically carried out at home. Table 9–2 shows that the size of the benefits are substantial.

The effects of family intervention are broad, benefiting both the patient and the family. Lam (1991), reviewing five major family intervention studies with 2-year outcomes, concluded that family therapy effects 1) the patient's mental state (family intervention is effective in preventing relapse at 9 months or a year with relapse rates of family treatment groups ranging from 6% to 23% compared with 40%–53% in comparison groups); 2) the patient's social functioning (family therapy–treated patients had longer periods of employment at 9 months); and 3) the relatives' burden of distress (which improved at 9 months and at 2-year follow-up) as well as effecting a reduction of EE in the family.

Two kinds of family intervention have been carried out in these studies. Leff et al. (1982) aimed to reduce EE and/or social contact. The techniques used varied from dynamic interpretations to behavioral interventions. Attention was paid to boundary making and the gradual resumption of responsibility for the patient (Berkowitz 1988). Behavioral family therapy has been used by other investigators to reduce EE, and techniques have included problem solving, relaxation, and attention to enhancing the clarity of family communications (Falloon et al. 1982; Tarrier et al. 1988). Teaching new ways to communicate may be by direct instruction or by methods such as role-playing, record keeping, and guided practice (Tarrier et al. 1988).

The principles of psychoeducation and improving family relationships by reducing EE have been shown to be useful for chronically ill patients. In one study, all relatives of patients in contact with a clinical team in a local day care facility were offered an educational intervention aimed at reducing the EE level (Kuipers et al. 1989; MacCarthy et al. 1989). A session at home was followed by a monthly group session with the relatives. Patients and their relatives in routine care with mental health teams in the same facility comprised the control group. The families who had the educational session and monthly groups showed reduced EE and improved family relationships. It was felt that this type of support for the families of long-term mentally ill patients may contribute to the quality of life of both families and patients.

Despite the importance of these developments in the family management of schizophrenia, there are a number of drawbacks. First, most of

Table 9–2. Percentage of relapses in treatment studies that preselected for high expressed emotion

	0–9 months		0–24 months	
Study	Family intervention	Routine or individual treatment	Family intervention	Routine or individual treatment
Leff et al. (1982, 1985)	8	50	50[a]	75[a]
Falloon et al. (1982, 1985)	6	44	17	83
Köttgen et al. (1984)	33	50	—	—
Hogarty et al. (1986, 1987)[b]	19	28	32	66
Tarrier et al. (1988, 1989)	12	48[c]	33	59[c]
Leff et al. (1989, 1990)	8	—	33	—
Median	10	48	33	71

[a]The percentages include subjects who stopped medication; suicides are counted as relapses. If those subjects are omitted, the outcomes are 20 (family treatment), 78 (routine care).

[b]Social skills training to individual clients produced a 9-month relapse rate of 20 and a 2-year rate of 42. A combined intervention of family and social skills training gave 0 relapse in 9 months and 25 in 2 years.

[c]Combined results for the brief education and routine treatment conditions.

Source. Adapted from Kavanagh 1992.

the benefit has been shown to occur in high-EE families, but many patients come from low-EE families (Kavanagh 1992) for whom the goals of family management may be less clear. Second, many families do not wish to start in treatment, and others drop out after treatment has commenced. This is particularly likely to occur in families that have high EE, which are those that could most benefit from intervention (Tarrier 1991). Third, the demonstrated benefits have been obtained by research investigators; it is necessary to show that the skills required could be effectively taught and applied in clinical service settings. Finally, skepticism remains about EE, and some investigators have disputed the role of the family in schizophrenic relapse (MacMillan et al. 1986) despite the impressive evidence for supporting this hypothesis. Others fear that involvement of the family will lead to the family members being blamed (Kanter et al. 1987).

The exact nature of EE remains unclear. It reflects certain aspects of family communication style, and is not fixed but rather changes over time (Falloon 1988b). It may be a reflection of coping. The concept of EE was developed as a theoretical measure of family life, and has not been linked to a particular model of individual or family functioning. It continues as an important predictor of schizophrenic relapse that is valid cross-culturally (Kavanagh 1992). This can best be explained by the interactional model that incorporates the interplay between biological, psychological, and family factors. High levels of criticism and over-involvement are stresses that may lead to relapse in those biologically predisposed to schizophrenia (Kavanagh 1992).

The family therapy that has been evaluated for schizophrenia has been related to EE research. However many therapists have used systems family therapy for schizophrenia, particularly that developed by Selvini-Palazzoli et al. (1978). These approaches differ in many ways from the empirically derived family therapy that has been described (Berkowitz 1988). Although they have become popular among some family therapists, they have not been evaluated and their effects are unknown.

Multiple Family Therapy

Multiple family therapy moves beyond the single-family model. O'Sheay and Phelps (1985) reviewed a number of reports on this modality and noted that multiple family therapy was regarded as a "sheltered workshop in family communication." Some have considered long-term multiple family therapy as the optimal intervention with schizophrenic patients for active restructuring of family interaction patterns. Falloon et al. (1984), using a multiple family format to evaluate 15-week behavioral coping-skills training programs, suggested that multiple family therapy combined with a single family therapy is useful. However, it must be noted that very few outcome studies that allow a reliable assessment of the effectiveness of this treatment modality have been carried out. Although multiple family therapy is not widely used, it may have economic advantages over treating one family at a time.

Marital Therapy

Many of the ideas that underlie marital therapy are the same as the ideas that underlie family therapy. This is because understanding the marital relationship, rather than simply considering two individuals' psychological functioning (e.g., mental states), requires understanding the pattern of that relationship. One way of doing this is the application of systems theory (Gorell Barnes 1985), which is influential in both family and marital therapy.

The same schools or approaches exist in the two kinds of therapy, although how they are used may require modification. The psychodynamic perspective explores the marriage as a system in which unconscious mental processes contribute to discord and unhappiness in the relationship. Particularly important is the projection of parts of the self onto the partner, and the way in which each individual may unconsciously seek in the partner aspects of earlier relationships (e.g., relationships with parents). Life-cycle and intergenerational issues are also important. The formation of mature relationships requires appropriate separation from the family of origin so that there can be appropriate emotional investment in the new relationship and preparation for the new life-cycle tasks such as child rearing. The intergenerational approach of Bowen and others stresses these issues (Bowen 1978).

The structural perspective of Minuchin emphasizes the need for an appropriate distance for healthy functioning, the modification of enmeshment that prevents healthy functioning, and the fostering of appropriate intergenerational alliances. The strategic approach emphasizes the need for problem solving, and, like the structural approach, deals with functioning in the present (Stanton 1981). The fourth approach is behavioral marital therapy (BMT), which also concentrates on the present. It aims for the relearning of communication and behavior in a way that is reinforcing and gratifying. BMT has been integrated with many aspects of systems thinking and is a commonly practiced kind of marital therapy (Crowe and Ridley 1990).

The term marital therapy is rather old-fashioned in that it implies that the therapy is for a married couple. In fact, the same therapeutic principles can be used with people whether or not they are married or even cohabiting, including among homosexual men (Butler and Clarke 1991) and lesbian women (Simons 1991). In view of this, the term couples therapy is preferred by some (Hooper and Dryden 1991).

Couples therapy can be carried out by people from many backgrounds who have the appropriate training, but usually psychiatrists, psychologists, and social workers are the therapists. It may be offered in a variety of settings such as hospitals, clinics, or offices. Marriage guidance is a movement developed to reduce the levels of marital distress, employing laypeople with some training.

Marital therapy is mostly offered for people who report distress in their marital or intimate relationships. Its efficacy has been extensively investigated, with most of these studies being carried out with BMT. A recent meta-analysis (Hahlweg and Markman 1988) indicated that BMT is better than no treatment in reducing marital distress. Furthermore, BMT is equally effective in United States and European settings and so is useful in many cultures. However, despite this conclusion, there is still controversy about the process of change and whether psychoanalytic, insight-oriented marital therapy (IOMT) is preferable to BMT. Snyder and Wills (1989) carried out a treatment trial that showed no difference between IOMT and BMT. Furthermore, at 4-year follow-up, they found on self-report measures of marital satisfaction, as well as from divorce rates, that IOMT was superior (Snyder et al. 1991). For example, whereas 38% of the BMT couples had divorced by the 4-year follow-up, only 3% of the IOMT couples had split up. However, certain aspects of the study have been questioned (Jacobson 1991).

Marital therapy has been used in the treatment of a variety of psychiatric disorders. Perhaps the most common situation is marital therapy for depression. The rationale for this is provided by research findings that the quality of the marital relationship is related to the onset of depression. A confiding relationship has been shown to be a protective factor against adversity that may lead to depression (Brown and Harris 1978). Furthermore, many studies have shown that the quality of communication, as measured by EE, is related to depression. In particular, high levels of criticism are related to the disorder (Florin et al. 1992; Hooley et al. 1986; Vaughn and Leff 1976). These findings are consistent with behavioral systems formulations of marital difficulties that aim to modify communication style by reducing conflict and increasing the level of mutually rewarding interchanges (which may be verbal interchanges) (Crowe and Ridley 1990). One trial evaluating the efficacy of marital therapy for depression (Bloch et al. 1991) confirmed clinical impressions that marital therapy is effective, especially when depression occurs in the presence of marital discord (Jacobson et al. 1991).

Other problems that may be treated by marital therapy include agoraphobia, marital violence, sexual problems, and substance and alcohol abuse. These problems may be understood in terms of the pattern of interchanges, including verbal exchanges, that occur between spouses and that need to be modified to reduce distress (Crowe and Ridley 1990). Marital therapy may also be used as an adjunct to medication in the management of the psychotic disorders, schizophrenia, and manic-depressive psychosis. The research on relapse in schizophrenia and EE includes a considerable number of patients who returned to their spouses (Leff et al. 1982). In these cases, the principles of psychoeducation and marital therapy to reduce levels of criticism and overinvolvement are as relevant as when patients return to their parents.

Group Psychotherapy

The rationale for group psychotherapy is that meetings of people who previously had not known each other can provide the opportunity for an improvement in psychological health. Although this improvement may be brought about in a number of different ways, it has been suggested that 11 specific factors are involved in the effectiveness of group therapy (Yalom 1985). These are listed in Table 9–3, with a brief explanation of each factor.

Psychotherapy groups vary considerably in their approach, but the constituents are those described by Yalom (1985). The variations between groups can be understood as different combinations of these constituents. Groups can be divided based on psychodynamic, social skills, behavioral and cognitive-behavioral, educational, and support orientations. Self-help groups are distinct from these in a number of ways. Social skills groups will be described elsewhere (see Chapter 10), but the others will be discussed here.

In *psychodynamically oriented groups*, psychoanalytic principles are applied to the group process. Key concepts are free association, resistance, transference and countertransference, acting out, interpretation, and working through (Shaffer and Galinsky 1989; Yalom 1985). The

Table 9–3.   Therapeutic factors in group psychotherapy

1. Installation of hope
2. Universality—the experience of not being alone in distress, and perhaps meeting people with very similar difficulties
3. Imparting of information
4. Altruism—others in the group will try to help the patient, and this behavior may be reciprocated
5. The corrective recapitulation of the primary group—previous family relationships will be reenacted in the group and better understood
6. Development of socializing techniques—social learning (i.e., the opportunity for learning new ways of relating)
7. Imitative behavior
8. Interpersonal learning—including the group as an emotional and corrective experience
9. Group cohesiveness—the experience of being part of, and connected to, the group, including the group therapist
10. Catharsis—the feeling of relief from disclosing experiences
11. Existential factors—consideration and acceptance of the vicissitudes and realities of life

Source.   Adapted from Yalom 1985.

therapist adopts a nondirective, neutral stance and offers interpretations to facilitate the acquisition of insight from the experience of participating in the group. There are many developments from this basic model, including groups that last much longer than the usual session (e.g., residential groups). More modern derivatives include encounter groups, which are much more confrontational. They are more related to the human potential movement (Shaffer and Galinsky 1989) and less to the treatment of psychiatric disorders.

Psychodynamic groups have been used frequently for the treatment of symptoms of anxiety and depression. Many studies have shown that they are beneficial for these symptoms (see Kaul and Bednar 1985). However, this type of group therapy generally has not been shown to be superior to other treatments for these symptoms. Psychodynamic groups have been used for most other psychiatric disorders, but with less evidence for their efficacy. Some (e.g., Horwitz 1977, 1987) has advocated their use for the treatment of borderline personality disorders, sometimes in combination with individual psychotherapy, although the difficulties of having more than one or two such patients in a group is readily acknowledged. In a recent review, Higgitt and Fonagy (1992) concluded that there is no compelling evidence that group therapy is preferable to individual psychotherapy for people with borderline personality disorders, other than for reasons of practicality and economy.

Behavioral group therapy is based on the principles of learning theory. It has been developed largely for reasons of practicality. As with many behavioral treatments, such therapy has been used for a large number of well-defined problems and disorders and has been well evaluated (Shaffer and Galinsky 1989). Principles of systematic desensitization and relaxation have been used in groups for the treatment of phobias. Specific behavior control therapy improves the patients' awareness of their own behavior, including feelings or situations that precipitate the undesired behavior. Such techniques have been used extensively for behaviors such as smoking, substance and alcohol abuse, and overeating.

Cognitive-behavior therapy, which has also been used in groups, was developed from behavior therapy. Probably the group therapy that has been best evaluated for a psychiatric disorder is behavioral therapy (which may include cognitive and educational components) for bulimia nervosa. High quality studies (Freeman et al. 1988) have indicated that this treatment is as effective as individual psychotherapy, and meta-analysis of a range of studies has also indicated the benefits from this treatment (Fettes and Peters 1992).

Educational and support groups may be used for many problems. There may be overlap between this kind of group and groups run on behavioral principles. Of particular interest is the application of educational and support groups in the prevention of relapse in schizophrenia. It has been shown that they may contribute to a reduction of EE in high-EE households (Leff et al. 1989). They have also been used extensively in the management of physical illness. One area that has attracted much research is the place of the group in facing life-threatening illnesses, particularly cancer, for which its usefulness has been established (Heinrich and Schag 1985; Spiegel et al. 1981).

The concept of self-help groups is well known in many countries and cultures. The best known example is Alcoholics Anonymous (AA), established over 50 years ago. The self-help movement has grown to encompass many other illness categories. Galanter (1988) estimated that there are now one-half million self-help groups involving several million members in the United States.

Self-help groups are composed of people who share a common condition, are largely self-governing, emphasize consensus rather than coercion, advocate self-reliance, minimize referrals to professionals, and offer face-to-face or telephone networks, usually without charge. They include organizations known as *self-help, mutual-help,* or *peer-help* services. They use professionals as consultants, supervisors, or resources, but the professionals do not deliver the service. Nevertheless, professionals may be active in founding self-help groups and may take a collaborative or cooperative role.

Self-help groups have some common ground with group psychotherapy and some differences (Lieberman 1990). The elements common to both are an expression of need (manifested by joining the groups), sharing of personal information, and the real or perceived similarity in the participants' suffering. These elements generate a sense of belonging, and are associated with group cohesiveness. There are also differences between self-help groups and group psychotherapy and among the different self-help groups. Self-help groups vary with regard to the emphasis on cognitive mechanisms (e.g., increasing understanding, putting things into perspective, and providing insight into personal problems). For example, these are important in women's consciousness-raising groups, but not for Compassionate Friends (a group for parents who have experienced the death of a child), for whom inculcation of hope and existential concerns are more important. Another aspect of the specificity of these groups concerns their ideology. It has been suggested that each has a specific ideology closely linked to the underlying psychological problem associated with the affliction (Antze 1976).

Clearly, it is not possible to evaluate the efficacy of self-help groups using standard research designs. Nevertheless, studies that have been done have suggested that many people obtain relief from distress by participating in the groups. In their review, Lieberman and Borman (1979) described significant benefits with women's consciousness-raising groups, showing increases in self-esteem and self-concept and alterations in life-style. Members of Mended Hearts (those forced to retire for health reasons) reported fewer somatic symptoms and experienced higher levels of self-esteem and coping. Widows and widowers in They Help Each Other Spiritually (THEOS) reported increased activity and more participation in groups compared to those who did not participate. Compassionate Friends members found significant help in coping with the death of a child.

Regarding the area for which self-help groups reach large numbers of people (i.e., alcoholism), Galanter et al. (1987) reported a study comparing a hospital-based alcoholism program with two ambulatory programs, one operated by professional staff and one experimental, based on self-help. The self-help group was staffed by half as many primary therapists as the other two groups yet its members scored higher on social adjustment. Drinking rates and the use of AA or disulfiram were no different from controls. Galanter et al. (1987) also quoted other studies showing that self-help groups may be effective for persons involved in natural disasters or war.

Therapeutic Communities

The therapeutic community represents a development of the principles of group psychotherapy. While in group psychotherapy participants have only brief contact with each other, although this may be over an extended time period, the therapeutic community is a residential group so that there is a high degree of face-to-face contact. In the therapeutic community all relationships, activities, and interchanges are potentially therapeutic and may be structured to realize this potential. The important components have been described by Rapoport et al. (1960):

1. The total social organization is viewed as affecting the therapeutic outcome.
2. The social organization is seen as a vital force, not background.
3. The core element is the opportunity of patients to take an active part in the affairs of the organization.
4. All relations within the hospital are seen as potentially therapeutic.
5. The emotional climate is seen as important.
6. High value is placed on communications.

The themes that are seen as most important for therapeutic communities are democratization, permissiveness, communalism, and reality-confrontation.

Early developments in therapeutic communities were influenced by psychoanalytic principles. The leaders of the institutions were often psychoanalytically trained psychiatrists and the institutions were part of the psychiatric services. Although only a small number of therapeutic communities were established, their influence spread to other settings, such as psychiatric wards and day hospitals; these are also considered here.

The Therapeutic Community and Personality Disorders

From the early days in the history of therapeutic communities, patients who were psychotic, alcohol or substance abusers, or in need of medication were generally considered not suitable for admission. Mostly the patients who were considered suitable had personality disorders. Patients need to have a considerable degree of reality orientation and be willing to participate in, and contribute to, the community. Patients are usually admitted after long assessments, and in some communities other patients participate in the decision-making process about who should be admitted. Admission may be for long periods of time (e.g., 12–15 months).

The rationale for such intensive and long-term treatment is that time is required for the healing process in view of the damage that is believed to have occurred in psychological development. Main, who coined the term *therapeutic community*, believed "it has the immediate aim of full participation of all its members in its daily life and the eventual aim of resocialization of the individual" (Main 1946).

Systematic evaluation of the benefits of therapeutic communities has not been carried out. However, some reports are available that indicate who might benefit the most and what the significance of change is. Denford et al. (1983), in a retrospective study at the Cassel Hospital in London, reported on the progress of 28 patients. They found that patients with neurotic rather than borderline psychopathology, those who were considerably depressed, those with little previous outpatient treatment, and those of superior intelligence made a better response to living in a therapeutic community. Dolan and Evans (1991) investigated symptom change. Patients reported symptom levels at preadmission assessments for entry into a therapeutic community and, when followed up 8 months after treatment, showed a significant reduction in symptoms.

Therapeutic communities within psychiatric services have been in decline in recent years (Trauer 1984). The reasons appear to be the loss of charismatic leadership, the medicalization of psychiatry, and the trend to shorter inpatient lengths of stay. The paucity of relevant research evaluating efficacy is another important factor, and may become more relevant as the demand for cost control in psychiatric care increases.

Therapeutic Communities and Substance Abuse

A different kind of therapeutic community has emerged for helping people with drug and alcohol dependence. These communities have tended to develop outside the existing service delivery systems. They were set up by people who had been substance abusers themselves, and so have much in common with self-help groups. They have flourished in the United States, and also exist in Europe and Australia (Rosenthal 1989). The daily regimen is full and may include encounter group therapy, tutorial learning sessions, and formal educational classes (De Leon 1985). These types of communities do not give the same emphasis to understanding and reflection as the more psychoanalytically oriented ones.

The effectiveness of therapeutic communities for substance abusers has been studied primarily through follow-up studies (De Leon 1984, 1985). The general conclusions are that among those who enter the communities, successful outcome is directly related to retention. However, many people leave after only a brief stay, without having received any significant benefit. There are few consistent predictors of successful outcome other than duration of treatment; but, when present, beneficial effects can be seen in the decline in drug use and criminality and in the improvement in employment or education.

The Therapeutic Milieu

The principles of therapeutic communities have been applied to psychiatric wards, day hospitals, and mental health centers. This is because many psychiatrists, while accepting that psychiatric disorders are heterogeneous and have varied etiologies, believe their patients can be helped in an appropriate social environment. The quality of relationships are important in reducing distress. The patient's separation from the family environment where relationships may be fraught, and participation in a regimen where there are clear rules but also warmth in relationships with staff are important.

A number of studies have investigated the beneficial and detrimental aspects of the therapeutic milieu (Watson and Bouras 1988). It has been shown that the number of patients on the ward is positively correlated with perception of aggression and anger. More staff on the ward is correlated with more interaction with patients. It would also seem that patterns of interaction between staff and patients and between patients are important, but the qualities of these interactions have not been well explored. One area that has been investigated is participation in ward discussion groups by acute patients, for whom groups were not found to be helpful (Fairweather 1964).

Psychosocial Interventions in Practice

The potential for effective treatment of psychiatric disorders has substantially increased in recent years. This is because of the development of many pharmacological, psychotherapeutic, and psychosocial treatments, and selective combinations of these. When so many options for intervention are available, it is useful to have some way of choosing between them. In this section we consider principles that influence the appropriate use of the psychosocial treatments.

First, the choice of treatment will obviously be influenced by the nature of the problem. It has been stated already that psychosocial interventions may be an adjunct to other treatments, such as drug treatments and inpatient care. The choice of psychosocial treatment should be influenced by the available empirical evidence concerning efficacy. In situations where the research findings are unclear, it will be necessary to make the best inferences from what is available. The increase in research in this area means that current areas of uncertainty are likely to be reduced.

Second, in selecting a particular psychosocial intervention for a patient, the therapist will need to consider that person's life-cycle stage. For most people family are the most significant relatives, and which family members to involve will be related to family and life-cycle stage. For children and adolescents, parents and siblings and other relatives living at home are the people who may be usefully involved in treatment. The nature of that involvement will depend on other factors such as the kind of disorder and whether inpatient treatment is also needed. Young adults who have stopped living with their family of origin and who may be living alone or with friends without having established close relationships, are frequently seen alone. Individual or group psychotherapy may be appropriate. Later in life, when adults are married or have formed close relationships, marital or couples therapy may be appropriate, especially when the relationship is discordant. The next life-cycle stage is parenthood, and for parents with psychological difficulties, especially when these involve their children, family therapy may be beneficial.

The third issue that needs to be considered in the provision of treatment is the patient's culture and value system. Obviously there needs to be some agreement between the views of the therapist and the patient for treatment to be acceptable and successful. Furthermore, because psychosocial treatments occur through the medium of language, they are all intimately related to culture. For most patients, care and support will come from family. Relatives in many societies will expect to be involved in treatment, and for this reason family therapy will be an appropriate psychosocial intervention. It may be unacceptable to many patients to meet strangers with difficulties in a group therapy setting.

Finally, it is always important to plan interventions on the basis of available resources. This refers both to available human skills as well as financial provision. On cost grounds, therapeutic communities in the forms described above will not be feasible in many societies, and indeed even in Britain where they began, cost is one factor leading to the contraction of their numbers. Marital and family therapies are economical in that usually a small number of sessions is provided, but still one therapist is needed for each family or couple. An important advantage of group psychotherapy is that treatment can be provided to many people simultaneously with a small amount of professional time.

Conclusions

It is now evident that there are a number of psychosocial interventions that provide effective treatment for many psychiatric disorders and behavior problems. They may also be useful in the management of physical illness. Continuing theoretical and research developments in this area make it difficult to be highly competent in each type of intervention. However, existing research findings and local cultural and resource factors should make it possible to plan appropriate psychosocial treatments.

References

Altschuler J, Black D, Tampeyer R, et al: Adolescents in end-stage renal failure: a pilot study of family factors in compliance and treatment considerations. Family Systems Medicine 9(3):229–247, 1991

Antze P: The role of ideologies in peer group organizations: some theoretical considerations and three case studies. Journal of Applied Behavioral Science 12:300–310, 1976

Asen K, George E, Piper R, et al: A systems approach to child abuse: management and treatment issues. Child Abuse Negl 13:45–57, 1989

Barrowclough C, Tarrier N: A behavioral family intervention with a schizophrenic patient: a case study. Behavioral Psychotherapy 15:252–271, 1987

Bateson G, Jackson DD, Haley J, et al: Toward a theory of schizophrenia. Behavioral Sci 1:251–264, 1956

Berger M, Jurkovic GJ, and Associates: Practicing Family Therapy in Diverse Settings. San Francisco, CA, Jossey-Bass, 1984

Berkowitz R: Family therapy and adult mental illness: schizophrenia and depression. Journal of Family Therapy 10:339–356, 1988

Berkowitz R, Eberlein-Fries R, Kuipers L, et al: Educating relatives about schizophrenia. Schizophr Bull 10:418–429, 1984

Bises A: After infarct: a pilot study. Family Systems Medicine 8:339–348, 1990

Black D: Life-threatening illness, children and family therapy. Journal of Family Therapy 11:81–101, 1989

Black D, Urbanowicz MA: Family intervention with bereaved children. J Child Psychol Psychiatry 28:467–476, 1987

Bloch S, Sharpe M, Allman P: Systemic family therapy in adult psychiatry: a review of fifty families. Br J Psychiatry 159:357–364, 1991

Bor R, Miller R, Perry L: Systemic counseling for patients with AIDS/HIV. Family Systems Medicine 6(1):21–39, 1988

Bowen M: Family Therapy in Clinical Practice. New York, Jason Aronson, 1978

Brendler J, Silver M, Haber M, et al: Madness, Chaos and Violence: Therapy With Families at the Brink. New York, Basic Books, 1991

Brown GW, Harris T: The Social Origins of Depression. London, Tavistock, 1978

Brown GW, Rutter M: The measurement of family activities and relationships: a methodological study. Human Relations 19:241–263, 1966

Brown GW, Carstairs GM, Topping G: Post hospital adjustment of chronic mental patients. Lancet ii:685–689, 1958

Brown GW, Birley JLT, Wing JK: Influence of family life on the course of schizophrenic disorders: implications. Br J Psychiatry 121:241–258, 1972

Butler M, Clarke J: Couple therapy with homosexual men, in Couple Therapy. Edited by Hooper D, Dryden W. Milton Keynes, England, Open University Press, 1991, pp 196–206

Clarkin JF, Glick ID, Haas GL, et al: A randomized trial of inpatient family intervention. J Affective Disord 18:17–28, 1990

Crowe M, Ridley J: Therapy With Couples. Oxford, England, Blackwell Scientific, 1990

Dare C: Family therapy. In Child and Adolescent Psychiatry: Modern Approaches, 2nd Edition. Edited by Rutter M, Hersov L. Oxford, England, Blackwell Scientific, 1985

Dare C, Eisler I, Russell GFM, et al: Family therapy for anorexia nervosa: implications from the results of a controlled trial of family and individual therapy. Journal of Marital and Family Therapy 16(1):39–57, 1990

De Leon G: The Therapeutic Community: Study of Effectiveness. National Institute on Drug Abuse Treatment Research Monograph Series. Washington, DC, US Government Printing Office, 1984

De Leon G: The therapeutic community: status and evolution. Int J Addict 20 (6–7):823–844, 1985

Denford J, Schacter J, Temple N, et al: Selection and outcome in in-patient psychotherapy. Br J Med Psychol 56:225–243, 1983

Doherty WJ: Family interventions in health care. Family Relations 34:129–137, 1985

Dolan BM, Evans C: Therapeutic community treatment for personality disordered adults: a prospective follow-up study. Psychiatric Bulletin, supplement 4, 15:87, 1991

Fairweather GW: Social Psychology in Treating Mental Illness: An Experimental Approach. New York, John Wiley, 1964

Falloon IRH (ed): Handbook of Behavioral Family Therapy. London, Hutchinson, 1988a

Falloon IRH: Expressed emotion: current status. Psychol Med 18:269–274, 1988b

Falloon IRH, Boyd JL, McGill CW, et al: Family management in the prevention of exacerbations of schizophrenia: a controlled study. N Engl J Med 306:1437–1440, 1982

Falloon IRH, Boyd J, McGill C: Family Care of Schizophrenia. New York, Guilford Press, 1984

Falloon IRH, Boyd JL, McGill CW, et al: Family management in the prevention of morbidity of schizophrenia: clinical outcome of a two-year longitudinal study. Arch Gen Psychiatry 42:887–896, 1985

Fettes PA, Peters JM: A meta-analysis of group treatments for bulimia nervosa. International Journal of Eating Disorders 11(2):97–110, 1992

Fishman-Havstad L, Marston AR: Weight loss maintenance as an aspect of family emotion and process. Br J Clin Psychol 23:265–271, 1984

Florin I, Nostadt A, Reck C, et al: Expressed emotion in depressed patients and their partners. Fam Process 31:163–172, 1992

Frank J: Persuasion and Healing. Baltimore, Johns Hopkins University Press, 1973

Frank J: Non-specific aspects of treatment: the view of a psychotherapist, in Non-Specific Aspects of Treatment. Edited by Shepherd M, Sartorius N. Toronto, Hans Hüber, 1989, pp 95–114

Freeman CPL, Barry F, Dunkeld-Turnbull J, et al: Controlled trial of psychotherapy for bulimia nervosa. BMJ 296:521–525, 1988

Galanter M: Research on social supports and mental illness. Am J Psychiatry 145:1270–1272, 1988

Galanter M, Castaneda R, Salamon I: Institutional self-help therapy for alcoholism: clinical outcome. Alcohol Clin Exp Res 11:424–429, 1987

Glick I, Clarkin JF, Spencer JH: A controlled evaluation of inpatient family intervention: I. preliminary results of the six months follow-up. Arch Gen Psychiatry 42:882–886, 1985

Goldberg D, Huxley P: Mental Illness in the Community—The Pathway to Psychiatric Care. London, Tavistock, 1980

Gorell Barnes G: Systems theory and family therapy, in Child and Adolescent Psychiatry: Modern Approaches, 2nd Edition. Edited by Rutter M, Hersov L. Oxford, England, Blackwell Scientific, 1985

Graham H, Senior R, Lazarus M, et al: Family therapy in general practice: views of referrers and clients. Br J Gen Prac 42:25–28, 1992

Gurman AS, Kniskern DP: Family therapy outcome research: knowns and unknowns, in Handbook of Family Therapy. Edited by Gurman AS, Kniskern DP. New York, Brunner/Mazel, 1981, pp 742–775

Gurman AS, Kniskern DP, Pinsof WM: Research on the process and outcome of marital and family therapy: progress, perspective and prospect, in Handbook of Psychotherapy and Behavioral Change. Edited by Garfield SL, Bergin EA. New York, Brunner/Mazel, 1986, pp 565–624

Haas GL, Glick I, Clarkin JF: Inpatient family intervention: a randomized clinical trial. Arch Gen Psychiatry 45:217–224, 1988

Hahlweg K, Markman HJ: Effectiveness of behavioral marital therapy: empirical status of behavioral techniques in preventing and alleviating marital distress. Journal of Counselling and Clinical Psychology 56:440–447, 1988

Hazelrigg MD, Cooper HM, Borduim CM: Evaluating the effectiveness of family therapy: an integrated review and analysis. Psychol Bull 101:428–442, 1987

Heinrich RL, Schag CC: Stress and activity management: group treatment for cancer patients and spouses. J Consult Clin Psychol 53:439–446, 1985

Higgitt A, Fonagy P: Psychotherapy in borderline and narcissistic personality disorder. Br J Psychiatry 161:21–43, 1992

Hodes M, Le Grange D: Expressed emotion in the investigation of eating disorders: a review. International Journal of Eating Disorders (in press)

Hodes M, Eisler I, Dare C: Family therapy for anorexia nervosa in adolescence: a review. Journal of the Royal Society of Medicine 84:359–362, 1991

Hogarty GE, Anderson CM, Reiss DJ, et al: Family psychoeducation, social skills training, and maintenance chemotherapy in the aftercare treatment of schizophrenia. I. one-year effects of a controlled study on relapse and expressed emotion. Arch Gen Psychiatry 43:633–642, 1986

Hogarty GE, Anderson CM, Reiss DJ: Family psychoeducation, social skills training, and medication in schizophrenia: the long and the short of it. Psychopharmacol Bull 23:12–13, 1987

Hooley JM, Orley J, Teasdale DJ: Levels of expressed emption and relapse in depressed patients. Br J Psychiatry 148:642–647, 1986

Hooper D, Dryden W: Why couple therapy? in Couple Therapy. Edited by Hooper D, Dryden W. Milton Keynes, England, Open University Press, 1991, pp 3–11

Horwitz L: A group-centered approach to group psychotherapy. Int J Group Psychother 27:423–439, 1977

Horwitz L: Indications for group psychotherapy with borderline and narcissistic patients. Bull Menninger Clin 51:288–295, 1987

Jacob T, Rickey T, Evit Kovic JF, et al: Communications styles of alcoholic and nonalcoholic families when drinking and not drinking. J Stud Alcohol 42:466–482, 1981

Jacobson NS: Towards enhancing the efficacy of marital therapy research. Journal of Family Psychology 4:373–393, 1991

Jacobson NS, Dobson K, Fruzzetti AE, et al: Marital therapy as a treatment for depression. J Consult Clin Psychol 59:547–557, 1991

Kanter J, Lamb HR, Loeper C: Expressed emotion in families: a critical review. Hosp Community Psychiatry 38:374–380, 1987

Kaufman E: Family systems and family therapy of substance abuse: an overview of two decades of research and clinical experience. Int J Addict 20:897–916, 1985

Kaul TJ, Bednar RL: Experiential group research: results, questions, and suggestions, in Handbook of Psychotherapy and Behavioral Change. Edited by Garfield SL, Bergin EA. New York, Brunner/Mazel, 1985, pp 671–714

Kavanagh DJ: Recent developments in expressed emotion and schizophrenia. Br J Psychiatry 160:601–620, 1992

Kennedy R: The treatment of child abuse in an in-patient setting. Bulletin of the Royal College of Psychiatrists 12:361–366, 1988

Köttgen C, Sonnichsen I, Mollenhauer K, et al: Group therapy with families of schizophrenic patients: results of the Hamburg Camberwell Family Interview Study III. International Journal of Family Psychiatry 5:83–94, 1984

Kuipers L, Bebbington P: Expressed emotion research in schizophrenia: theoretical and clinical implications. Psychol Med 18:893–909, 1988

Kuipers L, MacCarthy B, Hurry J, et al: Counselling the relatives of the long-term adult mentally ill. II. a low-cost supportive model. Br J Psychiatry 1154:775–782, 1989

Lam DH: Psychosocial family intervention in schizophrenia: a review of empirical studies. Psychol Med 21:423–441, 1991

Langsley DG, Machotka P, Flomenhaft K: Avoiding mental hospitalization: a follow-up study. Am J Psychiatry 127:1391–1394, 1971

Langsley DG, Barter JT, Yarvis RM: Deinstitutionalization: the Sacramento story. Compr Psychiatry 19:479–490, 1978

Lansky M: Organic brain disease in the family: illness, personality and family system. Family Systems Medicine 6:290–303, 1989

Lasegue EC: De l'anorexie hysterique. Archives Generales de Medicine 21:384–403, 1873. Reprinted in Evolution of Psychosomatic Concepts. Anorexia Nervosa: A Paradigm. Edited by Kaufman RM, Heiman M. New York, International Universities Press, 1964 (1873)

Lask B: Physical illness, the family and the setting, in Family Therapy: Complementary Frameworks of Theory and Practice. Edited by Bentovim A, Gorell Barnes G, Cooklin A. London, Academic Press, 1987, pp 319–344

Lask B, Matthews D: Childhood asthmas: a controlled trial of family psychotherapy. Archives of Disease in Childhood 55:116–119, 1979

Leff J, Kuipers L, Berkowitz R, et al: A controlled trial of intervention in the families of schizophrenic patients. Br J Psychiatry 114:121–134, 1982

Leff J, Kuipers L, Berkowitz R, et al: A controlled trial of social intervention in the families of schizophrenic patients: two year follow-up. Br J Psychiatry 146:594–600, 1985

Leff J, Berkowitz R, Shavit N, et al: A trial of family therapy versus a relatives group for schizophrenia. Br J Psychiatry 154:58–66, 1989

Leff J, Berkowitz R, Shavit N, et al: A trial of family therapy versus a relatives group for schizophrenia. Two-year follow-up. Br J Psychiatry 157:571–577, 1990

Le Grange D, Eisler I, Dare C, et al: Family criticism and self-starvation: a study of expressed emotion. Journal of Family Therapy 14:177–192, 1992a

Le Grange D, Eisler I, Dare C, et al: Evaluation of family treatments in adolescent anorexia nervosa: a pilot study. International Journal of Eating Disorders 12:347–357, 1992b

Lieberman MA: A group therapist perspective on self-help groups. Int J Group Psychother 40:251–277, 1990

Lieberman MA, Borman LA: Self-Help Groups for Coping With Crises: Origins, Members, Processes and Impact. San Francisco, CA, Jossey Bass, 1979

Lin T: Mental health in the third world. J Nerv Ment Dis 171:71–78, 1983

MacCarthy B, Kuipers L, Hurry J, et al: Counselling the relatives of the long-term adult mentally ill: I. evaluation of the impact on relatives and patients. Br J Psychiatry 154:768–775, 1989

MacMillan JF, Gold A, Crow TJ, et al: The Northwick Park study of first episodes of schizophrenia. IV. expressed emotion and relapse. Br J Psychiatry 148:133–143, 1986

Main TF: The hospital as a therapeutic institution. Bull Menninger Clin 10:66–70, 1946

Markus E, Lange A, Pettigrew J: Effectiveness of family therapy: a meta-analysis. Journal of Family Therapy 12:205–221, 1990

Minuchin S: Families and Family Therapy. London, Tavistock, 1974

Minuchin S, Fishman CH: Family Therapy Techniques. London, Tavistock, 1981

Minuchin S, Montalvo B, Guerney BG, et al: Families of the slums. New York, Basic Books, 1967

Minuchin S, Rosman BL, Baker BL: Psychosomatic Families: Anorexia Nervosa in Context. Cambridge, MA, Harvard University Press, 1978

Murberg MM, Price LH, Jalali B: Huntington's disease: therapy strategies. Family Systems Medicine 6:290–303, 1988

Neighbour R: Family therapy by family doctors. Journal of Royal College of General Practitioners 32:737–742, 1982

Nicol AR, Smith J, Kay B, et al: A focused casework approach to the treatment of child abuse: a controlled comparison. J of Child Psychol Psychiatry 29:703–711, 1988

O'Sheay MD, Phelps R: Multiple family therapy: current status and critical appraisal. Fam Process 24:555–582, 1985

Patterson G: Coercive Family Process. Eugene, OR, Castilia, 1982

Patterson G, Dishion TJ: Multilevel family process models: traits, interactions, and relationships, in Relationships Within Families. Mutual Influences. Edited by Hinde RA, Stevenson-Hinde J. Oxford, England, Clarendon Press, 1988

Patterson JM: Illness beliefs as a factor in the patient-spouse adaptation to treatment for coronary artery disease. Family Systems Medicine 7:428–442, 1989

Prabhu LR, Desai NG, Raghuram A, et al: Outcome of family therapy: two year follow-up. Int J Soc Psychiatry 34:112–117, 1988

Rapoport TN, Rapoport R, Rosow I: Community as Doctor: New Perspectives on a Therapeutic Community. London, Tavistock, 1960

Robins LN: Conduct Disorder. J Child Psychol Psychiatry 32:193–212, 1991

Rose-Itkoff C: Lupus: an interactional model. Family Systems Medicine 5:313–321, 1987

Rosenthal MS: The therapeutic community: exploring the boundaries. British Journal of Addiction 84:141–150, 1989

Roy R: Annotation: chronic pain and the family: a review. Journal of Family Therapy 11:197–204, 1989

Russell GF, Szmukler G, Dare C, et al: An evaluation of family therapy in anorexia nervosa and bulimia nervosa. Arch Gen Psychiatry 144:1047–1056, 1987

Rutter M, Brown GW: The reliability and validity of measures of family life and relationships in families containing a psychiatric patient. Soc Psychiatry 1(1):38–53, 1966

Selvini-Palazzoli M, Boscolo L, Cecehin G, et al: Paradox and Counterparadox: A New Model in the Therapy of the Family in Schizophrenic Transactions. New York, Jason Aronson, 1978

Shaffer J, Galinsky MD: Models of Group Therapy, 2nd Edition. Englewood Cliffs, NJ, Prentice-Hall, 1989

Simons S: Couple therapy with lesbians, in Couple Therapy. Edited by Hooper D, Dryden W. Milton Keynes, England, Open University Press, 1991, pp 207–216

Snyder DK, Wills RM: Behavioral versus insight-oriented marital therapy. J Consult Clin Psychol 59:138–141, 1989

Snyder DK, Wills RM, Grady-Fletcher A: Long-term effectiveness of behavioral versus insight-oriented marital therapy. J Consult Clin Psychol 59:138–141, 1991

Spencer JH, Glick I, Haas G, et al: A randomized clinical trial of inpatient family interventions. III: effects at 6-month and 18-month follow-ups. Am J Psychiatry 145:1115–1121, 1988

Spiegel D, Bloom JR, Yalom ID: Group support for patients with metastatic cancer. Arch Gen Psychiatry 38:527–533, 1981

Stanton MD: Marital therapy from a structural/strategic viewpoint, in Handbook of Marriage and Marital Therapy. Edited by Sholevar GP. Jamaica, NY, SP Medical and Scientific Books, 1981

Stanton MD, Todd JC: The Family Therapy of Drug Addiction. New York, Guilford, 1982

Stratton P: Spirals and circles: potential contributions of developmental psychology to family therapy. Journal of Family Therapy 10:207–231, 1988

Strober M, Humphrey LL: Familial contributions to the etiology and course of anorexia nervosa and bulimia. J Consult Clin Psychol 55(5):654–659, 1987

Szmukler GI, Eisler I, Russell GFM, et al: Anorexia nervosa, parental "expressed emotion" and dropping out of treatment. Br J Psychiatry 147:265–271, 1985

Tal D, Gil-Spielberg R, Antonovsky H, et al: Teaching families to cope with childhood asthma. Family Systems Medicine 8:135–144, 1990

Tarrier N: Some aspects of family interventions in schizophrenia. I. adherence to intervention programs. Br J Psychiatry 159:475–480, 1991

Tarrier N, Barrowclough C, Vaughn C, et al: The community management of schizophrenia: a controlled trial of a behavioral intervention with families to reduce relapse. Br J Psychiatry 153:532–542, 1988

Tarrier N, Barrowclough C, Vaughn C, et al: Community management of schizophrenia: a two-year follow-up of a behavioral intervention with families. Br J Psychiatry 154:625–628, 1989

Tolan PH, Cromwell RE, Brasswell M: Family therapy with delinquents: a critical review of the literature. Fam Process 25:619–649, 1986

Trauer, T: The current status of the therapeutic community. British Journal of Medical Psychology 57:71–79, 1984

Vaughn C, Leff J: The influence of family and social factors on the course of psychiatric illness. Br J Psychiatry 129:125–137, 1976

Vaughn C, Snyder KS, Jones S, et al: Family factors in schizophrenic relapse: replication in California of British research on expressed emotion. Arch Gen Psychiatry 41:1169–1177, 1984

Walker GE: Pediatric AIDS: towards an ecosystemic treatment model. Family Systems Medicine 9:221–227, 1991

Watson JP, Bouras N: Psychiatric ward environments and their effects on patients, in Recent Advances in Clinical Psychiatry—6. Edited by Granville-Grossman K. Edinburgh, Scotland, Churchill Livingstons, 1988, pp 135–160

Webster-Stratton C: Strategies for helping families with conduct disordered children. J Child Psychol Psychiatry 32:1047–1062, 1991

Wells KC, Egan J: Social learning and family systems therapy for childhood oppositional disorder: a comparative treatment outcome. Compr Psychiatry 29:138–146, 1988

Yalom ID: The Theory and Practice of Group Psychotherapy, 3rd Edition. New York, Basic Books, 1985

CHAPTER 10

Procedures Used in Rehabilitation

Lorenzo Burti, M.D.
Vasily S. Yastrebov, M.D.

Introduction

According to World Health Organization (WHO) estimates, psychiatric disability accounts for up to two-fifths of all disability worldwide, affects younger people especially, and shows the lowest percentage of recovery to full working and social capacity (Jablensky et al. 1980). Therefore, it is not surprising that chronic mental illness and its related disability and their management, treatment, and rehabilitation attracts the growing attention of clinicians, researchers, public health officers, and nongovernmental organizations (Amiel and Dubuis 1989). However, while a great deal of clinical experience and scientific data has been accumulated about psychiatric rehabilitation, its definition, scope, and processes remain insufficiently established. Watts and Bennett (1983) stated that "much of what passes as psychiatric rehabilitation betrays little understanding of the processes involved. . . . What is generally lacking is a broad conception of its aims and objectives" (p. 1).

A Selective Review of Psychiatric Rehabilitation

History

The basic tenets of psychiatric rehabilitation may be traced back to the liberation of insane people from the chains and the moral treatment of the nineteenth century. However, modern psychiatric rehabilitation started in close association with physical rehabilitation after World War I, and especially after World War II, when society had to reconcile the problem of a large number of disabled veterans with a public commitment to full employment (Neff 1971). This explains the common features in the underlying principles of the two forms of rehabilitation, and explains the initial emphasis on vocational functioning. However, over time, psychiatric rehabilitation has become concerned with the client's functioning in all areas of his or her life (Watts and Bennett 1983).

Psychiatric rehabilitation was greatly propelled by the deinstitutionalization movement and concurrent needs for resettlement (Bachrach 1983). This promoted the search for new techniques to improve the social performance of mental patients and broadened the aims of rehabilitation, stressing the importance of residential adjustment and the mutual accommodation of both handicapped and nonhandicapped people within and outside of the family (Bennett 1983). Today psychiatric rehabilitation is acquiring an ever increasing scope and is actually becoming more of an approach to psychiatric care than a set of specific techniques (Watts and Bennett 1983).

Current Definitions and Goals

In the English language *to rehabilitate* means 1) to restore to a former right, rank, or privilege lost or forfeited, and 2) to restore to a condition of health by a process of medical rehabilitation, or to a useful and constructive place in society through social rehabilitation (Gove et al. 1976). Both meanings are equally relevant in psychiatric rehabilitation; in fact, long-term psychiatric patients suffer because of enduring disabilities (i.e., they lack the skills to cope successfully in society) and handicaps (the relative disadvantage of the individual compared with others) caused by stigma and discrimination. Handicap does not necessarily derive from disability; it may start from prejudice and be raised by the social mechanisms of persistent exaggeration of differences (Allport 1954). Therefore, the mission of rehabilitation is to remedy disabilities through skill development in the individual, compensate for disabilities by providing a supportive environment (Frey 1984; Wood 1980), and fight stigma and discrimination by, *inter alia*, seeking the support of official health bodies, governmental and otherwise, for the recognition that public stigma is both a hazard to normal health and a source of additional economic cost in chronic health care needs and reduced productivity.

Conceptual Base

A conceptual base for rehabilitation implies a theory of disability. In fact, Jablensky et al. (1980) stressed "the inherent weakness of clinical psychiatry to distinguish between symptoms of disease and psychosocial consequences of disease." Follow-up studies have shown that symptoms and disability follow different future courses, while clinical diagnosis has poor predictive value for their course. Yet traditional psychiatric diagnosis is still used in rehabilitation, and training in behavioral skills is considered most effective when the learning process is infused by knowledge of psychopathology (American Psychiatric Association 1989c), thus denoting a state of uncertainty, disagreement, or ambiguity, even among the experts.

World Health Organization Classification

The *International Classification of Impairments, Disabilities, and Handicaps* (World Health Organization 1980) included a set of operational definitions that represented an important step toward a more solid theoretical base for rehabilitation.

Rehabilitation Versus Treatment

The WHO classification also helped to differentiate between treatment and rehabilitation. Clinical treatment focuses on reducing the symptoms of pathology; rehabilitation focuses on the disability and societal handicap (Farkas and Anthony 1987; Gittelman and Blumberg 1975). Rather than focusing on deficits, rehabilitation addresses and emphasizes positive capabilities of the individual and tries to build upon that person's individual, functional, and social resources to allow the development that was halted by the illness and to transfer improvement to new areas. However, by helping with the basic process of reintegration, rehabilitation may play a major part in the healing, and perhaps even recovery, of the person (Strauss 1986).

An interactional perspective is also fundamental in rehabilitation. As stated by Watts and Bennett (1983), "How a person functions will invariably be the result of the interaction between the capacities and dispositions he possesses as an individual and the environment in which he lives and operates" (p. 3).

Current Models of Psychiatric Rehabilitation

In 1968, WHO proposed dividing rehabilitation into medical, social, and occupational components. Kabanov (1985) distinguished rehabilitative therapy from readaptation and rehabilitation proper. Specific classifications apart, at least three general models of rehabilitation may be identified in the literature and in current clinical practice:

1. Rehabilitation is meant as an addition to treatment, with conservative goals. Maintenance and prevention of further secondary disability, rather than *restitutio in integrum* of the patient, are considered the goals of intervention. Occupational therapy and entertainment are relevant components of this model.
2. Rehabilitation is intended as a highly specialized treatment with relatively ambitious goals. The target population is described in terms of the need to develop specific skills, while goals and interventions are carefully planned. This approach is represented, for example, by social skills training and psychosocial rehabilitation.
3. Rehabilitation is meant as long-term aftercare. Integration of services and interventions is emphasized; patients' needs are highly considered, and support (as much and as long as needed) is recommended. According to this approach, there is no "once and forever" cure for chronicity; changes may ensue in the long run. Thus rehabilitation consists of longitudinal, comprehensive community care.

However, it should be noted that many in the field of psychosocial rehabilitation would see themselves in a category that combines the two latter approaches, working with persons with "ambitious" goals and "support" goals, depending of course on the person's needs.

Characteristics of Patients

The target population of psychiatric rehabilitation is represented by those who have become disabled as a consequence of a psychiatric illness. Operational definitions share a diagnosis of mental illness of prolonged duration, with a resulting functional or role incapacity (Farkas and Anthony 1987). It is estimated that 1.7–2.4 million persons in the United States are severely psychiatrically disabled (Goldman et al. 1981).

Data regarding competitive employment rates are reasonably consistent: 20%–25% of all persons discharged from a psychiatric hospital are in full-time competitive employment, independent of the length of follow-up (Anthony et al. 1972, 1978). If only severely psychiatrically disabled persons are studied, the rate falls to 15% or below (Farkas and Anthony 1987); in recent studies a 0% employment rate has been reported for long-term patients targeted for deinstitutionalization (Farkas et al. 1987). Recidivism rates also prove quite similar in different reviews and over time: 30%–40% at 6 months, 35%–50% at 1 year, and 67%–75% at 5 years (Farkas et al. 1987).

Assessment

A number of instruments are available for assessing disabilities; some provide a global assessment while others provide specific information on individual behavior or skills. Data are collected through questionnaires, semistructured interviews, and direct observation; the informant may be the patient, significant others (usually a relative), or staff members. Clinical needs and research pose different demands as to the instruments to be used; research is especially demanding in terms of standardization and reliability, while clinical work needs instruments specifically related to treatment procedures whose effects have to be measured over time. Evaluation in this sense is no different from treatment (Shepherd 1983). Unfortunately, this distinction is far from being currently acknowledged and applied, and many rehabilitators trouble themselves with forms and ratings that will eventually prove of little clinical value. For example, the instruments listed below (described in Wallace 1986; Weissman 1975; Weissman et al. 1981) are excellent for research purposes, but their clinical use should be considered conservatively:

- Disability Assessment Schedule (DAS; World Health Organization 1988)
- Katz Adjustment Scale (KAS)
- Personal Adjustment and Role Skills Scale (PARS)
- Psychiatric Status Schedule (PSS)
- Social Adjustment Scale (SAS)
- Social Behavior and Adjustment Scale (SBAS)

Predictors

Predictors of recidivism and employment have been reviewed by Anthony et al. (1978). The best predictor of rehospitalization is previous hospitalization (Lorei and Gurel 1973; McGlashan 1986; Miller and Willer 1976; Rosenblatt and Mayer 1974; Strauss and Carpenter 1977) and the best predictor of employment is employment history (Lorei and Gurel 1973; Strauss and Carpenter 1977; Watts and Bennett 1977). Psychiatric diagnosis is not related to recidivism (Buell and Anthony 1973; Lorei and Gurel 1973; Rosenblatt and Mayer 1974).

In the study of Ciompi et al. (1979), the following factors predicting unfavorable outcome were found: having spent 5 years or more in hospital, having poor social contacts, being older than 65 years, having an IQ of less than 90, having stayed in a locked ward, being female, or having attended work therapy (a finding also reported by Bennett 1970; Hamilton 1964; Simons 1965). In summary, risk factors were social and situational instead of diagnostic and psychopathological. Thus results in rehabilitation seem to depend little on the illness; on the contrary, sociodemographic variables and social factors (e.g., personal relationships at work; expectations of family, staff, and patients; or duration of time off work) seem to be more important.

In an extensive review of the research literature on the vocational capacity of the psychiatrically disabled, Anthony and Jansen (1984) listed the following conclusions. Psychiatric symptomatology and diagnosis are poor predictors of future work performance (Green et al. 1968; Gurel and Lorei 1972). While the schizophrenic/nonschizophrenic dichotomy accounts for only 2% of variance (Buell and Anthony 1973), some studies found more neurotic people than psychotic people employed (Watts and Bennett 1977). A person's ability to function in one environment is not predictive of a that person's ability to function in a different one, and work activity in the hospital has no correlation with subsequent community employment. Recidivism and posthospital employment have only a slight relationship or no relationship at all. The best clinical predictor of future work performance is work adjustment (getting along with co-workers and supervisors and being dependable).

Measures of Outcome

The measures used to determine outcome of early studies were recidivism, relapse, and employment, which are all measures of handicap. Today these simple outcome measures are usually complemented by more refined and qualitative measures of individual functioning, employment, and social life (e.g., community adjustment, independent living, social skills, type of employment, salary, satisfaction, productivity, work skills) (Dion and Anthony 1987). Change in a measure of outcome does not imply that other apparently related measures have changed accordingly, and a positive effect on one measure may have an associated negative effect on another (Anthony and Farkas 1982). Interestingly, the refinement of measurement strategies has revealed more positive effects of rehabilitation (see below).

Staffing and Training

A client's rehabilitation is not a function of either the professional's credentials or the cost of intervention. The most significant factor is not the role of personnel, but rather their ability to perform the functions that are helpful in rehabilitation: skills teaching, resource coordination, personal support, and, above all, establishing a therapeutic alliance (Anthony et al. 1990). Research has shown that nonprofessionals can be as effective or even more effective than professionals in promoting change in their clients (Anthony and Carkhuff 1978; Carkhuff 1968). These findings are of special importance for those countries where mental health professionals are lacking, while needs for health promotion strategies in community-based rehabilitation programs are tremendous, as in the developing countries (Gittelman et al. 1990). The WHO Collaborative Study showed that primary health care workers can effectively deliver mental health care to patients with severe mental illness (e.g., schizophrenia) (Sartorius 1987). Most practitioners, even in developed countries, do not receive formal training in rehabilitation as students; instead they have developed skills while actually working with mentally disabled clients. In recent years, curricula based on sound empirical and experiential data have been designed, successfully implemented, and evaluated (Anthony et al. 1988; Anthony and Liberman 1986). Books, multimedia packages, and courses are available to train both practitioners and trainers.

Relative Success of Rehabilitation in Various Conditions

Schizophrenia

There is growing evidence that acute onset and exacerbations are precipitated by stress-inducing factors. A factor extensively studied is the presence of a particularly critical, dominating, and intrusive family environment, measured by expressed emotion (EE) (Brown et al. 1972; Vaughn and Leff 1976). Using medications, reducing the amount of face-to-face contact between patient and family, and counseling relatives have proven effective in reducing the relapse rate in schizophrenic patients living in stressful environments. Putting too much pressure on the patient or ignoring his or her need for support are also considered responsible for exacerbations (Wing 1983).

The *clinical poverty syndrome,* once thought of as primary and permanent, has now been shown to be associated with the social poverty of the (institutional) environment and the resulting understimulation (Wing and Brown 1970). Unfortunately, improvements do not seem to originate from a learning effect but from social stimulation from a trusted person. Thus these improvements do not become generalized nor do they tend to persist when stimulation is withdrawn (O'Connor et al. 1956).

The effective components of rehabilitation of schizophrenia include assessment, planning, integration of services and interventions in order to provide continuity of care, prevention or correction of social disadvantage (poverty, unemployment, or homelessness or inadequate housing), restitution of morale and self-confidence, avoiding or reducing over-stimulation and understimulation (Creer 1978; Wing 1983), and counseling both patients and relatives. Patients may be involved in taking their medications, recognizing early signs of relapse, and reducing stress. Relatives should create an accepting and noncritical environment, keep expectations realistic, accept and cope with cognitive and emotional impairments, know effects and limits of medications, and learn to use medical and social services and voluntary and consumer organizations (Wing 1983).

Nonpsychotic Conditions

Problems of social adjustment of nonpsychotic patients are not so severe and prolonged as in the case of schizophrenic patients, nor do they require specific rehabilitation interventions because they usually improve spontaneously when symptoms recede. But this is not always the case. There is also growing evidence of interrelationships between primary psychiatric problems and difficulties in social adjustment (Watts and Bennett 1983).

Depression

Depressive patients continue to have poor self-esteem, low confidence, and helplessness after recovery from a depressive episode (Altman and Wittenborn 1980); may have long-lasting difficulties in establishing intimate relationships; tend to be more abnormal in their response to failure than to success; and may lack the skills necessary to establish new social contacts and sources of satisfaction (Costello 1972). Some typical symptoms of depression seem secondary to basic cognitive impairments: memory deficits and deficits in concentration and registration (Henry et al. 1973; Mueller 1976) and retardation and cognitive interference (Payne and Hewlett 1960). Therefore, distracting patients from their internal preoccupations (Foulds 1952) or training them to stop self-talk (Meichenbaum 1977) actually improves performance. Restoring a sense of mastery, a core concept of rehabilitation theory, is essential in a behavioral approach to the treatment of depression (Beck et al. 1979). The importance of the environment is also established: single people are more prone to depression (Pearlin and Johnson 1977) and must rely more on the social network (Watts and Bennett 1983). Studies on families with high EE show that depressed patients are very vulnerable to the effects of relatives' criticism (Vaughn and Leff 1976).

Phobic and Obsessive-Compulsive Disorders

Primitive cognitive impairments are also hypothesized with obsessive patients, like slow performance (Rachman 1974) and difficulty in dividing attention (Spelke et al. 1976). Behavioral rehabilitation techniques should be supplemented especially in areas of sexual, family, and other relationships (Watts and Bennett 1983).

Disorders of Personality and Behavior

In the case of disorders of personality and behavior, insufficient social adjustment is the presenting problem. The rehabilitation of these patients has to deal with modifying attitudes, developing personal motivation, increasing self-esteem, and providing support and understanding rather than with teaching skills (Watts and Bennett 1983).

Alcohol and Drug Addiction

Outcome criteria have changed in the case of alcoholic patients in the recent past from abstinence alone to a number of social aspects, including social effectiveness, accommodation stability, and employment (Costello 1980; Heather and Robertson 1981). Experimental programs that teach controlled drinking to alcoholics who refuse abstinence have been described (Sobell and Sobell 1976). However, studies of the effectiveness of this method are still inadequate and abstinence from alcohol should be regarded as a major treatment goal (American Psychiatric Association 1989b). A 50% success rate at 1-year follow-up is expected with programs offering an adequate array of treatment modalities (Costello et al. 1977).

Outcomes in different services were reviewed by Thorley (1983), who noted the following: detoxification services show little influence on later drinking behavior; hospital services are of little value to the patient and are probably not cost-effective; virtually all treatment modalities are possible in an outpatient or day care setting; research on residential communities is still poor—there is modest evidence of effectiveness, apparently for nonspecific factors; an integrated rehabilitative system is required for the *skid row* alcoholics; Alcoholics Anonymous is estimated to have a 34% success rate; company alcohol policies have high success rates and are extremely cost-effective; and a community alcohol team is becoming an important element in any network of services. However, differences in improvement rates seem to depend more on the kind of patient than the kind of treatment; in addition, different settings actually follow distinct populations. This makes generalizations questionable and explains why success rates go up with the number of treatment options offered (Baekeland et al. 1975).In a study by McLellan et al. (1983) on 460 male alcoholic and 282 drug addicted patients, the rating of overall psychiatric severity was the best general predictor at follow-up; it showed differential effectiveness from different treatments and from matching patient and treatment. Family characteristics are also related to treatment outcome (Moos et al. 1979; Pattison 1965).

In the case of patients who are addicted to drugs (opiates), Thorley (1981a) reported outcome rates of "primitive treatment strategies and virtually no coordination" (a condition of quasi-spontaneous remission rate [Waldorf and Biernacki 1979]) as follows: 10% drug free at 1 year; 25% after 5 years; 40% after 10 years; each year 2%–3% of a sample die of a drug-related cause. The patterns of "careers of recovery" are characterized by social stability (i.e., significant personal relationships, accommodation, and employment) before abstinence is achieved. Treatment is better than no treatment. In a review of British longitudinal studies, Thorley (1981b) found a significant improvement compared to spontaneous remission. As to differential effectiveness, although detoxification services have only limited influence on long-term outcome, therapeutic communities with an active reentry program and drug clinics that use both inpatient and outpatient settings and teamwork prove to be the most effective.

Mental Retardation

For mentally retarded patients, individual and group psychotherapy are used, both in their traditional forms (Cotzin 1948; K.R. Davis and Shapiro 1979; Ringelheim and Polotsek 1955; Sternlicht 1966) and using behavioral methods (R. R. Davis and Rogers 1985; Matson and Senatore 1981). In general the therapist should be concrete, active, flexible, supportive, and reassuring; he or she should engage patients in activities because of difficulties with verbal communication (American Psychiatric Association 1989a; Cytryn and Lourie 1975). Parental counseling is essential and marital and family therapy may be helpful in some cases. There are examples in various countries of family organizations that are also instrumental in developing services.

Education of mentally retarded individuals has a long tradition; there has been much debate over the issue of placement either in segregated or regular classes. In recent years the latter orientation has prevailed, although its effectiveness is still controversial (Dunn 1968; Gottlieb 1981). Vocational rehabilitation, neglected in the past, is recently gaining more recognition, especially when academic achievements are disappointing. There has also been a shift in vocational goals from sheltered to competitive employment. Within an ecological perspective (Karan and Shalock 1983), two complementary approaches have emerged: one focuses on developing individual social competency and skills (Chadsey-Rusch 1986) and the other focuses on identifying socially accessible environments that compensate for individual deficits and make competitive employment possible (Karan and Berger 1986).

Rehabilitation in Various Ages

Childhood and adolescence. Illness in childhood and adolescence always affects personality development and maturation. Thus rehabilitation must aim at restoring the natural process of mental and social development of the maturing organism and should also include pedagogical interventions: regular school lessons supplemented with lessons in rhythmics, speech therapy, psychomotor rehabilitation, and so on. Parents should be closely involved in the rehabilitative plan.

Advanced years. The majority of elderly people have chronic, at times multiple, somatic illnesses. A combination of somatic illness, involutive processes, and a sense of helplessness and dependence on others predisposes an individual to the development of chronic mental conditions. Hospitalization is undesirable with this population because of the risk of precipitating reactive confusional states. Home care and day care should be easily available; effective case management and service coordination are mandatory.

Rehabilitation Approaches: Living Goals

Ward-Based Rehabilitation

Psychiatric hospital wards are often the site of rehabilitation, either to prepare patients for community placement or to prevent further deterioration. Because of their large size, psychiatric hospitals usually have many resources that can be profitably reused for rehabilitation. However, patients in the wards tend to have serious disabilities, staff are relatively untrained, and institutional constraints work against rehabilitation efforts (Watts and Bennett 1983).

The degree of structural change the ward can afford determines the number and quality of different skills in which patients can be trained. A hostel-like organization, even on the hospital grounds, is more effective in teaching social skills by fostering independence, responsibility, and self-esteem in patients. The structure of the ward may be thoroughly modified to better serve the purposes of rehabilitation. Two specific models have become widely known and extensively studied: the *milieu therapy* model and the *token economy* model.

Milieu Therapy Model

Milieu therapy aims at creating a therapeutic setting per se. It draws on the findings of social psychology studies regarding the impact of the environment on individual behavior and the related concept of environmental press (Murray 1938). Maxwell Jones's (1953) therapeutic community served as a model and became the flag of an alternative treatment approach in psychiatry. The key concepts in this model are the diffusion of authority; an emphasis on sharing, discussing, and understanding individual difficulties together; and stress on group interaction (Van Putten and May 1976). The milieu-therapy inpatient program described by Paul and Lentz (1977) in their classical comparative study was based on living groups of 9–10 patients sharing daily tasks and group discussions. The major vehicle for promoting change was the social and group pressure of the group on its members. The program was based on three laws: expectancy (staff's use of positive feedback), involvement (responsibility in making decisions, solving problem, "trying again"), and group cohesion (Glynn and Mueser 1986).

Token Economy Model

The token economy model is a behavior modification approach named for the kind of reinforcers used in the program (i.e., plastic tokens received by patients after performing the desired behavior, to be used like currency in exchange for goods or privileges within a small-scale, closed economic system). Originally introduced by Ayllon and Azrin (1968), the model has been replicated in various settings. In a typical social-learning program (Paul and Lentz 1977), tokens could be earned by grooming appropriately, attending meetings and classes, engaging in appropriate informal conversation, and so on. A shift to internal, verbal, and social reinforcers of behavior was also actively sought. Other principles of learning theory were integrated into the program, like shaping (leading to desired behavior by progressive approximations), chaining (conditioning complex behaviors response after response), prompting, demonstrating, and modeling (showing the desired behavior).

The identification of rehabilitative components of the token economy has been the target of several studies (Baker et al. 1977; Liberman et al. 1977; Turner and Luber 1980; Woods et al. 1984). Findings from these studies supported the theory that human influences, rather than tokens, may well account for the results.

Comparative Effectiveness

Paul and Lentz (1977) compared the effectiveness of traditional hospital treatment with a milieu program and with a social-learning program. The subjects, chronic mental hospital inpatients who had spent an average of 17 years in psychiatric hospitals, were randomly assigned to the three forms of treatment: milieu therapy, social-learning program, and routine inpatient care commonly applied in state mental hospitals at that time.

The two psychosocial programs did better than traditional hospital treatment on all the following counts: release rate, days in the community, cost per patient, weeks in the program, use of medication, and ward behavior. The social-learning program was superior to the milieu one on all counts. Results were independent of individual characteristics, pretreatment level of functioning, and diagnosis. Specifically, social-learning almost eliminated all dangerous and aggressive acts, increased communicative and interpersonal skills by 1,200%, and improved those patients who had failed in the milieu treatment program; 25% of those severely disabled patients were not distinguishable from the "normal" population by the end of the program.

The effects of the two psychosocial programs in reducing the need for psychotropic medications were impressive: while 92% of patients took medications at outset, 3.5 years later 89% of those in the social-learning program and 82% in the milieu program were off medication; none in the control group was drug-free. Half the patients in each group, randomly selected, were given placebo during a 17-week double-blind trial. No difference was found between those on drugs and those on placebo, except that those on neuroleptics were slower to improve.

Institutional Psychotherapies

In France after World War II, several treatment methods derived from group psychotherapy were implemented in psychiatric hospitals with the intent of making the hospital "therapeutic." A number of then-current political (especially Marxist), sociological, and psychological (psychoanalytical) ideas contributed to the development of the movement of *institutional psychotherapy* (Daumezon and Koechlin in 1952; Vidon et al. 1989), which had a great success in France, Switzerland, Italy, and other countries for more than a decade, thus anticipating deinstitutionalization. The fathers of the movement (Daumezon, Koechlin, Oury, Sivadon, Tosquelles, etc.) were superintendents of psychiatric hospitals. Besides introducing psychodynamic psychotherapy as a major treatment modality, they strove to change and humanize the rigid organization of their hospitals by starting social and recreational group activities with patients, connecting the hospital with the neighborhood, and developing aftercare and community facilities. Their contribution to the understanding of institutional dynamics is also important, as is their contribution to the development of concepts like teamwork, continuity of care, contextualization, support, and other notions of rehabilitation (Vidon et al. 1989).

Community Rehabilitation

Deinstitutionalization

In a critical review of experimental studies of the outcomes for psychiatric patients, Braun et al. (1981) found that experimental alternatives to hospital care led to psychiatric outcomes not different from and occasionally superior to those of control inpatients, especially in trials regarding alternatives to admission and modifications of conventional hospitalization. Deinstitutionalization is likely to be unsuccessful in the absence of continuing care in the community (A. E. Davis et al. 1974; Test and Stein 1978).

Studies of brief versus long hospitalization (see Glick and Hargreaves 1979) have shown no clear advantage of long hospitalization for nonschizophrenic patients and for poor-prognosis schizophrenic patients who tend to stay in aftercare; only good-prognosis schizophrenic patients, who are likely to drop out of aftercare, may benefit from longer hospitalization.

In their evaluation of Italian deinstitutionalization, Mosher and Burti (1989) reported that the 1978 Italian law that mandated the gradual phasing down of mental hospitals, prohibited new admissions to mental hospitals, and the established general hospital psychiatric wards and community mental health centers for any specific catchment area was being widely, but not uniformly, implemented. However, other researchers (Debernardi 1980; Frisanco 1989; Misiti et al. 1981; Tansella and Williams 1987; Tansella et al. 1987; Williams et al. 1986) found that where both hospital and community services have been developed (which was in a vast part of the country), the reform was successful. The number of mental hospital inpatients has decreased from about 60,000 before the reform to less than 30,000. The closing of the front doors of the state mental hospitals prevented the institutionalization of new patients or the reinstitutionalization of those discharged. In addition, no increase in the number of admissions to private hospitals or in the number of short-term admissions to general hospital units was found. The overall inpatient care rate (including admissions) actually remained fairly stable after the reform. The literature on the Italian reform has been reviewed in detail by de Girolamo (1989).

Community Support Systems

The United States–based, National Institute of Mental Health–funded Community Support Program (CSP) is a well-known, comprehensive community system. In their review of studies on the CSP, Anthony and Blanch (1988) provided a general synopsis of present knowledge in all the relevant areas of a community mental health system: client identification and outreach, mental health treatment, health and dental services, crisis response services, housing, income support and entitlements, peer support, family and community support, rehabilitation services, protection and advocacy, case management, and system integration.

Client identification and outreach. This is a necessary prerequisite for the treatment of disabled patients, in fact, one-fourth to two-thirds of such patients do not follow through on referrals and 30%–40% quickly drop out of treatment. A more personal and informative referral procedure may substantially increase referral compliance (Anthony and Blanch 1988). Compliance also increases when clients perceive that services will meet their needs. Lipton et al. (1988) showed that homeless mental patients who were offered supportive housing at discharge accepted and successfully maintained their placement, spent significantly fewer nights in hospitals or undomiciled, and were more satisfied.

Health and dental services. Health and dental services seem to be an important component of community care of mental patients. Many psychiatric patients have a major medical illness that is generally unrecognized and can cause or exacerbate psychiatric symptoms (Anthony and Blanch 1988).

Crisis response services. A number of alternative services are known to be effective and to prevent hospitalization in cases of crises or exacerbations. A mobile crisis team reduces hospitalization by at least 50% (Hoult 1986; Hoult and Reynolds 1984; Hoult et al. 1984; Langsley and Kaplan 1968; Rueveni 1977; Schoenfeld et al. 1986; Stein and Test 1978; Test and Stein 1978). Residential alternatives to hospitalization cover a *surrogate parent model* and a *surrogate peer model*. The former model, developed in Denver, Colorado (Polak and Kirby 1976; Polak et al. 1979), is based on the combination of accommodating acute psychiatric patients in foster families and an intense use of mobile teams to supervise and support these families. The latter method is based on the model developed by Laing (1967) and Mosher and Menn (1978), in which patients live in a house where a familylike, supportive, therapeutic milieu is provided by specially trained nonprofessionals, with a minimum use of medications. Both models have proven to be at least as effective as standard hospital treatment, but are less expensive: a bed in a foster family costs $800–$900 per month; in the therapeutic community, it is less than $100 a day.

Housing. Decent, affordable housing is an essential support to effective rehabilitation, but it is rarely available because of the decreasing supply of cheap housing, the inadequacies of social services, and widespread discrimination against mental patients.

The concept of a *residential continuum* refers to a graded array of living environments (psychiatric hospital, nursing home, general hospital ward, crisis alternatives [crisis house, surrogate family, intensive on-site outreach], halfway house, group home, apartment program, and independent living). This model has been criticized for its naive belief that people with severe and persistent disabilities may benefit from transitional help of limited duration and for the fact that the continuum is practically never complete: long-term housing options, in particular, are generally unavailable in most communities. Thus the transitional accommodation tends to become permanent. Recent approaches (e.g., community residential rehabilitation developed by Bradley et al. 1986) have included the idea that transition should not imply a movement from one facility to another, which produces dislocation, but should occur in the person as he or she learns the necessary skills while living in a normal home (i.e., "normalization"; Wolfensberger 1970), with the support of the rehabilitation team.

Income support and entitlements. According to current estimates, 482,000 people with a psychiatric disability received welfare benefits in the United States in 1986, at a cost of $2.24 billion (Anthony and Blanch 1988); however, these recipients accounted for only 28% of those with severe, long-term mental disability. Budgetary constraints have produced cuts in welfare provisions. Reviews of cases, such as the Continuing Disability Investigation of 1981 in the United States (Anthony and Blanch 1988), have been severely criticized for their adverse effects on and discrimination against mentally impaired people. This was the consequence of the (wrong) assumption that limited or no symptoms indicate an ability to work, which is far from being true for mental patients

(Anthony and Jansen 1984). Unfortunately there seems to be no incentive to work; most clients who successfully obtain work in entry-level jobs do not earn enough to make it worth going off welfare (Mosher and Burti 1989).

Social security, sick-fund pensions, temporary subsidies, and financial aids to patients and families are available in several European countries (Gittelman and Black 1987), but their impact on the quality of life has not been reviewed.

Peer, family, and community support. People are dependent upon a social network to receive support for both their practical and their emotional needs and to cope against stress. There is evidence of a relationship between social ties and mortality rates in the general population, the absence of social support and increased psychological distress, and reduced social networks and schizophrenia (Anthony and Blanch 1988). The increased vulnerability to mental illness in the absence of a confiding intimate relationship has also been well established (Brown and Harris 1978). Disabled mental patients are no exception: they need continuing support as much as anybody else; unfortunately they are often estranged (at least emotionally, if not physically) from their natural support system and have to rely on the artificial support system provided by mental health services (Bennett and Morris 1983). There is plenty of evidence of the decisive influence on outcome of one support person (Cannady 1982), of a supportive environment (Stickney et al. 1980), and of a support team (Witheridge et al. 1982), especially if coupled with assertive outreach and advocacy (Stein and Test 1978).

Support may be provided by self-help and mutual-support groups. This approach has been followed in some rehabilitation programs, such as in the Fairweather Lodge programs (Fairweather et al. 1969), the clubhouse movement (see section on psychosocial rehabilitation centers, below), and, in general, in all programs characterized by group homes. The development of spontaneous self-help initiatives has been reported, even in the squalid environment of single-room occupancy hotels (Cohen and Sokolovsky 1979).

Protection and advocacy. Discrimination is known to be widespread, and either ignored or even fostered by the law. Historically, the state has placed restrictions on the liberty and privacy of mentally disabled citizens, with prohibitions on marriage, childbearing, voting, driving, holding public office, professional licensure, and so on. In addition, the state has failed to protect mental patients from discrimination by private parties in areas such as housing, employment, and public accommodations (Melton and Greenberg-Garrison 1987).

Advocacy directly addresses the handicap (in the sense of the WHO classification). The term *societal rehabilitation* (Anthony 1972) has also been introduced to describe interventions to remedy this handicap.

Current civil rights issues pertain to commitment, inappropriate and involuntary medication, use of electroconvulsive therapy, seclusion and restraint, as well as the denying of child custody to mentally ill women (Anthony and Blanch 1988). Advocacy then has to deal with both civil rights and the right to better services. In Italy, advocacy for the mentally ill became a major national concern in the 1970s and resulted in the 1978 mental health reform that virtually banned psychiatric hospitals (Mosher and Burti 1989). Unfortunately, studies on the effects of advocacy are still scant.

Case management. There are still few studies on the effects of case management on patients, and data from those are contradictory. Goering et al. (1988) found that case management; this result seemed due to the shortcomings of the services system, the lack of control the case manager had on the patient's medical care, and hospitalization being a poor measure of outcome. However, at the 2-year follow-up they found that patients in the case manager program had better occupational functioning and more independence and were less socially isolated than the control patients. Because these differences did not appear at the 6-month follow-up, the authors strongly suggested that a difficult population should not be studied over a short period. Average case management costs were estimated at $5,200 per year out of a total program cost of $15,000, a community mental health center cost of $47,000, and an inpatient cost of $82,000 (Anthony and Blanch 1988).

Mosher and Burti (1989) stressed that functions usually ascribed to case managers (i.e., case finding, assessment, services planning, linkage, coordination, monitoring, and advocacy) should be the responsibility of the mental health center team. A core team, rather than a "key worker"

(Watts and Bennett 1983), is most effective in ensuring coordination and continuity of interventions to individual patients.

Systems integration. Teamwork is considered essential in community mental health in general and in rehabilitation in particular. It suits the need for flexibility, a multidisciplinary focus, broad participation in the decision-making process, ongoing supervision, and training that such demanding, innovative community work entails (Burti and Mosher 1986).

Lack of coordination between services is often seen as the factor responsible for failures in community mental health programs. Decentralization of clinical and fiscal responsibility, so that the particular agency has control of its resources, has been reported to be effective, as well as capitation payment and outcome-based bonus systems. Coordination provided through a CSP has been shown to decrease hospital bed-days in an Oregon study (Anthony and Blanch 1988); assignment of responsibility for specific clients can reduce dropout rates and hospitalization while increasing employment and social activity (Mosher and Burti 1989).

Medication Issues

In spite of the almost universal use of neuroleptics with long-term, psychotic patients, their role in terms of outcome is still questionable and concern is growing about the high incidence of permanent side effects, like tardive dyskinesia (5% incidence per year; Kane et al. 1984). Approximately 70% of schizophrenic patients respond satisfactorily to medications in terms of reductions of symptoms and relapse; but 20%–40% of patients improve on placebo and about half of schizophrenic patients maintained on neuroleptics relapse within 2 years (J. M. Davis 1980). This relapse rate is not due to noncompliance; patients randomly assigned to injectable depot neuroleptics and to oral medication showed the same relapse rates (Hogarty et al. 1979; Rifkin et al. 1977). Unfortunately, it is impossible to predict who needs maintenance medication. Some researchers (Bleuler 1968; Huber et al. 1980; Mosher and Menn 1978) have suggested that the vast majority of newly diagnosed psychotics can recover without neuroleptics; moreover, researchers (Bleuler 1968; Ciompi 1980a, 1980b; Harding et al. 1987a, 1987b; Huber et al. 1980; Niskanen and Achte 1972) have found that the long-term prognosis for these patients has not been affected by neuroleptics.

Psychotherapy

Individual psychotherapy is at present rather discredited as a treatment for the severely mentally ill. A number of studies have provided contrasting results, but, in general, have shown limited effects for psychotherapy (Grinspoon et al. 1972; Gunderson et al. 1984; Karon and Vandenbos 1972; May 1968; Rogers et al. 1967). These results contributed to a widespread negative attitude about psychotherapy, in spite of warnings against premature conclusions because of serious design shortcomings (Mosher and Keith 1980). No major difference in the effects of insight-oriented and supportive psychotherapies in the treatment of schizophrenia was found (Gunderson et al. 1984); the latter is recommended, combined with the minimum essential amount of medication (Hogarty et al. 1974). However, a recent study (Glass et al. 1989) revealed the advantages of skillfully conducted psychodynamic exploration in terms of the 2-year outcome of the negative symptoms of schizophrenia. Group therapy alone offered few advantages, but increased the effect of another treatment approach when offered in combination (Mosher and Keith 1980).

Social Skills Training

Social skills training (SST) is a recently developed behavioral technique proposed to teach basic cognitive skills to regressed, disorganized, and distractible patients in preparation for further training of social skills. The rationale is that poor coping and competence skills have an important part in maintaining the disability of such patients, and that appropriate techniques may infuse the patients with certain abilities in spite of severe symptoms. Training addresses the area of social cognitive skills, like attentional skills, basic conversational skills, and, in some cases, social and independent living skills.

After an accurate assessment, using either naturalistic observation, self-reports (or reports made by significant others), or role-play performance, the therapist and patient together target the goals of training. Several procedures typical of the behavior modification approach are then used (role-play, coaching, shaping, modeling). Generalization (i.e., the transferring of new skills into the patients' natural environment) is sought through rehearsal, in vivo training, and home assignments. However, generalization is a major difficulty in SST, and SST should be embedded in a comprehensive program of rehabilitation that features continuity of care, supportive community services, therapeutic relationships, and judicious prescription of psychotropic drugs. Similar techniques are used for vocational rehabilitation.

Training in spare-time skills is also relevant, especially for patients with severe disabilities who are incapable of working; in fact, recreation is shown to remove psychopathology (Liberman et al. 1974; Paul and Lentz 1977; Wing and Brown 1970). However, simple access to recreation is not enough; prompting is necessary rather than reinforcement.

SST has proven effective with mentally retarded patients (Matson and Senatore 1981; Thompson and Grabowski 1972), with depressed patients (Bellack et al. 1981, 1983; Lewinsohn 1974), with psychiatric outpatients (Falloon et al. 1977), with psychiatric inpatients, in association with other psychosocial programs (Hersen 1979; Monti et al. 1980, 1979; Paul and Lentz 1977), and in association with family treatment (Falloon et al. 1982, 1985; Hogarty et al. 1986).

Family Interventions

Initial interest in the role of the family in the etiology of schizophrenia (Bateson et al.1956; Laing and Esterson 1967; Lidz et al. 1963; Singer and Wynne 1965; Wynne and Singer 1963) and in the outcome of nonbehavioral methods (Wells and Dezen 1978) has led to more rewarding (in terms of sound data) studies regarding the influence of behavioral family interventions on the course of the illness.

Review on outcome of family therapy. Short-term life events and long-term family pressures have been recognized as producing stress, which may precipitate a relapse. As a measure of family interaction, the EE score has been shown to be positively correlated to relapse. Brown et al. in 1972 found a 58% relapse rate in patients with high-EE families compared to a 16% relapse rate in patients with low-EE families. In a replication of this study, Vaughn and Leff (1976) found similar results and identified two protective factors: reduction of face-to-face contact and the use of neuroleptic medication. Further replications confirmed these latter findings (Leff and Vaughn 1981, 1985; Leff et al. 1983; Vaughn et al. 1984).

Strachan (1986) reviewed four experimental studies focusing on family interventions (Falloon et al. 1982, 1985; Goldstein et al. 1978; Hogarty et al. 1986; Leff et al. 1982, 1985) inspired by these concepts, all using medications plus various aggregates of education about mental illness (psychoeducation), skills training, and family management and treatment. In his conclusion, Strachan (1986) stressed the need to tailor treatment to the family; families with a patient at his or her first psychotic breakdown seem to benefit from a crisis-oriented approach, according to Goldstein and associates (1978), while they would be shocked by education on schizophrenia. For families with long-term patients, on the other hand, psychoeducation plus involving the family in a program of long-term aftercare seems appropriate; individual and family skills training is an effective supplement. Family treatment allows lower dosages of medications and *targeted medication* (patients are off drugs until prodromal signs of exacerbation are recognized [Carpenter and Heinrichs 1983; Carpenter et al. 1987; Herz 1984; Hirsch et al. 1987]).

Tarrier et al. (1988, 1989) assessed the effectiveness of psychoeducation and behavioral family intervention in comparison with routine treatment at 9-month and 2-year follow-up. Results were similar to those of studies mentioned before (an 8%–17% relapse rate in the experimental group versus 53% in the control group at 9 months, and a relapse rate of 33% and 59%, respectively, at 2 years), but the psychoeducation program proved ineffective at both follow-ups; at 2-year follow-up, the relapse rate was identical to that of the control group. According to the authors, these results should discourage the implementation of education programs as an alternative to long-term behavioral family management in the community treatment of schizophrenia.

Day Programs

Services offering rehabilitation include programs varying in size, schedule, goals, and techniques. All programs address clients' personal, relational, and instrumental disabilities and provides specific opportunities to overcome them and experience success within a supportive environment.

Day hospitals.   These are generally more medical in terms of staffing and orientation. They offer medication monitoring, consultation, group and family psychotherapy, and resocialization activities, as well as an alternative to inpatient care (Glasscote et al. 1969; Herz et al. 1971; Washburn et al. 1976; Wilder et al. 1966; Zwerling and Wilder 1964).

Psychosocial rehabilitation centers. Psychosocial rehabilitation centers follow the model of Fountain House, a clubhouse established in New York in the late 1940s, still very active and extensively imitated. The term *club* stresses the idea that members (clients) own the facility; the members feel they are wanted and needed in the program. The setting provides a prevocational day program (actually run by members and staff working together), a transitional employment program (see section on this subject, below), an evening and weekend social program, an apartment program, an outreach program, a thrift shop program, and an evaluation program (Beard et al. 1982). The overall program aims at providing a comprehensive approach in a context of self-help. Thresholds in Chicago and Horizon House in Philadelphia use a more structured and demanding model in terms of working behavior, but their overall philosophy is the same. The model of the Moadon Shalom of Jerusalem (Spivak 1977) relies on an optimal balance of theoretical postulates, program structure, and treatment dimensions. Rehabilitation services have proven effective in shortening inpatient stays and reducing relapse rates (as low as 10% a year versus an expected 40%–50%) of previously hospitalized patients (Anthony et al. 1972; Beard et al. 1982; Bond et al. 1985; Dincin and Witheridge 1982; Malamud 1985).

In two studies (see Beard et al. 1978), severely disabled mental patients, mostly schizophrenic, were randomly assigned to the Fountain House rehabilitation (experimental) program and to other community facilities (control). Fountain House members had significantly lower rates at 6-, 12-, and 24-month follow-up; rates remained lower up to 9 years, although differences were not significant. It emerged that rehospitalization was not prevented but delayed. Those experimental subjects who received outreach services had the lowest rehospitalization rates over the 9-year period, as well as spending two to three times longer in the community before rehospitalization and having 40% less time in hospital than the control subjects. Attendance was closely related to the incidence of rehospitalization: those with low or no attendance showed a rehospitalization rate equal to that of control subjects. But those who attended 100 or more times had rehospitalization rates of 37% at 5-year follow-up, the same rate as control subjects at the same interval. An evaluation of cost per patient, per day by Mosher and Burti (1989) showed psychosocial rehabilitation centers ($20–30) to be more cost-effective than day hospitals ($100–150).

Self-Help Groups

Family organizations. A number of family organizations have grown up in several countries (e.g., the National Alliance for the Mentally Ill [NAMI] in the United States, the National Schizophrenia Fellowship in the United Kingdom, Unione Tutela Salute Mentale in Italy), basically out of dissatisfaction with the outcome of psychiatric treatment and the lack of services. They provide reciprocal support, education, dissemination of knowledge, and fund-raising. Especially in the United States, they are becoming politically influential and advocate enhanced inpatient services and psychiatric research (usually biological). There are some reports in the literature on their effectiveness (Hatfield 1984, 1985), but no longitudinal or comparative studies are available.

User and former-user organizations. Organizations such as the National Alliance of Mental Patients [NAMP], the National Mental Health Consumer Association [NMHCA], the Manic-Depressive Association, Recovery, the Mental Patient Liberation Front, Mental Patients' Association [MPA], GROW started in the early 1970s and are spreading in the United States and, recently, in Europe. They provide support, education, advocacy and political action, and run walk-in centers. They have been described by Chamberlin (1978), Zinman (1986), and Zinman et al. (1987). GROW is currently being studied in depth; preliminary results indicate beneficial effects for people actively involved for 9 months or more, and point to the low cost of such programs, which are mostly staffed by volunteers (Anthony and Blanch 1988).

Rehabilitation Approaches: Work Goals

Work and Rehabilitation

Rehabilitation is connected to the working environment because we live in a strongly work-oriented society; the ability to perform remunerated employment is a *sine qua non* of full citizenship and has also been internalized as an indispensable requirement for becoming an autonomous and independent adult (Neff 1968).

An important point that needs to be immediately emphasized is that within the past 5 or 6 years, the field has begun to recognize that many of the problems in the area of work rehabilitation have come from the fact that practitioners have focused on the notion of a person with a psychiatric disability getting a job—any kind of job or activity that is like a job. And many who did get work lost that work fairly rapidly. What we have learned is that there is a distinction between getting a job and learning to select a career path for oneself, whether it be a manual labor career or a more intellectual pursuit. Many people had their psychotic breaks at the very time when, developmentally speaking, they would be in the process of developing a sense of themselves in relation to the world of work and understanding what career direction they would like to take. Career development interventions have therefore become one of the major trends in work rehabilitation.

Assessment

Vocational rehabilitation has striven to improve assessment techniques and to study the ways people adapt to work. Industrial or vocational tests have low predictive validities with disabled persons who may have no previous work experience and very low motivation (Neff 1966, 1970). Other evaluation techniques, like the Work Sample (Institute for the Crippled and Disabled 1967; Leshner and Snyderman 1965; Overs 1964a, 1964b, 1968) and the Situational Assessment (Gellman 1961; Gellman et al. 1957; Neff 1968), and related rating scales (Cheadle and Morgan 1972; Gellman et al. 1963; Soloff and Bolton 1969; Watts 1978) have proven valid and reliable.

Theory of Work Behavior

Work adjustment, including tenure, depends on both satisfaction (i.e., liking the job) and satisfactoriness (i.e., meeting work requirements) (Lofquist and Dawis 1969). Empirical findings have shown little or no relationship between ability-requirement scores and satisfactoriness (Betz et al.1966). Job tenure seems unrelated to either variable for most workers, and probably depends more on the characteristics of the job market (Warner 1985).

Neff (1971) uses the notion of *work personality*, a distinct part of the general personality that is built up during middle childhood and adolescence, especially in relation to school, but also in relation to parental influence and that of the mass media and teenage subculture. An implication of this theory is that maladaptation to work depends little on task competence; instead, it reflects some inability to cope with one or another of the complex, especially interactional demands (relating to peers, supervisors, and subordinates) of work as a social situation. In fact, enthusiasm, response to supervision, and social relationships make it possible to predict a return to work, while task competence does not (Watts 1983). A long history of unemployment or a total absence of previous employment and low expectation in the family—two conditions very common among mental patients—also tend to reduce motivation to work (Alfano 1973; Ciompi et al. 1979).

Given the serious psychosocial handicaps and low morale of mental patients, the rehabilitator cannot restrict himself or herself to those who are already motivated to work; he or she has to "motivate the unmotivated," becoming an active therapeutic agent who brings about psychological change in the maladapted individual (Neff 1971). Basically two techniques are classically used: therapeutic counseling (akin to conventional psychotherapy) and rehabilitative workshops (akin to milieu therapy). In more recent years there has been a substantial advance in behavioral techniques (social skills training), various forms of transitional employment, and combined techniques (see below).

Resettlement

Resettlement in employment depends on a number of factors independent of those already seen. Potential employers are less likely to offer a job if the person is a mental patient, mostly because of prejudices (Farina and Felner 1973; Hartlage 1965; Olshansky et al. 1958; Whatley 1964). However, a patient who has already worked in a certain job is likely to be reemployed (Cole et al. 1964; Olshansky et al. 1958). Mental patients seem to have difficulties in obtaining employment because of poor interview skills (Barbee and Kiel 1973; Searls et al. 1971), thus they may benefit from appropriate training (Kiel and Barbee 1973). Azrin et al. (1975) devised a *job-finding club* that provides skills training, supervision, and practical encouragement and support. A controlled study revealed that the program was effective (Azrin and Phillip 1979).

Job Tenure

The amount of work in the previous 2 years predicted return to work, but not job tenure. On the other hand, occupational stability in the past predicted job tenure, but not return to work (Watts and Bennett 1977). One of the difficulties with work resettlement is the gap between a rehabilitation workshop and open, free employment. That is why a scaled variety of intermediate job opportunities is advisable.

Work Therapy, Industrial Therapy, and Sheltered Workshops

The importance of work to prevent or reverse the adverse effects of institutionalization was conceptualized by Simon (1927, 1929), based on his experience at Gutersloh in Germany. The approach became very popular in mental hospitals in different countries. It has been criticized because of the frequent exploitation of patients and for providing work activities within the closed system of the asylum.

Industrial therapy introduced the innovation of subcontracted work. In Britain the first workshop was set up in 1956 (Carstairs et al. 1956); by 1967 workshops existed in 100 out of 122 hospitals examined in England (Wansbrough and Miles 1968). Eventually, industrial therapy became a classic setting for vocational rehabilitation, and has been extensively used in practically all industrialized countries ever since (Gittelman and Black 1987). Industrial workshops are common practice in Eastern Europe, especially in the former Soviet Union and Poland, where comprehensive multistage systems of work training and placement (cooperatives, workshops, ordinary industries) are also reported. There is a vast body of literature on the principles, practices, and environment of industrial therapy (Bennett and Wing 1963; Early 1968, 1973; Wadsworth et al. 1962). Industrial therapy has shown itself to provide protection against breakdown on discharge and facilitate resettlement in open employment (Wing et al. 1964), to improve self-care and enhance morale (Esser and Chamberlain 1965), to ameliorate poor intellectual performance (Hamilton 1964), and even to bring about changes in primary handicaps (Wing and Brown 1970). The problem with sheltered workshops is that, while providing a minimal level of remunerated and productive employment, they may easily become an institutionalized, maintenance program.

The Rehabilitative Workshop

The model of the rehabilitative workshop, which shares the principles of the therapeutic community, was initiated by the Jewish Vocational Service of Chicago (Gellman et al. 1957). Unlike the sheltered workshop, where maintenance is not discarded as a goal, at least for a number of regressed patients, the rehabilitative workshop is designed to be transitional. The patient's length of stay is fixed to prevent dependency, but length may be highly individualized according to the patient's needs (Neff 1971). It simulates real working conditions, though fairly permissive ones, at least initially. The key person is the work supervisor, who inconspicuously acts both as a supervisor and as an observer/therapist.

Work Cooperatives

Work cooperatives in Italy are self-run business organizations that list a number of former mental patients besides other handicapped and marginally functioning individuals among their members. Members' activities are usually cleaning, gardening, and running restaurants. The cooperatives have been relatively successful in providing job opportunities and group affiliation to patients discharged from mental hospitals. Initially they are offered work by the public authorities, but they may easily become competitive in the open market. Only descriptive data are available. In the United States, the Fairweather Lodge program (Fairweather et al. 1969) and its numerous replications have some similarities, but also offer housing opportunities in a group situation to members.

Transitional Employment Program

The transitional employment program (TEP), a model devised at Fountain House in New York, has gained increasing popularity and recognition for its effectiveness. It consists of regular job positions contracted between the rehabilitation agency and the employer. Usually two patients share a full-time job; if a patient does not show up, another patient, or even a staff member, will take over to ensure the work is completed. The patient will be supervised and supported by staff to increase his or her chances of success, but failure is not viewed as a devastating event.

In a major follow-up study performed at Fountain House (Farkas and Anthony 1987), employment outcome increased as a function of the time since initial participation in a TEP. For those who initially participated in a TEP at least 42 months earlier, 36% were competitively employed, while those who participated 12 and 24 months earlier had employment rates of 11% and 19%, respectively.

In a study at Thresholds rehabilitation center in Chicago, an accelerated form of TEP proved more effective than a regular one: 20% in the accelerated program versus 7% in the regularly paced one were employed at the 15-month follow-up (Bond and Dincin 1986). Moreover, TEPs seem to have a significant impact on employment as the follow-up period increases.

Job-Finding Club

The job-finding club approach, originally developed by Azrin and associates (Azrin and Besalel 1980; Azrin and Phillip 1979), essentially addresses patients' lack of interviewing skills, but actually combines a number of techniques. It addresses three phases: training in job-seeking skills (through a training workshop), the job search proper (the club provides information, facilities, and support), and follow-up and job maintenance (weekly sessions on strategies and problem solving related to co-workers, boss, symptoms, and so on). Liberman and colleagues (American Psychiatric Association 1989c; Liberman et al. 1986) found at 8-month follow-up that 66% of patients had successfully found a job; patients with positive symptoms had greater difficulty.

Supported Employment

Vocational programming, consistent with the philosophy and principles of rehabilitation in general, is moving toward the concept of ongoing job support. Supported employment is akin to TEP, though it differs in that it is not transitional and it includes non–entry-level jobs, possibly with career ladders. Support is guaranteed as needed; however, it may take place on the job site or elsewhere; lowering stress in the nonworking environment is also considered important (Anthony and Blanch 1988).

Summary on Outcome

Using outcome criteria of hospital recidivism and posthospital employment, Anthony et al. (1972, 1978) reviewed the effects of rehabilitation and concluded that traditional inpatient treatment (i.e., individual and group therapy, work therapy, and drug therapy) does not affect recidivism and employment. Even innovative techniques do not in themselves affect posthospital adjustment. Only comprehensive programs improve future community functioning.

Outpatient drug maintenance without periodic outpatient contacts does not affect recidivism or employment (Anthony et al. 1972; Engelhardt and Rosen 1976; Franklin et al. 1975). Studies on maintenance medication (J. M. Davis et al. 1976; Hogarty et al. 1974) showed that 20%–50% on placebo did not relapse, while even 20%–50% maintained on drugs did, thus throwing doubt on this established practice.

Aftercare clinics were found to reduce recidivism of the more chronic patients (Anthony and Buell 1973; Kirk 1976), if attendance is fostered. Transitional facilities are effective as long as patients remain members (Beard et al. 1978; Rog and Raush 1975). Rehabilitation programs that use different settings and joint planning, as well as providing social and vocational rehabilitation and community support, without arbitrary time limits, produce better outcomes (Anthony and Farkas 1982).

With the refinement of outcome measures regarding the gains of psychiatric rehabilitation, more positive findings have emerged. Dion and Anthony (1987) gave the example of a study that, although not showing the desired effect on recidivism, showed positive results in community tenure (Beard et al. 1978) and instrumental functioning (Wasylenki et al. 1985). Length of follow-up is also critical in outcome studies. A longer follow-up may reveal striking effects that were less visible or even nonexistent in a short-term evaluation. This is true of role functioning (Goering et al. 1988), employment (Bond and Dincin 1986), living arrangements and employment (Farkas et al. 1987), and symptomatology and overall functioning (Bleuler 1968; Ciompi 1980a, 1980b; Harding et al. 1987a, 1987b; Huber et al. 1980; Tsuang et al. 1979).

Transfer of skills is a critical component of rehabilitation interventions. Because behavior is contingent upon the environment, social skills do not transfer easily from the rehabilitation setting to the person's own environment and to the natural environment. Improvements may be just a temporary response to the rehabilitative setting. For instance, Walker and McCourt (1965) found no significant relationship between patients' occupational therapy in hospital and postdischarge employment. Ellsworth et al. (1968) found that the most obnoxious and combative patients in the hospital eventually had the best friendship skills at discharge. Thus a rehabilitation program must be designed to prepare people for the environment in which they will eventually function and specific steps must be taken to allow the transfer of skills (Watts and Bennett 1983).

In conclusion, reviews of outcome studies have suggested that psychiatric rehabilitation has a positive impact on outcome and that people with severe psychiatric disabilities, long histories of institutionalization or abandonment, and even with active psychiatric symptoms can learn social and vocational skills and achieve better adjustment; the proviso is that interventions must be integrated, that community support be granted without limits of time, and that stigma and discrimination be challenged.

References

Alfano AM: A scale to measure attitudes towards working. Journal of Vocational Behavior 3:329–333, 1973

Allport GW: The Nature of Prejudice. Cambridge, MA, Addison-Wesley, 1954

Altman JH, Wittenborn JR: Depression-prone personality in women. J Abnorm Psychol 89:303–308, 1980

Amiel R, Dubuis J (eds): La réhabilitation des malades mentaux à l'horizon de l'an 2000. Actualités Psychiatriques 19(3):2–67, 1989

American Psychiatric Association: Mental retardation: psychotherapy, in Treatments of Psychiatric Disorders: A Task Force Report of the American Psychiatric Association, Vol 1. Washington, DC, American Psychiatric Association, 1989a, pp 108–111

American Psychiatric Association: Psychoactive substance use disorders (alcohol): goals of treatment, in Treatments of Psychiatric Disorders: A Task Force Report of the American Psychiatric Association, Vol 2. Washington, DC, American Psychiatric Association, 1989b, pp 1072–1076

American Psychiatric Association: Rehabilitation in schizophrenic disorders, in Treatments of Psychiatric Disorders: A Task Force Report of the American Psychiatric Association, Vol 2. Washington, DC, American Psychiatric Association, 1989c, pp 1567–1583

Anthony WA: Societal rehabilitation: changing society's attitudes toward the physically and mentally disabled. Rehabilitation Psychology 19:117–126, 1972

Anthony WA, Blanch A: Research on community support services: what have we learned? Paper presented at the Community Support and Rehabilitation Services Research Meeting, Bethesda, MD, May 3–5, 1988

Anthony WA, Buell GJ: Psychiatric aftercare clinic effectiveness as a function of patient demographic characteristics. J Consult Clin Psychol 41:116–119, 1973

Anthony WA, Carkhuff RR: The functional professional therapeutic agent, in Effective Psychotherapy. Edited by Gurman A, Razin A. London, Pergamon, 1978

Anthony WA, Farkas MD: A client outcome planning model for assessing psychiatric rehabilitation interventions. Schizophr Bull 8:13–38, 1982

Anthony WA, Jansen MA: Predicting the vocational capacity of the chronically mentally ill: research and policy implications. Am Psychol 39:537–544, 1984

Anthony WA, Liberman RP: The practice of psychiatric rehabilitation: historical, conceptual, and research base. Schizophr Bull 12:542–559, 1986

Anthony WA, Buell GJ, Sharratt S, et al: The efficacy of psychiatric rehabilitation. Psychol Bull 78:447–456, 1972

Anthony WA, Cohen MR, Vitalo R: The measurement of rehabilitation outcome. Schizophr Bull 4:365–383, 1978

Anthony WA, Cohen MR, Farkas MD: Professional preservice training for working with the long-term mentally ill. Community Ment Health J 24:258–269, 1988

Anthony WA, Cohen MR, Farkas MD: Psychiatric Rehabilitation. Boston, Center for Psychiatric Rehabilitation, 1990

Ayllon T, Azrin N: The Token Economy. New York, Appleton-Century-Crofts, 1968

Azrin NH, Besalel VA: Job Club Counselors Manual: A Behavioral Approach to Vocational Counseling. Baltimore, University Park Press, 1980

Azrin NH, Phillip RA: The job club method for the job handicapped: a comparative outcome study. Rehabilitation Counseling Bulletin 23:144–155, 1979

Azrin NH, Flores T, Kaplan SJ: Job Finding Club: a group assisted program for obtaining employment. Behav Res Ther 13:17–27, 1975

Bachrach LL (ed): Deinstitutionalization. San Francisco, CA, Jossey-Bass, 1983

Baekeland F, Lundwall L, Kissin B: Methods for the treatment of chronic alcoholism: a critical appraisal, in Research Advances in Alcohol and Drug Problems, Vol. 2. Edited by Gibbins RH, Israel Y, Kalant H, et al. Toronto, Wiley, 1975

Baker R, Hall JK, Hutchinson K, et al: Symptom changes in chronic schizophrenic patients on a token economy: a controlled experiment. Br J Psychiatry 131:381–393, 1977

Barbee JR, Kiel EC: Experimental techniques of job interview training for the disadvantaged: videotape feedback, behavior modification and microcounselling. J Appl Psychol 58:209–213, 1973

Bateson G, Jackson DD, Haley J, et al: Toward a theory of schizophrenia. Behav Sci 1:251–264, 1956

Beard JH, Malamud TJ, Rossman E: Psychiatric rehabilitation and long-term rehospitalization rates: the findings of two research studies. Schizophr Bull 4:622–635, 1978

Beard JH, Propst R, Malamud TJ: The Fountain House model of psychiatric rehabilitation. Psychosocial Rehabilitation Journal 5:47–53, 1982

Beck AT, Rush AJ, Shaw BF, et al: Cognitive Therapy of Depression. Chicester, England, John Wiley, 1979

Bellack AS, Hersen M, Himmelhoch J: Social skills training compared with pharmacotherapy and psychotherapy in the treatment of unipolar depression. Am J Psychiatry 138:1562–1567, 1981

Bellack AS, Hersen M, Himmelhoch J: A comparison of social skills training, pharmacotherapy and psychotherapy for depression. Behav Res Ther 21:101–107, 1983

Bennett DH: The value of work in psychiatric rehabilitation. Soc Psychiatry 5:224–230, 1970

Bennett DH: The historical development of rehabilitation services, in Theory and Practice of Psychiatric Rehabilitation. Edited by Watts FN, Bennett DH. Chicester, England, John Wiley, 1983

Bennett DH, Morris I: Support and rehabilitation, in Theory and Practice of Psychiatric Rehabilitation. Edited by Watts FN, Bennett DH. Chicester, England, Wiley, 1983

Bennett DH, Wing JK: Sheltered workshops for the psychiatrically handicapped, in Current Trends in the Mental Health Services. Edited by Freeman H, Farndale J. New York, Macmillan, 1963

Betz E, Weiss DJ, Dawis RW, et al: Seven Years of Research on Work Adjustment. Minnesota Studies in Vocational Rehabilitation, no 20. Minneapolis, MN, University of Minnesota, 1966

Bleuler M: A 23-year longitudinal study of 208 schizophrenics and impressions in regard to the nature of schizophrenia, in The Transmission of Schizophrenia. Edited by Rosenthal D, Kety SS. Oxford, England, Pergamon, 1968

Bond GR, Dincin J: Accelerating entry into transitional employment in a psychosocial rehabilitation agency. Rehabilitation Psychology 31:143–154, 1986

Bond GR, Witheridge TF, Setze PJ, et al: Preventing rehospitalization of clients in a psychosocial rehabilitation program. Hosp Community Psychiatry 36:993–995, 1985

Bradley V, Allard MA, Spence R, et al: Providing Housing and Supports for People With Psychiatric Disabilities: A Technical Assistance Manual for Applicants for the Robert Wood Johnson Foundation Initiative to Improve Urban Mental Health Systems. Boston, MA, Human Services Research Institute and Center for Psychiatric Rehabilitation, 1986

Braun P, Kochansky G, Shapiro R, et al: Overview: deinstitutionalization of psychiatric patients, a critical review of outcome studies. Am J Psychiatry 138:736–749, 1981

Brown GW, Harris T: Social Origins of Depression: A Study of Psychiatric Disorder in Women. London, Tavistock, 1978

Brown GW, Birley JLT, Wing JK: Influence of family life on the course of schizophrenic disorders: a replication. Br J Psychiatry 121:241–258, 1972

Buell GJ, Anthony WA: Demographic characteristics as predictors of recidivism and post-hospital employment. Journal of Counseling Psychology 20:361–365, 1973

Burti L, Mosher L: Training psychiatrists in the community: a report of the Italian experience. Am J Psychiatry 143:1580–1584, 1986

Cannady D: Chronics and cleaning ladies. Psychosocial Rehabilitation Journal 5:13–16, 1982

Carkhuff RR: The differential functioning of lay and professional helpers. Journal of Counseling Psychology 15:117–126, 1968

Carpenter WT, Heinrichs DW: Early intervention, time-limited, targeted pharmacotherapy of schizophrenia. Schizophr Bull 9:533–542, 1983

Carpenter WT, Heinrichs DW, Hanlon TE: A comparative trial of pharmacologic strategies in schizophrenia. Am J Psychiatry 144:1466–1470, 1987

Carstairs GM, O'Connor N, Rawnsley K: Organization of a hospital workshop for chronic psychotic patients. British Journal of Preventive and Social Medicine 10:136–140, 1956

Chadsey-Rusch J: Identifying and teaching valued social behaviors, in Competitive Employment Issues and Strategies. Edited by Rusch FR. Baltimore, Brookes, 1986

Chamberlin J: On Our Own: Patient-Controlled Alternatives to the Mental Health System. New York, McGraw-Hill, 1978

Cheadle AJ, Morgan R: The measurement of work performance of psychiatric patients: a reappraisal. Br J Psychiatry 120:437–441, 1972

Ciompi L: The natural history of schizophrenia in the long term. Br J Psychiatry 136:413–420, 1980a

Ciompi L: Catamnestic long-term study of the course of life and aging of schizophrenics. Schizophr Bull 6:606–618, 1980b

Ciompi L, Dauwalder HP, Ague C: Ein Forschungsprogramm zur Rehabilitation psychisch Kranker: III. Laengsschnittuntersuchung zum Rehabilitationserfolg und zur Prognostik. Nervenarzt 50:366–378, 1979

Cohen CI, Sokolovsky J: Clinical use of network analysis for psychiatric and aged populations. Community Ment Health J 15:203–213, 1979

Cole NJ, Brewer DL, Allison RB, et al: Employment characteristics of discharged schizophrenics. Arch Gen Psychiatry 10:314–319, 1964

Costello CG: Loss of reinforcers or loss of reinforcer effectiveness. Behavior Therapy 3:240–247, 1972

Costello RM: Alcoholism treatment effectiveness: slicing the outcome variance pie, in Alcoholism Treatment in Transition. Edited by Edwards G, Grant M. London, Croom Helm, 1980

Costello RM, Biever P, Baillargeon JG: Alcoholism treatment programming: historical trends and modern approaches. Alcohol Clin Exp Res 1:311–318, 1977

Cotzin M: Group therapy with mentally defective problem boys. American Journal of Mental Deficiency 53:268–283, 1948

Creer C: Social work with patients and their families, in Schizophrenia: Towards a New Synthesis. Edited by Wing JK. London, Academic Press, 1978

Cytryn L, Lourie RS: Mental retardation, in Comprehensive Textbook of Psychiatry, 2nd Edition, Vol 1. Edited by Freedman AM, Kaplan HI, Sadock BJ. Baltimore, Williams & Wilkins, 1975, pp 1158–1197

Davis AE, Dinitz S, Pasamanick B: Schizophrenics in the New Custodial Community: Five Years After the Experiment. Columbus, Ohio State University Press, 1974

Davis JM: Antipsychotic drugs, in Comprehensive Textbook of Psychiatry, Vol 3. Edited by Kaplan HI, Freedman AM, Sadock BJ. Baltimore, Williams & Wilkins, 1980

Davis JM, Gosenfeld L, Tsai CC: Maintenance antipsychotic drugs do prevent relapse: a reply to Tobias and MacDonald. Psychol Bull 83:431–447, 1976

Davis KR, Shapiro LJ: Exploring group process as a means of reaching the mentally retarded. Social Casework 60:330–337, 1979

Davis RR, Rogers ES: Social skills training with persons who are mentally retarded. Ment Retard 23:186–196, 1985

Debernardi A: Suicidi e legge 180. Epidemiologia e Prevenzione 3–4(10–11):57–58, 1980

De Girolamo G: Italian psychiatry and reform law: a review of the international literature. Int J Soc Psychiatry 35:21–37, 1989

Dincin J, Witheridge TF: Psychiatric rehabilitation as a deterrent to recidivism. Hosp Community Psychiatry 33:645–650, 1982

Dion GL, Anthony WA: Research in psychiatric rehabilitation: a review of experimental and quasi-experimental studies. Rehabilitation Counseling Bulletin 30:177–203, 1987

Dunn LM: Special education for the mildly retarded: is much of it justifiable? Except Child 35:5–22, 1968

Early DF: The role of industry in rehabilitation, in The Treatment of Mental Disorders in the Community. Edited by Daniel GR, Freeman HL. London, Bailliere, Tindall and Cassell, 1968

Early DF: Industrial therapy organization, 1966–1970. Soc Psychiatry 8:109–116, 1973

Ellsworth RB, Foster L, Childers B, et al: Hospital and community adjustment as perceived by psychiatric patients, their families and staff. J Consult Clin Psychol 32 (monograph suppl):1–41, 1968

Engelhardt DM, Rosen B: Implications of drug treatment for the social rehabilitation of schizophrenic patients. Schizophr Bull 2:454–462, 1976

Esser AH, Chamberlain AS: Productivity of chronic schizophrenics in a sheltered workshop. Compr Psychiatry 6:41–50, 1965

Fairweather GW, Sanders D, Cressler D, et al: Community Life for the Mentally Ill: An Alternative to Institutional Care. Chicago, Aldine, 1969

Falloon IRH, Lindley P, McDonald R, et al: Social skills training of out-patient groups: a controlled study of rehearsal and homework. Br J Psychiatry 131:599–609, 1977

Falloon IRH, Boyd JL, McGill CW, et al: Family management in the prevention of exacerbations of schizophrenia. N Engl J Med 306:1437–1440, 1982

Falloon IRH, Boyd JL, McGill CW, et al: Family management in the prevention of morbidity of schizophrenia: clinical outcome of a two-year longitudinal study. Arch Gen Psychiatry 42:887–896, 1985

Farina A, Felner RD: Employment interviewer reactions to former mental patients. J Abnorm Psychol 82:268–272, 1973

Farkas MD, Anthony WA: Outcome analysis in psychiatric rehabilitation, in Rehabilitation Outcomes: Analysis and Measurement. Edited by Fuhrer MJ. Baltimore, Brookes, 1987

Farkas MD, Rogers ES, Thurer S: Rehabilitation outcome of long-term hospital patients left behind by deinstitutionalization. Hosp Community Psychiatry 38:864–870, 1987

Foulds GA: Temperamental differences in maze performance: II. the effect of distraction and electroconvulsive therapy on psychomotor retardation. Br J Psychiatry 43:33–41, 1952

Franklin J, Kittredge L, Thrasher J: A survey of factors related to mental hospital readmissions. Hosp Community Psychiatry 26:749–751, 1975

Frey WD: Functional assessment in the 80s: a conceptual enigma, a technical challenge, in Functional Assessment in Rehabilitation. Edited by Halpern AS, Fuhrer MJ. Baltimore, Brookes, 1984

Frisanco R (ed): Il Dopo 180: Primo Bilancio di una Riforma. Rome, Edizioni TER, 1989

Gellman WG: The vocational adjustment shop. Personnel and Guidance Journal 39:630–633, 1961

Gellman WG, Gendel H, Glaser NM, et al: Adjusting People to Work. Chicago, Jewish Vocational Service, 1957

Gellman WG, Stern D, Soloff A: A Scale of Employability for Handicapped Persons. Chicago, Jewish Vocational Service, 1963

Gittelman M, Black B: A cross-cultural perspective on psychiatric disability, in Psychiatric Disability: Clinical, Legal and Administrative Dimensions. Edited by Meyerson AT, Fine T. Washington, DC, American Psychiatric Press, 1987, pp 351–369

Gittelman M, Blumberg I: Rehabilitation, in Mental Health: The Public Health Challenge. Edited by Lieberman EJ. Apha, 1975

Gittelman M, Dubuis J, Nagaswami V, et al: Mental health promotion through psychosocial rehabilitation. International Journal of Mental Health 18(3):99–116, 1990

Glass LL, Katz HM, Schnitzer RD, et al: Psychotherapy of schizophrenia: an empirical investigation of the relationship of process to outcome. Am J Psychiatry 146:603–608, 1989

Glasscote RM, Kraft AM, Glassman SM, et al: Partial Hospitalization for the Mentally Ill: A Study of Programs and Problems. Washington, DC, Joint Information Service and National Association for Mental Health, 1969

Glick ID, Hargreaves WA: Psychiatric Hospital Treatment for the 1980s: A Controlled Study of Short Versus Long Hospitalization. Lexington, MA, Heath, 1979

Glynn S, Mueser KT: Social learning for chronic mental inpatients. Schizophr Bull 12:648–668, 1986

Goering PN, Wasylenki DA, Farkas M, et al: What difference does case management make? Hosp Community Psychiatry 39:272–276, 1988

Goldman HH, Gattozzi AA, Taube CA: Defining and counting the chronically mentally ill. Hosp Community Psychiatry 32:21–27, 1981

Goldstein MJ, Rodnick EH, Evans JR, et al: Drug and family therapy in the aftercare treatment of acute schizophrenia. Arch Gen Psychiatry 35:169–177, 1978

Gottlieb J: Mainstreaming: fulfilling the promise? American Journal of Mental Deficiency 86:115–126, 1981

Gove PB, Artin E, Bethel JP, et al: Webster's Third New International Dictionary of the English Language, Unabridged. Springfield, MA, Merriam, 1976

Green HJ, Miskimins RW, Keil EC: Selection of psychiatric patients for vocational rehabilitation. Rehabilitation Counseling Bulletin 11:297–302, 1968

Grinspoon L, Ewalt JR, Shader RI: Schizophrenia: Pharmacotherapy and Psychotherapy. Baltimore, Williams & Wilkins, 1972

Gunderson JG, Frank AF, Katz HM, et al: Effects of psychotherapy on schizophrenia: II. Comparative outcome of two forms of treatment. Schizophr Bull 10:564–598, 1984

Gurel L, Lorei TW: Hospital and community ratings of psychopathology as predictors of employment and readmission. Journal of Counseling and Clinical Psychology 34:286–291, 1972

Hamilton V: Psychological changes in chronic schizophrenics following differential activity programs: a repeat study. Br J Psychiatry 110:283–286, 1964

Harding CM, Brooks GW, Ashikaga T, et al: The Vermont longitudinal study of persons with severe mental illness, I: methodology, study sample and overall status 32 years later. Am J Psychiatry 144:718–726, 1987a

Harding CM, Brooks GW, Ashikaga T, et al: The Vermont longitudinal study of persons with severe mental illness, II: long-term outcome of subjects who retrospectively met DSM-III criteria for schizophrenia. Am J Psychiatry 144:727–735, 1987b

Hartlage LC: Expanding comprehensiveness of psychiatric rehabilitation. Mental Hygiene 49:238–243, 1965

Hatfield A: Coping With Mental Illness in the Family. National Alliance for the Mentally Ill, 1984

Hatfield A: Consumer Guide to Mental Health Services. National Alliance for the Mentally Ill, 1985

Heather N, Robertson I: Controlled Drinking. London, Methuen, 1981

Henry GM, Weingartner H, Murphy DL: Influence of affective states and psychoactive drugs on verbal learning and memory. Am J Psychiatry 130:966–971, 1973

Hersen M: Modification of skill deficits in psychiatric patients, in Research and Practice in Social Skills Training. Edited by Bellack AS, Hersen M. New York, Plenum, 1979

Herz MI: Intermittent medication and schizophrenia, in Drug Maintenance Strategies in Schizophrenia. Edited by Kane JM. Washington, DC, American Psychiatric Press, 1984

Herz MI, Endicott J, Spitzer R, et al: Day versus inpatient hospitalization: a controlled study. Am J Psychiatry 127:1371–1382, 1971

Hirsch SR, Jolley AG, Manchanda R, et al: Early intervention medication as an alternative to continuous depot treatment in schizophrenia: preliminary report, in Psychosocial Treatment of Schizophrenia. Edited by Strauss JS, Böker W, Brenner HD. Toronto, Huber, 1987

Hogarty GE, Goldberg SC, Schooler NR, et al: Drug and sociotherapy in the aftercare of schizophrenic patients: II. Two-year relapse rates. Arch Gen Psychiatry 31:603–608, 1974

Hogarty GE, Schooler NR, Ulrich R, et al: Fluphenazine and social therapy in aftercare of schizophrenic patients: relapse analyses of a two-year controlled study of fluphenazine decanoate and fluphenazine hydrochloride. Arch Gen Psychiatry 36:1283–1294, 1979

Hogarty GE, Anderson CM, Reiss DJ, et al: Family psychoeducation, social skills training and maintenance chemotherapy in the aftercare treatment of schizophrenia: I. one year effects of a controlled study on relapse and expressed emotion. Arch Gen Psychiatry 43:633–642, 1986

Hoult J: The community care of the acutely mentally ill. Br J Psychiatry 149:137–144, 1986

Hoult J, Reynolds I: Schizophrenia: a comparative trial of community-oriented and hospital-oriented psychiatric care. Acta Psychiatr Scand 69:359–372, 1984

Hoult J, Rosen A, Reynolds I: Community oriented treatment compared to psychiatric hospital oriented treatment. Soc Sci Med 11:1005–1010, 1984

Huber G, Gross G, Schuttler T, et al: Longitudinal studies of schizophrenic patients. Schizophr Bull 6:592–605, 1980

Institute for the Crippled and Disabled: TOWER: Testing, Orientation and Work in Rehabilitation. New York, Institute for the Crippled and Disabled, 1967

Jablensky A, Schwartz R, Tomov T: WHO collaborative study on impairments and disabilities associated with schizophrenic disorders. Acta Psychiatr Scand 62 (suppl 285):152–159, 1980

Jones M: The Therapeutic Community: A New Treatment Method in Psychiatry. New York, Basic Books, 1953

Kabanov MM: Rehabilitation of the Mentally Ill. Leningrad, 1985

Kane JM, Woerner M, Weinhold P, et al: Incidence of tardive dyskinesia: five year data from a prospective study. Psychopharmacol Bull 20:382–386, 1984

Karan OC, Berger C: Developing support networks for individuals who fail to achieve competitive employment, in Competitive Employment Issues and Strategies. Edited by Rusch FR. Baltimore, Brookes, 1986, pp 241–255

Karan OC, Shalock RL: An ecological approach to assessing vocational and community living skills, in Habilitation Practices with the Developmentally Disabled Who Present Behavioral and Emotional Disorders. Edited by Karan OC, Gardner WI. Madison, WI, Rehabilitation Research and Training Center in Mental Retardation, 1983, pp 121–173

Karon BP, Vandenbos GR: The consequences of psychotherapy for schizophrenic patients. Psychotherapy: Theory, Research and Practice 9:111–119, 1972

Kiel EC, Barbee JR: Training the disadvantaged job interviewee. Vocational Guidance Quarterly 22:50–56, 1973

Kirk SA: Effectiveness of community services for discharged mental patients. Am J Orthopsychiatry 46:646–659, 1976

Laing RD: The Politics of Experience. New York, Ballantine, 1967

Laing RD, Esterson S: Families and schizophrenia. International Journal of Psychiatry 4:65–71, 1967

Langsley DG, Kaplan DM: The Treatment of Families in Crisis. New York, Grune & Stratton, 1968

Leff JP, Vaughn CE: The role of maintenance therapy and relatives' expressed emotion in relapse of schizophrenia: a two year follow-up. Br J Psychiatry 139:102–104, 1981

Leff JP, Vaughn CE: Expressed Emotion in Families. New York, Guilford, 1985

Leff JP, Kuipers L, Berkowitz R, et al: A controlled trial of social intervention in the families of schizophrenic patients. Br J Psychiatry 141:121–134, 1982

Leff JP, Kuipers L, Berkowitz R, et al: Life events, relatives' expressed emotion and maintenance neuroleptics in schizophrenic relapse. Psychol Med 13:799–806, 1983

Leff JP, Kuipers L, Berkowitz R, et al: A controlled trial of social intervention in the families of schizophrenic patients: two year follow-up. Br J Psychiatry 146:594–600, 1985

Leshner S, Snyderman G: A new approach to the evaluation and rehabilitation of the vocationally handicapped, in Counseling and Guidance—A Summary View. Edited by Adams J. New York, Macmillan, 1965

Lewinsohn PM: A behavioral approach to depression, in The Psychology of Depression: Contemporary Theory and Research. Edited by Friedman RJ, Katz MM. Washington, DC, Winston, 1974

Liberman RP, De Risi WJ, King LW, et al: Behavioral measurement in a community mental health center, in Evaluating Behavioral Programs in Community, Residential and Educational Settings. Edited by Davidson P, Clark F, Hamerlynck L. Champaign, IL, Research Press, 1974

Liberman RP, Fearn CH, De Risi WJ, et al: The credit incentive system: motivating the participation of patients in a day hospital. Br J Soc Clinical Psychology 16:85–94, 1977

Liberman RP, Mueser KT, Wallace CJ, et al: Training skills in the psychiatrically disabled: learning coping and competence. Schizophr Bull 12:631–647, 1986

Lidz T, Fleck S, Alanen YO, et al: Schizophrenic patients and their siblings. Psychiatry 26:1–18, 1963

Lipton FR, Nutt S, Sabatini A: Housing the homeless mentally ill: a longitudinal study of a treatment approach. Hosp Community Psychiatry 39:40–45, 1988

Lofquist LH, Dawis RV: Adjustment to Work: A Psychological View of Man's Problems in a Work-Oriented Society. New York, Appleton-Century-Crofts, 1969

Lorei TW, Gurel L: Demographic characteristics as predictors of posthospital employment and readmission. J Consult Clin Psychol 40:426–430, 1973

Malamud TJ: Evaluation of Clubhouse Model—Community-Based Psychiatric Rehabilitation. Washington, DC, National Institute of Handicapped Research, Office of Special Education and Rehabilitation Services, US Department of Education, 1985

Matson JL, Senatore V: A comparison of traditional psychotherapy and social skills training for improving interpersonal functioning of mentally retarded adults. Behavior Therapy 12:369–382, 1981

May PRA: Treatment of Schizophrenia: A Comparative Study of Five Treatment Methods. New York, Science House, 1968

McGlashan TH: The prediction of outcome in chronic schizophrenia: IV. the Chestnut Lodge follow-up study. Arch Gen Psychiatry 43:167–176, 1986

McLellan AT, Luborsky L, Woody GE, et al: Predicting response to alcohol and drug abuse treatments. Arch Gen Psychiatry 40:620–625, 1983

Meichenbaum D: Cognitive and Behavior Modification: An Integrative Approach. New York, Plenum, 1977

Melton GB, Greenberg-Garrison E: Fear, prejudice, and neglect: discrimination against mentally disabled persons. Am Psychol 42:1007–1026, 1987

Miller GH, Willer B: Predictors of return to a psychiatric hospital. J Consult Clin Psychol 44:898–900, 1976

Misiti R, Debernardi A, Gerbaldo C, et al: La Riforma Psichiatrica. Prima Fase di Attuazione. Rome, Italy, Il Pensiero Scientifico, 1981

Monti PM, Fink E, Norman W, et al: The effect of social skills training groups and social skills bibliotherapy with psychiatric patients. J Consult Clin Psychol 47:189–191, 1979

Monti PM, Curran JP, Corriveau DP, et al: Effect of social skills training groups and sensitivity training groups with psychiatric patients. J Consult Clin Psychol 48:241–248, 1980

Moos RH, Bromet E, Tsu V, et al: Family characteristics and the outcome of treatment for alcoholism. J Stud Alcohol 40:78–88, 1979

Mosher LR, Burti L: Community Mental Health: Principles and Practice. New York, Norton, 1989

Mosher LR, Keith SJ: Psychosocial treatment: individual, group, family, and community support approaches. Schizophr Bull 6:10–41, 1980

Mosher LR, Menn AZ: Community residential treatment for schizophrenia: two-year follow-up. Hosp Community Psychiatry 29:715–723, 1978

Mueller JH: Anxiety and cue utilization in human learning and memory, in Anxiety: New Concepts, Methods and Application. Edited by Zuckerman M, Spielberger CD. New York, Erlbaum, 1976

Murray H: Explorations in Personality. New York, Oxford University Press, 1938

Neff WS: Problems of work evaluation. Personnel and Guidance Journal 44:682–688, 1966

Neff WS: Work and Human Behavior. Chicago, Atherton Press, 1968

Neff WS: Vocational assessment—theory and models. Journal of Rehabilitation 36:27–29, 1970

Neff WS: Rehabilitation and work, in Rehabilitation Psychology. Edited by Neff WS. Washington, DC, American Psychological Association, 1971, pp 109–142

Niskanen P, Achte KA: Course and Prognosis of Schizophrenic Psychoses in Helsinki: A Comparative Study of First Admissions in 1950, 1960, and 1965. Monographs from the Psychiatric Clinic of the Helsinki University Central Hospital, No 4, 1972

O'Connor N, Heron A, Carstairs GM: Work performance of chronic schizophrenics. Occupational Psychology 30:1–12, 1956

Olshansky S, Grob S, Malamud IT: Employers' attitudes and practices in the hiring of ex-mental patients. Mental Hygiene 42:391–401, 1958

Overs R: Evaluation for Work by Job Sample Tasks. Cleveland, OH, Vocational and Rehabilitation Service, 1964a

Overs R: Obtaining and Using Actual Job Samples in a Work Evaluation Program. Cleveland, OH, Vocational and Rehabilitation Service, 1964b

Overs R: The Theory of Job Sample Tasks. Milwaukee, WI, Curative Workshop of Milwaukee, 1968

Pattison EM: Treatment of alcoholic families with nurse home visits. Fam Process 4:75–94, 1965

Paul GL, Lentz RJ: Psychosocial Treatment of Chronic Mental Patients: Milieu Versus Social-Learning Programs. Cambridge, MA, Harvard University Press, 1977

Payne RW, Hewlett JHG: Thought disorders in psychotic patients, in Experiments in Personality, Vol 2. Edited by Eysenck HJ. London, Routledge and Kegan, 1960

Pearlin LI, Johnson JS: Marital status, life strains and depression. American Sociological Review 42:704–715, 1977

Polak PR, Kirby MW: A model to replace psychiatric hospitals. J Nerv Ment Dis 162:13–22, 1976

Polak PR, Kirby MW, Deitchman W: Treating acutely psychiatric patients in private homes, in New Directions for Mental Health—Alternatives to Acute Hospitalization, Vol 1. Edited by Lamb HR. San Francisco, CA, Jossey-Bass, 1979

Rachman SJ: Primary obsessional slowness. Behav Res Ther 12:9–18, 1974

Rifkin A, Quitkin F, Rabiner C, et al: Fluphenazine decanoate, fluphenazine hydrochloride given orally, and placebo in remitted schizophrenics. I. Relapse rates after one year. Arch Gen Psychiatry 34:43–47, 1977

Ringelheim D, Polotsek I: Group therapy with a male defective group. American Journal of Mental Deficiency 60:157–162, 1955

Rog DJ, Raush HL: The psychiatric halfway house. How is it measuring up? Community Ment Health J 11:155–162, 1975

Rogers CR, Gendlin EG, Kiesler DJ, et al: The Therapeutic Relationship and Its Impact. Madison, WI, University of Wisconsin Press, 1967

Rosenblatt A, Mayer JE: The recidivism of mental patients: a review of past studies. Am J Orthopsychiatry 44:697–706, 1974

Rueveni J: Family network intervention: mobilizing support for families in crisis. International Journal of Family Counseling 5:77–83, 1977

Sartorius N: Solving the conundrum of schizophrenia: WHO's contribution, in Schizophrenia: Recent Biosocial Developments. Edited by Stefanis CN, Rabavilas AD. New York, Human Sciences Press, 1987, pp 23–38

Schoenfeld P, Halvey J, Hemley-van der Velden E, et al: Long-term outcome of network therapy. Hosp Community Psychiatry 37:373–376, 1986

Searls DJ, Wilson LT, Miskimins RW: Development of a measure of unemployability among restored psychiatric patients. J Appl Psychol 55:223–225, 1971

Shepherd GW: Planning the rehabilitation of the individual, in Theory and Practice of Psychiatric Rehabilitation. Edited by Watts FN, Bennett DH. Chicester, England, Wiley, 1983

Simon H: Aktiviere Krankenbehandlung in der Irrenanstalt. I. Allgemeine Zeitschrift für Psychiatrie 87:97, 1927

Simon H: Aktiviere Krankenbehandlung in der Irrenanstalt. II. Allgemeine Zeitschrift für Psychiatrie 90:69, 1929

Simons OG: Work and Mental Illness. New York, John Wiley, 1965

Singer MT, Wynne LC: Thought disorders and family relations of schizophrenics. III. methodology using projective techniques. IV. results and implications. Arch Gen Psychiatry 12:187–212, 1965

Sobell MB, Sobell LC: Second year treatment outcome of alcoholics treated by individualized behavior therapy: results. Behav Res Ther 14:195–215, 1976

Soloff A, Bolton BF: The validity of the CJVS scale of employability for older clients in a vocational adjustment workshop. Educational and Psychological Measurement 29:993–998, 1969

Spelke E, Hirst W, Neisser U: Skills of divided attention. Cognition 4:215–230, 1976

Spivak M: Towards a systematization of a social competency approach to rehabilitation: theory and definitions. The Israel Annals of Psychiatry and Related Disciplines 15:289–299, 1977

Stein LI, Test MA (eds): Alternatives to Mental Hospital Treatment. New York, Plenum, 1978

Sternlicht M: Psychotherapeutic procedures with the retarded, in International Review of Research in Mental Retardation, Vol 2. Edited by NR Ellis. New York, Academic Press, 1966

Stickney SK, Hall RL, Gardner ER: The effect of referral procedures on after-care compliance. Hosp Community Psychiatry 31:567–569, 1980

Strachan AM: Family intervention for the rehabilitation of schizophrenia: toward protection and coping. Schizophr Bull 12:678–698, 1986

Strauss JS: Discussion: what does rehabilitation accomplish? Schizophr Bull 12:720–723, 1986

Strauss JS, Carpenter WT: Prediction of outcome in schizophrenia. III. five-year outcome and its predictors. Arch Gen Psychiatry 34:159–163, 1977

Tansella M, Williams P: The Italian experience and its implications. Psychol Med 17:283–289, 1987

Tansella M, De Salvia D, Williams P: The Italian psychiatric reform: some quantitative evidence. Soc Psychiatry 22:37–48, 1987

Tarrier N, Barrowclough C, Vaughn C, et al: The community management of schizophrenia: a controlled trial of a behavioral intervention with families to reduce relapse. Br J Psychiatry 153:532–542, 1988

Tarrier N, Barrowclough C, Vaughn C, et al: Community management of schizophrenia: a two-year follow-up of a behavioral intervention with families. Br J Psychiatry 154:625–628, 1989

Test MA, Stein LI: Community treatment of the chronic patient: research overview. Schizophr Bull 4:350–364, 1978

Thompson T, Grabowski J (eds): Behavior Modification of the Mentally Retarded. New York, Oxford University Press, 1972

Thorley A: Longitudinal studies of drug dependence, in Drug Problems in Britain: A Review of Ten Years. Edited by Edwards G, Busch C. London, Academic Press, 1981a

Thorley A: Drug problems in the United Kingdom: retrospect and prospect. J R Soc Med 74:461, 1981b

Thorley A: Problem drinkers and drug takers, in Theory and Practice of Psychiatric Rehabilitation. Edited by Watts FN, Bennett DH. Chicester, England, John Wiley, 1983

Tsuang MT, Woolson RF, Fleming JA: Long-term outcome of major psychoses, I: schizophrenia and affective disorders compared with psychiatrically symptom-free surgical conditions. Arch Gen Psychiatry 36:1295–1301, 1979

Turner SM, Luber RF: The token economy in day hospital settings: contingency management or information feedback. J Behav Ther Exp Psychiatry 11:89–94, 1980

Van Putten T, May PRA: Milieu therapy of the schizophrenias, in Treatment of Schizophrenia: Progress and Prospects. Edited by West LJ, Flinn DE. New York, Grune and Stratton, 1976

Vaughn CE, Leff JP: The influence of family and social factors on the course of psychiatric illness. a comparison of schizophrenic and depressed neurotic patients Br J Psychiatry 129:125–137, 1976

Vaughn CE, Snyder KS, Jones S, et al: Family factors in schizophrenic relapse: a California replication of the British research on expressed emotion. Arch Gen Psychiatry 41:1169–1177, 1984

Vidon G, Petitjean F, Bonnet-Vidon B: Thérapeutiques institutionnelles, in Encyclopédie Médico-Chirurgicale, Psychiatrie. 37930G[10], 10-1989. Edited by Bach JF, Imbert JC, Jasmin C, et al. Paris: Editions Techniques, 1989, pp 1–14

Wadsworth WV, Wells BWP, Scott RF: The organization of a sheltered workshop. Journal of Mental Science 108:780–785, 1962

Waldorf D, Biernacki P: Natural recovery from heroin addiction: a review of the incidence literature. Journal of Drug Issues 2:281–289, 1979

Walker R, McCourt J: Employment experiences among 200 schizophrenic patients in hospital and after discharge. Am J Psychiatry 122:316–319, 1965

Wallace CJ: Functional assessment in rehabilitation. Schizophr Bull 12:604–630, 1986

Wansbrough N, Miles A: Industrial Therapy in Psychiatric Hospitals. London, King's Fund, 1968

Warner R: Recovery From Schizophrenia: Psychiatry and Political Economy. London, Routledge and Kegan, 1985

Washburn S, Vannicelli M, Longabaugh R, et al: A controlled comparison of psychiatric day treatment and inpatient hospitalization. J Consult Clin Psychol 44:665–678, 1976

Wasylenki DA, Goering PN, Lancee WJ, et al: Impact of a case manager program on psychiatric aftercare. J Nerv Ment Dis 173:303–308, 1985

Watts FN: A study of work behavior in a psychiatric rehabilitation unit. British Journal of Social and Clinical Psychology 17:85–92, 1978

Watts FN: Employment, in Theory and Practice of Psychiatric Rehabilitation. Edited by Watts FN, Bennett DH. Chicester, England, John Wiley, 1983

Watts FN, Bennett DH: Previous occupational stability as a predictor of employment after psychiatric rehabilitation. Psychol Med 7:709–712, 1977

Watts FN, Bennett DH (eds): Theory and Practice of Psychiatric Rehabilitation. Chicester, England, John Wiley, 1983

Weissman MM: The assessment of social adjustment. a review of techniques. Arch Gen Psychiatry 32:357–365, 1975

Weissmann MM, Sholomskas D, John K: The assessment of social adjustment. an update. Arch Gen Psychiatry 38:1250–1258, 1981

Wells RA, Dezen AE: The results of family therapy revisited: the nonbehavioral methods. Fam Process 17:251–274, 1978

Whatley CD: Employer attitudes, discharged patients and job disability. Mental Hygiene 48:121–131, 1964

Wilder J, Levin G, Zwerlin I: A two-year follow-up evaluation of acute psychiatric patients treated in a day hospital. Am J Psychiatry 122:1095–1101, 1966

Williams P, De Salvia D, Tansella M: Suicide, psychiatric reform, and the provision of psychiatric services in Italy. Soc Psychiatry 21:89–95, 1986

Wing JK: Schizophrenia, in Theory and Practice of Psychiatric Rehabilitation. Edited by Watts FN, Bennett DH. Chicester, England, John Wiley, 1983

Wing JK, Brown GW: Institutionalism and Schizophrenia. London, Cambridge University Press, 1970

Wing JK, Bennett DH, Denham J: The Industrial Rehabilitation of Long-Stay Schizophrenic Patients. Medical Research Council Memorandum No. 42. London, Her Majesty Stationery Office, 1964

Witheridge TF, Dincin J, Appleby L: Working with the most frequent recidivists: a total team approach to assertive resource management. Psychosocial Rehabilitation Journal 5:9–11, 1982

Wolfensberger W: The principle of normalization and its implications to psychiatric services. Am J Psychiatry 127:291–297, 1970

Wood PHN: Appreciating the consequences of disease—the classification of impairments, disability, and handicaps. The WHO Chronicle 34:376–380, 1980

Woods PA, Higson PJ, Tannahill MM: Token economy programs with chronic psychiatric patients: the importance of direct measurement and objective evaluation for long-term maintenance. Behav Res Ther 22:41–51, 1984

World Health Organization: International Classification of Impairments, Disabilities and Handicaps. Geneva, World Health Organization, 1980

World Health Organization: WHO Psychiatric Disability Assessment Schedule (WHO/DAS). Geneva, World Health Organization, 1988

Wynne LC, Singer MT: Thought disorder and family relations of schizophrenics. I. a research strategy. II. a classification of forms of thinking. Arch Gen Psychiatry 9:191–206:1963

Zinman S: Self-help: the wave of the future. Hosp Community Psychiatry 37:213, 1986

Zinman S, Harp H, Budd T (eds): Reaching Across: Mental Health Clients Helping Each Other. San Francisco, CA, California Network of Mental Health Clients, 1987

Zwerling I, Wilder JF: An evaluation of the applicability of the day hospital in treatment of acutely disturbed patients. Israel Annals of Psychiatry 2:162–185, 1964

Section V

Influence of Culture
on Treatment

Introduction to Section V

This section of the book brings in the use of traditional medical procedures relevant for psychiatry. These practices are based on oral traditions and not on a codified body of medical knowledge documented in historical texts and learned treatises. Not included in this overview are contemporary European folk medicine and modern Western "alternative" therapies, which are, to a large extent, idiosyncratic interpretations and variations of scientific medicine. On the other hand, traditional medicine is practiced in many countries of the world, and in some (e.g., China and India) it has official or semi-official status, with officially recognized teaching and research facilities. For these reasons, we thought that it deserves consideration in a book on psychiatric treatment.

In the following chapters, Jilek and Marsella and Westermeyer review the cultural factors that play a major role in all aspects of the treatment process, including assessment, diagnosis, and therapy content and process. There is in fact no aspect of the doctor-patient relationship that escapes cultural influence and determination. This is because both the patient and the doctor are members of ethnocultural traditions that encode and socialize various assumptions and premises regarding health and illness, and because the doctor belongs to a medical subculture that also has encoded and socialized various assumptions and premises about health and disease. A careful understanding of these factors can certainly help in the achievement of therapeutic objectives.

CHAPTER 11

Traditional Medicine Relevant to Psychiatry

Wolfgang G. Jilek, M.D.

Definition and Delimitation

The term *traditional medicine*, as used here, refers to folk therapy practices operating outside official health care systems. These practices are based on oral traditions and not on a codified body of medical knowledge as documented in historical texts and learned treatises. The latter is the case in classical Greco-Roman and medieval European schools of medicine, as well as in the ancient medical systems of China, India (Ayurvedic and Unani medicine), and the Arab countries (Greco-Arabic medicine). These written-down medical systems are not included in the present overview. They are categorically different from traditional ethnomedicine (cf. Bannerman 1982); in China and India they have official or semi-official status along with officially recognized teaching and research facilities. In some of these institutions research projects have been conducted with World Health Organization (WHO) technical collaboration (Bannerman et al. 1983). Also not included in this overview are contemporary European folk medicine and modern Western "alternative" therapies; they are demonstrably offshoots of medieval European schools of medicine or idiosyncratic interpretations and variations of scientific medicine.

The author would like to thank Louise Jilek-Aall, Ellen Corin, Gilles Bibeau, Alberto Perales, and Bernward Hochkirchen for their assistance in data collection.

341

Categories and Functions of
Traditional Practitioners

Traditional practitioners and ritualists explicitly or implicitly attend to the curing of illness, the relief of distress, the alleviation of anxiety, and the maximization of a feeling of well-being and security in individuals and groups. Unlike practitioners of scientific medicine and of codified traditional medical systems, traditional practitioners referred to in this overview do not qualify for their profession through examination after formal studies or training courses at schools or other institutions; they also usually follow other occupations in addition to their healing activity.

Traditional practitioners often enter the healing vocation after a culture-specific *calling* experience that frequently involves an altered state of consciousness, and in shamanic healers is typically associated with an *initiatory sickness* (Eliade 1964). Candidates are selected according to disposition, talent, and aptitude, and sometimes also by inheritance. They are usually apprenticed to an experienced senior practitioner and often go through a formal initiation process.

Different categories of traditional practitioners, as relevant to psychiatry, can be defined according to their predominant functions and to the types of procedures they employ. Among the practitioners of traditional medicine as defined in this overview, we find a considerable overlap of the above categories and of the therapeutic procedures used. Although most traditional practitioners are generalists, some specialize in the treatment of mental illness, as is found in parts of Africa (Makanjuola 1987; Peltzer 1988; Prince 1961).

Herbalists. Herbalists deal only or primarily with the therapeutic application of plant remedies. Although plants and animal items used in traditional medicine may often have symbolic or placebo functions, many plant remedies have not yet been identified botanically, much less been subjected to pharmacological and chemical investigations. A number of plants that have been examined have been shown to possess psychoactive principles (see Appendix 11–1).

Diviners. Diviners diagnose causes of illness and advise on remedial action through communication with supernatural beings or ancestral, guardian, or other spirits; by revelation in vision or dream; or through the interpretation of oracles. They are usually assisted by keen observation and by information elicited indirectly from patients and through the social network. Many diviners are also therapists.

Medicine men. Medicine men are believed to be authorized or empowered by supernatural, magical, or ancestral forces with which they engage in verbal and nonverbal (ritual-symbolic) therapeutic activities; they often also use herbal remedies and physical and physiotherapeutic applications.

Shamanic healers. Shamanic healers perform certain medicine man functions by entering into altered states of consciousness to communicate with supernatural beings in an ecstatic trance, to summon spirit powers and helpers, or to embody supernatural entities in possession states for the purpose of acting therapeutically with special powers. Typically, shamans are considered able to travel to the otherworld or to the spiritual or ancestral realm with the help of their spirit helpers and powers in order to retrieve aberrant or abducted souls and spirits belonging to patients made ill by this loss. Shamanic healers may also use plant hallucinogens to induce altered states of consciousness in themselves for divinatory and ritual performance, and in their clients to facilitate catharsis, abreaction, and suggestibility. Shamanic healers are primarily found in the Amazon region and along the northern Pacific coast of South America (Chiappe et al. 1985; Harner 1973; Hollweg 1991; Pineda 1986).

Therapeutic cult leaders and ritualists. Therapeutic cult leaders and ritualists operate in the context of traditional group ceremonials or cults that often involve altered states of consciousness.

Religious healers. In recent decades, Christian faith healers and "prophets" of fundamentalist Christian or Christian-derived syncretistic sects have taken over the functions of traditional practitioners among some populations in Africa and Latin America. Religious functionaries in Islam and Buddhism have always exercised healing functions. Today these are especially valuable in the rehabilitation of substance-dependent persons.

Principles Common to
Traditional Treatments

As Sartorius (1979) noted, "Traditional forms of mental health care contain important elements that have not been adequately studied and understood and therefore not fully utilized" (p. 717). In the following sections, I introduce several of the principles common to traditional treatments to elucidate the elements that might be applicable to more modern treatments of mental illness.

Culture-congeniality.   One major asset of traditional medicine practitioners is that they share, or at least are familiar with, the cultural value system of their clients.

Holistic approach.   As a rule, traditional practices integrate the physical, psychological, social, and spiritual aspects of healing.

Personality of the healer.   Traditional medicine recognizes the significance of the personality characteristics of the healer who, in order to be successful, has to be able to achieve and maintain a certain confidence-inspiring charisma.

Affective psychotherapy.   The traditional healer uses suggestive methods and altered states of consciousness and manipulates culturally validated symbols, working on the patient's affectivity to mobilize natural healing resources. This *affective psychotherapy* (Stumpfe 1983) can be considered complementary to modern somatic treatments and cognitive psychotherapy.

Relational approach.   Traditional treatment is never an exclusive matter between the therapist and patient, but is equally the concern of the patient's in-group. Often a *therapy management group* (Janzen 1978) is spontaneously formed—a therapy collective comprising kinspeople, friends, and community members who join forces with healer and patient in defining the nature of the problem and discerning the remedial action to be taken. In some tradition-directed societies, practitioner and assistants, patient and family, community members and ancestral spirits are all expected to be present at healing ceremonies, forming a *psychothera-peutic assembly* (Makang Ma Mbog 1969). Traditional medicine procedures therefore tend to be relational, involving the interaction of several people in the diagnostic and therapeutic enterprise, which fosters kin and community cohesion.

Ceremonial format. Traditional treatment usually takes place in the context of a healing ceremony composed of several ritual elements. It often entails the enactment of a therapeutic myth (Jilek and Jilek-Aall 1982) with the combined efforts of the healer, assistants, and members of the patient's in-group together with the patient, who is thereby re-anchored in the community of people from whom he or she may have become alienated.

Social engineering. In traditional psychotherapy, the practitioner does not assume a detached stance; rather there is a tendency toward social engineering by giving advice with authority and by direct or indirect manipulation of the client's immediate human environment. Traditional practitioners specializing in mental health care often temporarily accommodate the patient in their own home, or in a compound or healing shrine adjacent to their home, while the patient maintains close contact with his or her family. In traditional healing centers, shrines, or compounds, the patients are immersed in a daily ritual activity and household occupations, which constitutes effective milieu therapy (Field 1960; Peltzer 1987).

Traditional Therapeutic
Modalities and Their Effects

The Naming Process

In traditional medicine, the diagnostic process of naming the affliction and determining its causation often involves elaborate procedures in which a diagnostician-diviner, patient, and kinspeople participate. While designed to lead to the choice of appropriate remedial action, the naming process itself has significant therapeutic aspects (Bascom 1969; Corin

1979, 1985; Devisch 1978; Evans-Pritchard 1937; Guthrie and Szanton 1976; Jilek and Jilek-Aall 1967; Jilek and Knaub 1985; Levi-Strauss 1963; Peltzer 1987; Prince 1961; Prinz 1984; Reynolds 1963; Torrey 1972; Tseng 1976).

Although there is considerable cultural variation, it is possible to generalize from the available reports that the great majority of practitioners of noncodified traditional medicine do not see mental illness as an accident of nature but as stemming from three causes that can be categorized under three headings: 1) heredity (e.g., "in the blood"), 2) interpersonal intervention (e.g., by sorcery), and 3) supernatural intervention (e.g., by divine or demoniac powers, by spirits of the dead, or by other supernatural entities). It is the diviner's task to find or define the source of the trouble and to provide an answer to the vexing questions, Why am I afflicted? and Why is our kinsperson afflicted? In the divinatory naming process, traditional medicine has developed procedures to deal with and alleviate the anxiety and guilt aroused by these questions.

Traditional practitioners use a great variety of divining methods: divinatory devices and objects and oracles of many kinds. These methods are assumed to be controlled by supernatural powers, but may in fact be manipulated by the diviner who also relies on social network information, experience, and educated intuition. Depending on cultural traditions, the diviner may resort to hand trembling, gazing at reflecting surfaces, interpreting numbers, or using magico-religious words or verses. Moreover, the patient sometimes takes part in the selection or interpretation, comparable to projective testing. For the practitioner, divination procedures may facilitate concentration on the case and decision making.

The patient's dreams are nearly universally valued as diagnostic leads, whether they are considered vehicles of access to information from the supernatural or—as in Western psychotherapy—from the unconscious. The anxiety-generating role of certain dreams is recognized by some diviners who practice dream therapy or immunization against bad dreams (Jilek and Jilek-Aall 1967). The diviner's and healer's own dreams and visions are also chosen as modes of defining cause and remedial action in traditional indigenous medicine, particularly in Asia, North and South America, and Papua New Guinea (Jilek and Knaub 1985).

During the divination process, the practitioner may enter an altered state of consciousness induced by psychological and physiological means, and in some areas by hallucinogenic plants. The diviner is then seen by the audience as inspired or possessed by supernatural powers and therefore in a position of sanctioned authority.

In the naming process, the patient's feelings and experiences are restructured into a culturally validated image system. The patient is provided with a language in which ineffable psychic states can be expressed and chaotic experiences reorganized, thereby becoming intelligible and manageable (Levi-Strauss 1963). Once the problem is given an explanation and the offending agent or act identified, the patient and his or her group have an opportunity to commit themselves together to the recommended remedial or protective action within a culturally sanctioned framework, and to jointly involve themselves in the prescribed rituals or sacrificial offerings that are conducive to the alleviation of individual and collective anxiety and guilt.

Traditional Psychotherapies

Effective use of suggestion and catharsis are important aspects of traditional psychotherapy.

Therapeutic Suggestion

Traditional therapists use explicit suggestion by ego-strengthening reassurance and empathic assertion of successful cure; often they also skillfully use a metaphor, simile, parable, or illustrative story. However, therapeutic suggestion is mostly implicit and is based on collective suggestion; the shared culturally accepted belief in the healing powers of the therapist, ritual, and paraphernalia legitimizes the healer's role and methods. Implicit and collective suggestion are commonly operant in ritual-symbolic procedures, sacrificial rites, and the application of preventive devices.

Ritual-symbolic procedures. Traditional healers manipulate arcane, magical, or sacred images and objects (paraphernalia) under incantations, invocations, or recitations of magico-religious formulas in front of the patient and audience, who often participate by singing, chanting, and performing rhythmic movements. Patients respond to the suggestive power of culturally validated symbols—words, acts, and objects—by a reorganization of their emotions. A resolution of symptoms may then occur, especially after cathartic abreaction and when the patient is in an altered state of consciousness.

Sacrificial rites. Sacrificial rites are universally performed to appease and recompense supernatural or ancestral powers, and to urge their withdrawal of a punishing illness or to supplicate their intervention on behalf of the patient. Rituals of sacrifice are often associated with confession of having broken divine or ancestral rules (*taboos*) or with public admission of transgressions against community members, followed by promise of appropriate rectification.

Rites of scapegoating transfer the illness from the patient on to an animal to be sacrificed or on to a carved or modeled figure to be destroyed. Sprinkling with the sacrificial animal's blood establishes a blood covenant between the supernatural being and the patient.

The sacrificial ritual often ends with a communal meal in which the healer, patient, and kinspeople partake of the sacrificed animal's meat, a symbolic act sealing conciliation with supernatural beings or ancestors. These rites have a marked anxiety-alleviating and guilt-relieving effect and often lead to symptom resolution in neurotic-reactive conditions (Prince 1975).

Preventive devices. With appropriate suggestion, patients may be given objects that have culturally validated symbolism, such as amulets, charms, talismans, or medicine bundles, which have been blessed or otherwise "worked on" by the healer; patients may also receive special magico-religious formulas. Such objects and formulas are universally assumed to protect the bearer from illness and evil influence, affording him or her tranquility and peace of mind.

Catharsis

Triggered by adequate situational or sensory stimulation, or while in an altered state of consciousness induced by psychological, physiological, or phytochemical means, the patient may experience affective release in a psychodramatic abreaction, the therapeutic effect of which is increased by an accepting and empathic audience (Jilek 1989).

Traditional Physical Therapies

Physical restraint. Binding, shackling, or chaining patients to posts, or putting them into stocks or wooden blocks, are methods used in the management of severely agitated, aggressive psychotic patients. As a rule these measures are applied temporarily to prevent harm to self and others; such restraining contraptions are sometimes ingeniously constructed to allow for necessary body movements (Jilek-Aall 1964). However, certain patients may be kept in restraints for long periods resulting in muscular atrophy and skeletal deformity (W. G. Jilek, unpublished photographs, August 1985; Tan Pariaman 1983).

Physiotherapy and hydrotherapy. Various types of massage—deep pressure, light stroking, rubbing with oil, brushing with twigs, bathing, washing, sponging, and dousing—are procedures frequently applied in traditional medicine and are known to have somatopsychic effects of relaxation and stimulation.

External application of plant preparations. Various plant preparations are externally applied to the skin, especially to the head and its orifices because these are often believed to be the most direct route to the mind.

"Purification" measures. Herbal emetics and laxatives administered with copious amounts of fluid, sweat baths, steam baths, and fumigation with incense or smoke, are procedures intended by the healer, and understood by the patient, as purifying and cleansing measures to get rid of "polluting" or otherwise pathogenic substances. Consequently, they provide some relief from anxiety. Due to known physiological effects, drastic emetic purgation will also facilitate the entering of altered states of consciousness and open the patient to suggestive therapeutic influence (e.g., as is found in some traditional treatments of drug dependence).

Surgical procedures. Incisions (especially on the scalp), sucking, cupping, bloodletting, cauterization at the head, and trepanation (Margetts 1967) are usually performed in psychiatric patients in order to release, remove, or expel sick-making or "poisonous" agents, vapors, objects, or creatures. Such "psychosurgery" is infrequently practiced in traditional medicine today. Its obvious risks outweigh the therapeutic effect of implicit suggestion (a quick cure) on a somatizing patient.

Exorcism. The driving out of demons or evil spirits from psychiatric and epileptic patients is practiced in many cultures and religions and also has a venerable tradition in Christianity. It is often an impressive ritual with suggestive symbolism and, if pronounced successful by a charismatic exorcist, rarely fails to afford the believing patient some relief of anxiety. Unfortunately, exorcism may also entail such physical treatments as beating, flogging, whipping, smoking out, submersion in water, or partial burying—all supposedly directed at the sick-making spirit but often very harmful, even lethal, for the patient who may initially have accepted the procedure in order to be cured of evil spirit possession.

Phytotherapy. Phytotherapy is a therapy based on the administration of plants or substances derived from plants. A detailed description of the main phytotherapeutic methods appears in Appendix 11–1.

Tradition-Based Group Therapies
Involving Altered States of Consciousness

Altered states of consciousness (ASCs) are qualitative shifts in mental functioning that are subjectively and objectively recognizable as deviation from general norms of experience during alert waking consciousness. ASC can be induced by physiological techniques (e.g., rhythmic sensory stimulation) and by psychological influence (e.g., through individual and collective suggestion operant in a specific situation). ASCs correspond to M. Bleuler's (1961) concept of *Bewusstseinsverschiebung* (shifting of consciousness). Hypnotherapy is one of the few examples of the therapeutic use of an ASC in modern medicine.

It may be said that modern clinical psychiatry has neglected the therapeutic potential of ASCs and ignored the fact that entering an ASC is part of the normal capability of the human central nervous system. This capability may tend to be suppressed through the child rearing practices of modern Western and Westernized societies. The study of the therapeutic application of ASC has, in recent decades, been an important topic of ethnopsychiatric research (Dittrich and Scharfetter 1987; Ludwig 1966; Sargant 1967; Tart 1969; Torrey 1972; Ward 1989). In most non-Western cultures, and in premodern Western cultures, ASCs are interpreted either as states of possession in which a supernatural entity acts through the possessed individual, or as a special state of the individual allowing close interaction with supernatural entities, such as perceiving them in visions, receiving their messages, and imitating their actions. These two basic variations of culturally defined ASC have been designated *possession-trance* and *trance*, respectively, and their global distribution has been mapped (Bourguignon 1973).

In this section I consider only institutionalized, culturally patterned ASCs, which have societal sanction and are induced, without psychoactive plants or other agents, mainly for therapeutic purposes in the context of a traditional belief system. These ritualized ASCs, whether their cultural interpretation corresponds to possession-trance or trance states, manifest a normal dissociative capability of the mental apparatus and must be conceptually differentiated from psychopathological conditions. The latter usually occur outside a ceremonial context and are defined as pathological by indigenous experts, even when occurring as so-called culture-bound syndromes. The pathology labeling by Western observers of ASCs institutionalized in religious or therapeutic ceremonials of non-Western cultures constitutes a Eurocentric and positivistic fallacy that has for a long time promoted a distorted view of traditional practitioners (Jilek 1971).

Therapeutic Functions of Group Ceremonial Activities

The psychotherapeutic, psychohygienic, prophylactic, and socially adaptive functions of ceremonial group activities involving ASCs in non-Western societies have been attested to by several expert observers (Corin and Bibeau 1980; Kiev 1972; W. Pfeiffer 1971; Prince 1968, 1974; Walker 1972; Young 1975). Initiation to such ceremonials can be described as an often intensive therapeutic process in which an ASC is induced in the new client by ritualist leaders and by group influence through psychological and physiological methods, usually in conjunction with physical activity, especially dancing. The initiation process in some traditional group therapies involving ASC is geared toward personality depatterning with subsequent personality reorientation. Some examples are the initiation procedures in the revived North American Indian dance ceremonials that today successfully aim at the rehabilitation of Amerindian individuals whose sociocultural alienation has led to chronic dysphoria with alcohol and drug abuse and anomic depression (Jilek 1978, 1982).

The therapeutic functions of traditional group ceremonials with ritualized ASC, as reported by observers, can be summarized as follows. On the *psychological level*, cathartic abreaction is facilitated and tension relieved; frustrated emotional and interpersonal needs are often gratified in a supportive group milieu; shame, remorse, and guilt are deflected; and anxiety is alleviated. Ceremonials with psychodramatic role-playing permit symbolic expression of suppressed or repressed aspects of the personality in a socially acceptable fashion in front of an empathic audience and in a setting conducive to sociocultural learning. In possession-trance ceremonials, the possessed individual is amnesic and not held responsible for dramatic behavior in an ASC that is attributed to a supernatural entity. At the same time, the possessed individual in ritualized ASC is secure from harm or from overstepping the limits of decorum because of the caretaking of the ritualist leaders and other group members. Ritualist leaders exert therapeutic influence on new members through presented example and suggestive advice. Most importantly, like many other traditional healers, the leaders articulate and manipulate culturally validated images and symbols that in traditional group therapy can easily access the participant in an ASC. Clients who seek help contribute to their rehabilitation by their own actions, which strengthens their self-esteem. Many clients graduate to be ritualistic leaders (i.e., the initial sick role is converted into a health-providing role and into an identification model for novices).

On the *social level*, membership in a ceremonial group may help in the resolution of interpersonal, interfamily, and intergenerational conflicts by altering social relationships and by supporting the individual's demands on the social network. Group participation often leads to a restructuring of social existence, finding of a more adaptive sociocultural identity, and better sociocultural integration. The participant may acquire social status and prestige by virtue of being seen as having been chosen as the vehicle of supernatural powers manifested in an ASC. Possession-trance cults may serve not only as outlets for disadvantaged persons but also as channels for upward social mobility, which is especially the case for female ritualist leaders in a male-dominated society.

Africa. Examples of possession-trance cults with such identifiable psychotherapeutic and sociotherapeutic functions are found in Central and West Africa, the Zebola ritual in Zai Senegal (Gravrand 1966; Zempleni 1966), the Bori and Holey cults of Hausa-Songhai cultures (Lombard 1967; Nicolas 1970), and the Orisa cults of the Yoruba of Nigeria (Prince 1964). In Zambia and Malawi, culturally patterned neurotic and psychosomatic disorders are effectively treated in trance dances under the guidance of specialized healers, with participation of the entire village, and in therapeutic possession cults such as the Vimbuza (Kappa 1980; Peltzer 1987). In Somalia, possession cults like the Minghis, Numbi, and Borane, constitute a principal source of therapeutic assistance for those with emotional disturbance (Jaria 1985). In general it can be said that cult dances associated with altered states of consciousness are a key aspect of traditional African psychotherapy (Awanbor 1982). To some extent, the therapeutic functions of traditional trance and possession cults have been taken over by the syncretistic sects and prophetic-messianic churches in parts of Africa (Benz 1965; Daramola 1979; Jilek 1967a; Sundkler 1961), by *spiritist* healing cults among Puerto Ricans (Harwood 1977; Koss 1987; Ruiz 1979), and by spiritualist congregations in Mexico (Bourguignon 1976; Finkler 1981)—all with confirmed effectiveness in neurotic-reactive and psychosomatic conditions.

Brazil and Caribbean nations. The psychotherapeutic and psychohygienic functions of possession-trance cults of Caribbean and Brazilian populations have been well analyzed, especially Haitian Vodun (Jilek-Aall and Jilek 1983; Kiev 1968; Wittkower 1964), a syncretistic amalgamation of traditional West African and European (folk Catholicism, mesmerism) elements; Santeria (Babalu cult) in Cuba (Davidson 1966); Shango in Trinidad (Ward 1979); and the Brazilian Umbanda (Akstein 1966; Figge 1975, 1980; Pressel 1987; Richeport 1987; Stubbe 1979), which derived from traditional Afro-Brazilian cults (Candomble, Macumba, Xango), absorbed Kardecian spiritism, and some Amerindian culture traits to eventually develop into the most popular group therapeutic venture existing today.

North America. In North America, ancient Amerindian cult dance ceremonials have been revived and adjusted to current psychosocial needs. These indigenous group therapeutic endeavors use altered states of consciousness and are especially geared to the effective treatment and prevention of alcohol and drug dependence, cultural change–related dysthymic conditions (anomic depression; Jilek 1974), and psychosomatic disorders. Examples are the Sun Dance ceremonial of Amerindian tribes in Wyoming, Idaho, Utah, Colorado, North and South Dakota; the Winter Spirit Dance of the Salish Indians in British Columbia and Washington State; and the medicine societies of the Iroquois Indians in Canada (Ontario and Quebec) and New York State (False Face, Husk Face, Little Water medicine societies; Jilek 1978).

Arabic-Islamic states. Examples of trance and possession cults with attested group therapeutic functions in the Arabic-Islamic culture area are the Hamadsha of Morocco (Crapanzano 1973) and the Zar. The Zar cult is practiced in Ethiopia, its country of origin, among Moslems and Christians and in many Islamic countries (Somalia, Sudan, Egypt, the Gulf states, Iraq, and Iran), providing effective ritual therapy, especially for female patients with neurotic-reactive and functional disorders (Baasher 1967; El Islam 1967; El Sendiony 1974; Gharagozlou-Hamadani et al. 1981; Kennedy 1967; Messing 1959; Modarressi 1968; Nelson 1971; Okasha 1966; Torrey 1967; Young 1975).

East and Southeast Asia. Examples of effective traditional group therapy using ASC in Southeast and East Asia are the Phii Pha ceremonial in Thailand (Suwanlert and Visuthikosol 1983), Main Puteri in Malaysia (Chen 1979; Kramer 1970), traditional group trance rites in Indonesia (W. Pfeiffer 1971), and the "Salvation Cult" in Japan, which derived from an ancient Shintoist-Buddhist sect (Lebra 1976).

The general conclusion to be drawn from these reports is that the above cited traditional group therapies involving ASC are subjectively and objectively effective methods of symptom removal, restoration of functioning, and social rehabilitation, in the following conditions: 1) neurotic-reactive syndromes such as anxiety states, dysthymia, "hysterical" somatiform and "functional" psychophysiologic disorders; 2) reactive and anomic depression; and 3) alcohol and drug dependence. While patients with acute psychotic reactions have been reported to benefit from participation in certain group therapeutic ceremonials involving ASC, those with chronic schizophrenic processes are not likely to respond with significant remission; exacerbation of psychotic symptoms may in some patients be triggered by induction of ASC.

Indigenous Therapy and Prevention of Alcohol and Drug Dependence

Amerindian Culture

In North America psychosocial and physical problems associated with alcohol abuse have been prevalent among indigenous populations since alcoholic beverages were introduced by European traders in the eighteenth and nineteenth centuries. Commonly observed is the relatively poor response of Amerindian alcohol abusers to Western methods of treatment and rehabilitation, especially the limited appeal of Western-type Alcoholics Anonymous (AA) groups (Jilek-Aall 1978). However, there is evidence that revived traditional Amerindian ceremonials, redefined and adjusted to the therapeutic needs of the younger generation, are successful in combating alcoholism among certain aboriginal peoples of North America.

The success of the *peyote cult* (ritual group therapy using the hallucinogenic peyote cactus *Lophophora williamsii*, in the Native American Church of North America among Amerindian tribes in the United States and Canada east of the Rocky Mountains) in the rehabilitation of alcoholics has been confirmed by Professor K. Menninger and other experts (Albaugh and Anderson 1974; Bergman 1971; Jilek 1978). The observed positive results of the peyote cult with Amerindians dependent on alcohol and opiate drugs have been attributed to the hallucinogenic alkaloids and also to the isoquinoline alkaloids in the peyote cactus (Blum et al. 1977). However, the decisive factor in the anti-alcoholic and antidrug effectiveness of the peyote ritual is primarily due not to the bio- and psychoactive substances in the cactus but to the goal-directed group therapeutic process of the ceremonial. Under the suggestive guidance of the ritualist leaders, the subjective experiences of individual peyote eaters are channeled in a therapeutic ego- and group-strengthening direction.

Comparable results in the rehabilitation of alcohol and drug dependents have been achieved without any psychoactive agents in the revived North American Indian dance ceremonials, notably the Gourd Dance, the Sun Dance, and the Winter Spirit Dance (Jilek 1978). In the Sun Dance ceremonial of Amerindian tribes in Wyoming, Idaho, Utah, Colorado, and North and South Dakota, and in the Winter Spirit Dance of the Salish in British Columbia and Washington State, the initiation process involves the induction and effective utilization of altered states of consciousness. These are brought about by physiological and psychological shamanic techniques. The aim of the initiation is to help the candidate establish a healthy new existence without alcohol and drug use, and to build up a new personal and cultural identity. This is achieved in a symbolic process of ritualized death and rebirth, and through traditional methods of personality depatterning and subsequent resynthesis and reorientation under individual and collective suggestion and didactic guidance. The revived Winter Spirit ceremonial has become a most effective preventive and therapeutic program to combat alcohol and drug dependence among Amerindians in the Pacific Northwestern United States (Jilek 1981, 1982).

Other therapeutic movements among North American indigenous peoples that have been successful in fighting alcohol and drug dependence are the revived Amerindian Sweat Lodge Ceremonial for physical and spiritual fortification (Hall 1986), the Amerindian AA groups organized along traditional cultural patterns (Jilek-Aall 1981), the Alaska Eskimo Spirit Movement (Mala 1985), the still active Handsome Lake Movement Gaiwiio among the Iroquois (Heath 1983; Jilek-Aall 1978), and the Indian Shaker Church in the Pacific Northwestern United States (Barnett 1957; Collins 1950; Gunther 1949; Jilek-Aall 1978).

How can we explain that apparently effective, culture-congenial therapeutic responses to the Amerindian alcohol abuse problem co-exist with the seemingly undiminished problem? The answer has to be sought in the complex and varied sociocultural situation of the contemporary indigenous population of North America. Many Amerindian people have become strangers to their own culture through imposed Westernization, without, however, being fully integrated into the majority society. In this growing population of marginal Amerindians, anomie, relative deprivation, and cultural identity confusion are significant factors contributing to alcohol and drug abuse. The revival of indigenous ceremonials appeals to Amerindians who still maintain ties with their traditional culture and to those who make an effort to return to their aboriginal roots in search of a cultural identity. While the number of traditionally living people is steadily declining, the number of younger people finding their way back to traditional Amerindian spirituality depends on the local situation, on individual motivation, and on the readiness and ability of the native community to inaugurate and support the revival of traditional ceremonials for therapeutic purposes. Many socioculturally isolated and alienated indigenous people, at high risk of alcohol and drug dependence, are still quite removed from the spirit of Amerindian renaissance that has led to the revival of traditional activities in North America.

Latin American Cultures

Puerto Rican espiritismo healers in the United States have established therapeutic centers in which Hispanic alcoholics are effectively rehabilitated by a combination of individual and family counseling, magicoreligious suggestion rituals, and social manipulation (Singer and Borrero 1984). Mexican folk healers treat alcoholics by counseling, social engineering, symbolic ritual acts, and the administration of herbal sedatives (Arredondo et al. 1987; Trotter and Chavira 1978). The use of aversion therapy in alcohol dependence is also known in Latin American ethnomedicine. Herbalists in northern Mexico administer roasted seeds of *haba de San Ignacio* (*Hura polyandra L., Hura crepitans L.*), which contain toxalbumins, to induce nausea and vomiting in conjunction with subsequent consumption of alcohol (Trotter 1979). A similar example of Pavlovian-type deconditioning with emetic herbal teas, to be taken together with alcoholic drinks, is practiced in a healing compound of the Colorado Indians of Ecuador, frequented by rural and urban patients (Jilek-Aall and Jilek 1983). In northern Peru, *curanderos* also use aversion therapy with herbal emetics and laxatives. Prior to this procedure chronic alcoholic patients are admitted to a healing compound and undergo a process of emotional and physical fortification (Chiappe et al. 1972, 1985).

Buddhist Cultures

Traditional methods of detoxification and rehabilitation of opiate addicts are applied in four Buddhist monasteries in Thailand, while a fifth also treats alcoholics (Poshyachinda 1982). Candidates take a solemn vow of abstention upon admission to the treatment, which consists of herbal remedies, steam baths, and spiritual-didactic and work-oriented group therapy. Among these Buddhist addiction treatment centers, Wat Tam Kraborg is known internationally for successful rehabilitation of addicts from inside and outside Thailand, including non-Buddhists. Repeated administration of strongly emetic plant medicines with copious amounts of water, plus herbal steam baths, is purported to clean the patient from the harmful substances he or she was addicted to; it certainly may lead to collapse, induce an altered state of consciousness, and open the way for personality reorientation in a therapeutic milieu (Jilek-Aall and Jilek 1985; Poshyachinda 1980). Comparative case follow-up investigations conducted by the Drug Dependence Research Center of Chulalongkorn University, Bangkok showed that the overall success rates of this indigenous addiction treatment program equaled those of much more expensive modern medical methods. The same conclusion had been reached in a previous study (Westermeyer 1979) comparing long-term therapeutic results in Laotian opiate addicts treated at Wat Tam Kraborg with the results of a medical facility, although at that time (1972–1975) mortality among elderly patients was higher at the monastery (Westermeyer 1979, 1980). During visits in recent years, I (W. G. Jilek) have seen very few elderly patients at Wat Tam Kraborg and overall mortality has declined significantly. Laotian folk treatment of opium addicts by Buddhist monks and traditional herbalists during the 1970s has been described as successful (Westermeyer 1973, 1982).

More recently, the growing opium abuse problem among younger Laotian hill-tribe refugees in camps in northern Thailand has prompted the International Rescue Committee, in consultation with myself (W.G. Jilek) acting as the United Nations refugee mental health coordinator, to integrate traditional shamanic ceremonies into modern detoxification and rehabilitation programs. The active participation of traditional practitioners and the introduction of shamanic rites and sacrifices, with recourse to supernatural sanction of abstinence and ritual burning of opium utensils, has led to a significant increase in the success rate of these programs (Jilek and Jilek-Aall 1990).

In Japan, traditional practices of the Shinshu Buddhist sect have been adapted for the rehabilitation of alcoholics in the form of *naikan* (self-examination therapy), which, complemented by a culture-congenial group approach (*danshukai*) has become a valuable therapeutic resource in the management of alcohol dependence (Suwaki 1979, 1990).

Islamic Cultures

In Malaysia, traditional treatment of substance dependence—mostly opiate addiction but also alcohol abuse—is performed by Islamic Malay, Chinese-Taoist, and Hinduist-Ayurvedic practitioners (Heggenhougen 1984; Heggenhougen and Navaratnam 1979; Johnson 1983; Lee 1985; McGovern 1982; Spencer et al. 1980; Teo Hui Khian 1983; Werner 1979, 1984). The clientele of practitioners with a reputation in drug rehabilitation is not limited to co-religionists. Adaptations of rituals may be made in a tolerant manner to accommodate patients of other religious persuasions.

Islamic traditional healers in Malaysia specializing in drug dependence vary in their methods but follow a common therapeutic pattern. During the initial detoxification phase medicinal teas are given. Some of the herbal ingredients have purgative, astringent, diaphoretic, and sedative properties; others have analgesic and motor activity-decreasing effects conducive to the suppression of withdrawal symptoms. Religious teaching and Koranic texts are employed in symbolic and near-magical ways in the rehabilitation process, which is often buttressed by a solemn oath to abstain from drug use for a specified period. Evaluation of outcome has placed the results of drug addiction treatment by Islamic traditional healers on a par with those of the best modern medical programs offered in Malaysia or elsewhere (Spencer et al. 1980).

In the initial withdrawal phase, concoctions of medicinal plants with apparent calming effects are administered, combined with balneotherapeutic applications. The rehabilitation phase relies on didactic counseling and on rituals and sanctions of a religious or magical character in order to minimize the risk of relapse; all these factors appear to enhance the efficacy of traditional as compared to modern medical modalities of drug dependence therapy (Heggenhougen 1984; Teo Hui Khian 1983).

Traditional drug rehabilitation centers have been established in Malaysia with government encouragement. Treatment follows similar principles, whether the center is run by an Islamic Malay or by a Chinese traditional practitioner, but is adapted to the cultural-religious and medicinal traditions of the respective groups.

The integration of Islamic spiritual approaches in the therapy of drug addiction has been pioneered in Egypt (Abu El Azayem 1987; Baasher and Abu El Azayem 1980) and Saudi Arabia (Al Radi, unpublished manuscript, September 1990). In 1977, a treatment unit for drug addicts was established at Abu El Azayem Mosque in Cairo, in which the religious leader (*sheikh*) assumed special functions in the therapeutic team by holding group meetings, providing religious teaching with emphasis on Islamic injunctions regarding dependence-producing substance use, encouraging the strengthening of social ties, and encouraging mosque-centered activities such as counseling on personal matters and organizing social support. Propagation of anti-drug messages through religious media and during Friday mass prayers served preventive purposes and promoted the rehabilitation of drug addicts in the community. In subsequent years, the number of new cases reporting to the mosque clinic and the compliance rate was found to be significantly higher than at other city clinics without a religious component, while treatment at the mosque clinic was more cost-effective. A comparative double-blind study (Abu El Azayem 1987) showed that substance addicts treated at the mosque clinic realized a significantly higher score of therapeutic objectives than equivalent patients at a "normal" clinic.

The addiction unit at Shahar Hospital, Taif, Saudi Arabia, has for several years now integrated a program of religious therapy in which the mosque is the center of therapeutic activity. Behavioral changes are engendered in group therapy following prayer sessions with joint worship and recitation of the holy scriptures.

The importance of fostering religious motivation as distinct from other motivations in attaining abstinence in Saudi drug addicts was shown in a follow-up study (Al Radi, unpublished manuscript, September 1990) comparing relapse rates in patients of the Shahar Hospital Addiction Unit: 75% of probands with "inner religious considerations" maintained abstinence over 2 years, as compared to 33% of probands motivated by other considerations.

Black-African Religious Movements

The independent Black-African churches of Southern Africa, sometimes named *Zionist*, *Ethiopian*, or *Apostolic*, combine messianic Christianity and pan-African consciousness with traditional elements of Bantu culture and a mandate to heal spiritually, mentally, and physically (Benz 1965; Peltzer 1987; Sundkler 1961). In the Republics of South Africa, Malawi, and Namibia, these churches, often led by charismatic prophet-healers, have a large though rapidly changing membership and considerable sociopolitical influence. Members are subject to proscriptions, which usually include an injunction against the consumption of alcoholic beverages and in many cases against the use of other drugs. This religious prohibition is associated with a readiness to rehabilitate the substance-dependent repentant as a patient in the context of the church's healing mandate, usually without charge beyond general tithing. A confession with free admission of personal problems is expected. In many congregations this is combined with purification rites for the "elimination of all evil," both spiritual and material. Ritual vomiting and body cleansing is used. Counseling is conducted by faith healers and former alcoholic church members; often there is also dream interpretation by authorized leaders.

Summary: The Effectiveness of Traditional Medicine in Psychiatric Disorders

Difficulties of Scientific Evaluation

These referenced reports on the effectiveness of traditional medicine in psychiatric disorders are based on the observations and experience of their authors, rather than on hard scientific evidence, with the exception of the pharmacological action of certain plants used in traditional medicine, as established by scientific laboratory methods (see Appendix 11–1). The scarcity of reported evaluations satisfying the criteria of experimental science is not due to lack of effort or motivation. Rather it is due to the inherent constraints of scientific research in this field:

1. The ceremonies and ritual symbolic acts that are part of most traditional practices are often sacred or arcane. Their divulgence is usually taboo.
2. Experimental research into traditional practices may not only be rejected (as interference), but in many cases alters the situation and those procedural conditions that render a certain ritualized activity therapeutically effective (e.g., conducive to the induction of altered states of consciousness in a ceremonial framework).
3. In many tradition-directed societies, the healer's expertise and knowledge is considered private or family property and is not readily divulged; it is often thought to be ineffective or even dangerous if applied by outsiders.
4. The reluctance of traditional practitioners to reveal information might be based on past experience of discrimination, condemnation, and even prosecution, especially of shamanic healers by political or ecclesiastic authorities. It may also be a reaction to the pseudo-scientific labeling of traditional practitioners as sociopathic and psychologically abnormal (for documentation see Jilek 1971) or to still persisting negative attitudes among Western- and Soviet-trained health professionals.
5. Traditional practitioners commonly use several procedures in their management of a case, often at the same time. It is therefore not always possible to evaluate the merits of a single procedure in order to gauge the general outcome of treatment or the results of involvement in traditional group therapy.

Demonstrated Effectiveness of Tradition-Based Therapeutic Practices

The following conclusions are drawn from reports in the scientific literature cited in this text, and from my (W. G. Jilek) own observations:

1. In general, tradition-based practices provide effective therapeutic management for neurotic disorders (especially with dissociation and conversion symptoms), for psychosomatic and somatoform disorders, for psychosocial problems, and for reactive depressions, including self-destructive behavior (see Asuni 1979; Awanbor 1982; Baddeley 1985; Boyer 1964; Brautigam and Osei 1979; Cheetham and Cheetham 1976; Corin and Bibeau 1980; Dean and Thong 1972; El Islam 1982; Field 1960; Gelfand 1964, 1967; Harding 1975; Hartog and Resner 1972; Harvey 1976; Heinze 1988; Hidayat 1983; Hollweg 1985, 1991; Hooper 1985; Janzen 1978; Jilek 1967b, 1988; Jilek and Jilek-Aall 1983; Jilek and Todd 1974; Kaplan and Johnson 1964; Ketter 1983; Kinzie et al. 1976; Kortmann 1987; Kusumanto and Salan 1986; Lambo 1956; Lapuz 1983; Lebra 1982; Levy 1967; Mahania 1977; Makang Ma Mbog 1969; Makanjuola 1987; Muzaham 1983; Naka 1985; Peltzer 1987, 1988; Peters 1978; Polack-Eltz 1986; Ponce 1986; Prince 1961, 1964; Rappaport 1979; Roeder and Opalic 1987; Salan and Maretzki 1983; Sanua 1979; Seguin 1971, 1979; Shakman 1969; Sich 1980; Suwanlert 1976; Tan et al. 1980; Tan Pariaman 1983; Tella 1979; Tseng 1976; Werner 1984; Young 1976; Zarkasi 1983; Zolla 1982).

2. Traditional medicine practices, ritual procedures, and sedative herbal remedies are effective in the treatment of reactive and transient psychoses and psychosis-like, culture-bound syndromes. Traditional intervention by protective measures and by reassuring, anxiety-alleviating ceremonies involving kinspeople often avoids segregation of the patient from the family. This may prevent chronic psychotic developments, which are known to be less common in tradition-directed than in modern industrialized societies (see Cheetham and Cheetham 1976; Dean and Thong 1972; Field 1960; Harding 1975; Jilek 1988; Jilek and Jilek-Aall 1970; Kaplan and Johnson 1964; Ketter 1983; Kusumanto Setynegoro and Salan 1986; Makanjuola 1987; Ponce 1986; Salan and Maretzki 1983; Seguin 1971, 1979; Young 1976).

3. In the treatment, rehabilitation, and prevention of alcohol and drug dependence, therapeutic practices based on indigenous cultural and religious traditions have, in many instances, been as successful and sometimes more successful than "official" treatment and rehabilita-

tion programs (see Abu El Azayem 1987; Albaugh and Anderson 1974; Al Radi, unpublished manuscript, September 1990; E. N. Anderson, unpublished manuscript, November 1986; Baasher and Abu El Azayem 1980; Bergman 1971; Blum et al. 1977; Chiappe 1970; Chiappe et al. 1972; Hall 1986; Heath 1983; Heggenhougen 1984; Howard 1976; Jilek 1978, 1982; Jilek and Jilek-Aall 1990; Jilek-Aall 1978, 1981; Jilek-Aall and Jilek 1985; Lee 1985; Mala 1984; McGovern 1982; Pascarosa et al. 1976; Peltzer 1987; Poshyachinda 1980, 1982; Roy 1973; Seguin 1974; Singer and Borrero 1984; Spencer et al. 1980; Suwaki 1979, 1980; Trotter 1979; Trotter and Chavira 1978; Werner 1979, 1984; Westermeyer 1973, 1979).

However, because of their specific religious and ethnocultural aspects, the ceremonials involved are not readily accessible to many marginal persons who remain alienated from ethnocultural and religious traditions, although this alienation may be a major factor contributing to substance abuse.

Limited Effectiveness of Tradition-Based Therapeutic Practices

In schizophrenic and manic psychoses, effective tranquilization has been achieved in some areas of Africa and Asia by using medicinal plants with tranquilizing and sedative properties, such as *Rauwolfia spp.*, long before these substances became known in Europe and America (see Appendix 11–1). However, modern neuroleptic medications with specific indications and exact dosage would appear preferable.

Traditional milieu and occupational therapy has led to symptomatic improvement, facilitating the rehabilitation and social reintegration of schizophrenic patients admitted to a healer's house, healing shrine, or compound, instead of to the usually remote psychiatric hospital (Field 1960; Harding 1975; Jilek 1988; Peltzer 1987, 1988; Prince 1961, 1964). The same beneficial effects of traditional milieu therapy in healing shrines or compounds have been reported for some patients with major depression and involutional melancholia (Field 1960; Peltzer 1987).

Nevertheless, the risks of delayed medical treatment and of possible neglect of organic conditions limit the usefulness of traditional practices in most cases of schizophrenic and affective psychoses, if modern health care is locally available.

Negative Effects of Certain Tradition-Based Practices

Delay in establishing effective modern chemotherapy in cases of schizophrenia has been the concern of several authors (Kortmann 1987; Naka 1985; Tan et al. 1980; Tseng 1976; Yeoh 1980).

Some physical procedures carry obvious risks, such as long-term bodily restraint, a cruel treatment often leading to muscular atrophy and skeletal deformity (W. G. Jilek, unpublished photographs, August 1985; Tan Pariaman 1983); exorcism by beating and other aggressive physical means (Jilek 1986); and primitive psychosurgical operations on the head (though these rarely cause complications [Margetts 1967]). Certain herbal treatments entail relative risks due to imprecise dosage, inherent toxicity, or excessive purgation, especially of patients in poor physical condition.

In tradition-based treatments of epileptic seizure disorders, instances of appropriate use of anticonvulsive plant medicine (Watt 1967) are outweighed by many examples of inappropriate case management, leading to punitive isolation, physical harm, and psychiatric complications. Attitudes toward epileptic patients are often governed by the belief that epilepsy is an untreatable, guilt-associated, and contagious affliction (see Jilek and Jilek-Aall 1980; Orley 1970).

Consumer Use of Traditional Medicine

In most non-Western societies, traditional therapeutic resources are the consumers' first resort in mental health problems, and continue to be consulted along with available medical services. Preferential use of traditional medicine resources is a widespread phenomenon in non-Western countries, as documented in the reviewed literature. Reasons for this phenomenon include the following:

1. Traditional medicine is culture-congenial; traditional practitioners are easily accessible, foster kinship and community cohesion, and operate informally and without involving the authorities.

2. In most developing countries, and certainly in rural areas, the alternative to consulting traditional practitioners for mental health problems is not consulting anyone at all, as mental health professionals are not readily available. Local health staff tend to have very little psychiatric expertise and usually very little time to attend to psychiatric problems.

3. In many areas where adequate community mental health services have not been developed, psychiatric treatment is only available by removing the patient to remote or alien institutions where discharge may be delayed for reasons often unrelated to the patient's clinical condition. This erodes kin-group relations, creates or increases social stigma, makes resocialization difficult, and may contribute to chronicity.

Cost-Effectiveness of Traditional Medicine

Costs to the Public

In those psychiatric conditions for which traditional medicine provides effective therapeutic management, utilization of traditional resources is considerably more cost-effective for the general taxpaying public than the official health service system, as public funds need not be invested to maintain or expand it, nor to supply medication. However, traditional treatment is rarely free, and direct costs, often substantial, have to be met by the patient or the patient's family.

In those psychiatric conditions for which traditional medicine practices are relatively ineffective in comparison with modern psychiatric treatment, or where such psychiatric conditions are not recognized and are inappropriately treated by traditional practitioners, the public may have to bear the costs of delayed effective therapeutic management. In cases of damage caused by inappropriate or harmful procedures, the public will have to bear costs of secondary medical intervention, assistance, and rehabilitation.

Costs to the Consumer

Consumer costs of using traditional therapeutic resources vary and are usually individualized. There may be no obligatory fee but an expectation of donations, which may be in kind and according to one's means. Consumer cost is on the average lower than the cost of fees for private medical services. These are, however, often provided free or covered by state insurance schemes.

Cost considerations do not impede consumer use of traditional medicine for psychiatric problems wherever the traditional practices are congenial to the patient's culture and psychiatry is not (Jilek 1983, 1985, 1989). This is evidenced by the survival and revival of traditional healing among non-Western ethnic minorities in Western countries with government-sponsored health services. This is changing, however, because even the Western majority is turning increasingly away from government-sponsored care.

Relationship of Traditional Medicine and Formal Health Services

Official Acceptance or Toleration of Traditional Medicine

Prohibitive restrictions on nonprofessional health care, such as that provided by traditional practitioners, were introduced by European colonial authorities. These are no longer enforced in those countries formerly under French, Belgian, Spanish, and Dutch colonial jurisdiction that have not yet introduced new laws legalizing traditional medicine, and the current situation is one of de facto toleration, and in some countries even official promotion, of traditional healing, although the old laws have not yet been formally repealed (Stepan 1983).

Developing countries with legislation legalizing the practice of traditional medicine or exempting such practice from the prohibition of unauthorized health care under various defined conditions are Mali, Burkina Faso, Sierra Leone, Ghana, Uganda, Tanzania, Lesotho, South Africa, Malaysia, Singapore, Kiribati, Papua New Guinea, Tonga, and Fiji. Similar policies are planned by Algeria and Mongolia.

It is to be noted that in many developing countries legal obstacles to close collaboration between health professionals and traditional healers are still in existence due to unchanged regulations of professional conduct, notwithstanding proclaimed or planned legalization of traditional medicine practices, notwithstanding policy statements in national health plans, and notwithstanding the efforts made by WHO since the conference of Alma Ata 1978 to promote the integrated cooperation of modern and traditional health care resources (see Akerele 1987).

Countries with legally sanctioned co-existence of officially recognized traditional medicine systems and modern medical health care are India, which recognizes Ayurveda, Siddha, and Unani; Pakistan, which recognizes Unani and Ayurveda; Bangladesh, which recognizes Unani and Ayurveda; Sri Lanka, which recognizes Ayurveda; Myanmar, which recognizes "indigenous Burmese medicine"; and Thailand, which recognizes the "old-fashioned art of healing." Countries with a proclaimed policy of integrating officially recognized traditional medicine systems and modern medical health care are Nepal, which recognizes Ayurveda; China, which recognizes traditional Chinese medicine; and Democratic People's Republic of Korea, which recognizes traditional Korean and Chinese medicine.

It is noteworthy however, that, in the above-cited Asian countries, while there is official recognition of certain systems of traditional medicine, nonrecognized forms of traditional medicine, such as shamanic folk healing, have no official status or support.

Countries where the official health care system is based on licensed professionals with recognized academic qualifications and degrees, who enjoy certain exclusive privileges, but where healing by "nonscientific" methods is nevertheless not legally prohibited, are the United Kingdom, Germany, the Netherlands, the Scandinavian countries, the United States, Canada, Australia, and most Latin American lands.

Official Non-Acceptance of Traditional Medicine

Countries with prohibitive legislation reserving the right to provide health care exclusively to physicians, dentists, midwives, and nurses trained at recognized schools and licensed by state-authorized bodies are France, Belgium, Luxembourg, Austria, and the former socialist countries of Eastern Europe. However, in none of these countries are authorities likely to proceed against non-European traditional healers practicing among immigrant or migrant compatriots. The situation in the former Soviet republics is unclear; acceptance of Islamic traditional practices is now promoted in the Muslim republics.

Recommendations

The following recommendations are made regarding the relationship of traditional medicine and formal health services:

1. Universal implementation, at the local level, of a policy of close collaboration between the health/mental health system and traditional medicine in general, and between individual health/mental health professionals and traditional practitioners in particular. This has long been advocated by WHO (Akerele 1987) and has already been formulated in the national health plans of many countries.
2. Creation of local operational frameworks for the exchange of information and for the mutual referral of cases between health/mental health services and traditional medicine resources, based on the criteria of most effective management according to patient and type of disorder.
3. Development of practical guidelines for case screening and mutual referral from health/mental health services to traditional medicine resources and vice versa, in line with the general findings of this overview but adjusted to national, regional, and local situation.

References

Aberle DF: The Peyote Religion Among the Navaho. Chicago, Aldine, 1966

Abu el Azayem GM: A psycho-socio-religious approach to contain substance abuse in Egypt, in Congress Proceedings. Lahore, Pakistan, World Islamic Association for Mental Health, 1987, pp 409–415

Ahyi A: Ethnomedizin, Ethnobotanik und Ethnopharmakologie in Togo. Ethnomedizin/Ethnomedicine (Hamburg) 5:161–170, 1978

Akerele O: The best of both worlds: bringing traditional medicine up to date. Soc Sci Med 24:177–181, 1987

Akstein D: Les trances rituelles brasiliennes et les perspectives de leur application a la psychiatrie et a la medecine psychosomatique. Transcultural Psychiatric Research Review 3:156–158, 1966

Albaugh B, Anderson P: Peyote in the treatment of alcoholism among American Indians. Am J Psychiatry 131:1247–1250, 1974

Arredondo R, Weddige RL, Justice CL, et al: Alcoholism in Mexican-Americans: intervention and treatment. Hosp Community Psychiatry 38:180–183, 1987

Asuni T: Modern medicine and traditional medicine, in African Therapeutic Systems. Edited by Ademuwagun ZA. Waltham, MA, Brandeis University Crossroads Press, 1979, pp 176–181

Awanbor D: The healing process in African psychotherapy. Am J Psychotherapy 36:206–213, 1982

Baasher T: Traditional psychotherapeutic practices in the Sudan. Transcultural Psychiatric Research Review 4:158–160, 1967

Baasher T, Abu el Azayem GM: Egypt (2): the role of the mosque in treatment, in Drug Problems in the Sociocultural Context: A Basis for Policies and Program Planning. Edited by Edwards G, Arif A. Public Health Paper No 73. Geneva, World Health Organization, 1980, pp 131–134

Baddeley J: Traditional healing practices of Rarotonga, Cook Islands, in Healing Practices in the South Pacific. Edited by Parsons C. Honolulu, HI, University of Hawaii Press, 1985, pp 129–143

Baer G: Peruanische Ayahuasca-Sitzungen: Schamanen und Heilbehandlungen, in Ethnopsychotherapie. Edited by Dittrich A, Scharfetter C. Stuttgart, Ferdinand Enke, 1987, pp 70–80

Bannerman R: Traditional medicine in modern health care. World Health Forum 3:8–26, 1982

Bannerman R, Burton J, Wen-Chieh C (eds): Traditional Medicine and Health Care Coverage. Geneva, World Health Organization, 1983

Barnett HG: Indian Shakers: A Messianic Cult of the Pacific Northwest. Carbondale, Southern Illinois University Press, 1957

Bascom W: Ifa Divination: Communication Between Gods and Men in West Africa. Bloomington, Indiana University Press, 1969

Benz E (ed): Messianische Kirchen, Sekten und Bewegungen im heutigen Afrika. Leiden, EJ Brill, 1965

Benzi M: Les derniers adorateurs du Peyotl. Paris, Gallimard, 1972

Bergman R: Navaho peyote use: its apparent safety. Am J Psychiatry 128:695–699, 1971

Bleuler M: Bewusstseinstoerungen in der Psychiatrie, in Bewusstseinsstoerungen. Edited by Staub H, Thoelen H. Stuttgart, Germany, Thieme, 1961, pp 199–213

Blum K, Futterman S, Pascarosa P: Peyote, a potential ethnopharmacologic agent for alcoholism and other drug dependencies: possible biochemical rationale. Clinical Toxicology 11:459–472, 1977

Bourguignon E (ed): Religion, Altered States of Consciousness and Social Change. Columbus, OH, Ohio State University Press, 1973

Bourguignon E: The effectiveness of religious healing movements: a review of recent literature. Transcultural Psychiatric Research Review 13:5–21, 1976

Boyer LB: Folk psychiatry of the Apaches of the Mescalero Indian reservation, in Magic, Faith and Healing. Edited by Kiev A. New York, Free Press, 1964, pp 384–419

Brautigam W, Osei Y: Psychosomatic illness concept and psychotherapy among the Akan of Ghana. Can J Psychiatry 24:451–457, 1979

Burton-Bradley B: Arecaidinism: betel chewing in transcultural perspective. Can J Psychiatry 24:481–488, 1979

Cheetham RWS, Cheetham RJ: Concepts of mental illness amongst the rural Xhosa people in South Africa. Aust N Z J Psychiatry 10:39–45, 1976

Chen P: Main Puteri: an indigenous Kelantanese form of psychotherapy. Int J Soc Psychiatry 25:167–175, 1979

Chiappe M: El tratamiento curanderil del alcoholismo en la Costa Norte del Peru, in Psiquiatria en la America Latina: Anales del V Congreso Latinoamericano de Psiquiatria. Edited by Roselli A. Medicina, Bogota, Colombia, 1970, pp 542–548

Chiappe M: El empleo de alucinogenos en la psiquiatria folklorica, in Psiquiatria Folklorica. Edited by Seguin CA. Lima, Peru, Ermar, 1979, pp 99–108

Chiappe M, Campos Fuentes J, Dragunsky L: Psiquiatria folklorica peruana: el tratamiento del alcoholismo. Acta Psiquiatr Psicol Am Lat 18:385–394, 1972

Chiappe M, Lemlij M, Millones L: Alucinogenos y Shamanismo en el Peru Contemporaneo. Lima, Peru, El Virrey, 1985

Collins JM: The Indian Shaker church. Southwestern Journal of Anthropology 6:399–411, 1950

Corin E: A possession psychotherapy in an urban setting: Zebola in Kinshasa. Soc Sci Med 13B:327–338, 1979

Corin E: La question du sujet dans les therapies de possession. Psychoanalyse—Revue de l'Ecole Belge de Psychanalyse 3:153–166, 1985

Corin E, Bibeau G: Psychiatric perspectives in Africa; part II: the traditional viewpoint. Transcultural Psychiatric Research Review 17:205–223, 1980

Crapanzano V: The Hamadsha: A Study in Moroccan Ethnopsychiatry. Berkeley, University of California Press, 1973

Daramola SO: The traditional treatment of the psychiatric patient in Nigeria. Journal of Psychiatric Nursing and Mental Health Services 17:28–34, 1979

Davidson W: Psychiatric significance of trance cults. Transcultural Psychiatric Research Review 3:45–49, 1966

Dean S, Thong D: Shamanism versus psychiatry in Bali, isle of the gods. Am J Psychiatry 129:59–62, 1972

Devisch R: Towards a semantic study of divination. Bijdragen, Tijdschrift voor Filosofie en Theologie 39:173–189, 270–288, 1978

Dittrich A, Scharfetter C (eds): Ethnopsychotherapie. Stuttgart, Ferdinand Enke, 1987

Dobkin de Rios M: Hallucinogens: Cross-cultural Perspectives. Albuquerque, University of New Mexico Press, 1984

Edgerton R: A traditional African psychiatrist. Southwestern Journal of Anthropology 27:259–278, 1971

Eliade M: Shamanism: Archaic Techniques of Ecstasy. London, Routledge & Kegan Paul, 1964

El Islam MF: The psychotherapeutic basis of some Arab rituals. Int J Soc Psychiatry 13:265–268, 1967

El Islam MF: Arabic cultural psychiatry. Transcultural Psychiatric Research Review 19:5–24, 1982

El Sendiony M: The problem of cultural specificity of mental illness: the Egyptian mental disease and the Zar ceremony. Aust N Z J Psychiatry 8:103–107, 1974

Evans-Pritchard EE: Witchcraft, Oracles and Magic Among the Azande. Oxford, England, Oxford University & Clarendon Press, 1937

Fernandez JW: Tabernanthe iboga: narcotic ecstasis and the work of the ancestors, in Flesh of the Gods: The Ritual Use of Hallucinogens. Edited by Furst P. New York, Praeger, 1972, pp 237–260

Field MJ: Search for Security: An Ethnopsychiatric Study of Rural Ghana. Chicago, Northwestern University Press, 1960

Figge H: Spirit possession and healing cult among the Brasilian Umbanda. Psychother Psychosom 25:246–250, 1975

Figge H: Funktionen der Therapieversuche in der brasilianischen Umbanda. Curare (Heidelberg) 3:159–164, 1980

Finkler K: Non-medical treatments and their outcomes; part two: focus on adherents of spiritualism. Cult Med Psychiatry 5:65–103, 1981

Gelfand M: Witch Doctor: Traditional Medicine Man of Rhodesia. London, Harvill Press, 1964

Gelfand M: Psychiatric disorders as recognized by the Shona. Cent Afr J Med 13:39–46, 1967

Gharagozlou-Hamadani H, Foulks E, Sherif M, et al: Zar healing in South Iran. Journal of Operational Psychiatry 12:127–131, 1981

Gravrand H: Le "Lup" Serer. Psychopathologie Africaine 2:195–226, 1966

Gunther E: The Shaker religion of the Northwest, in Indians of the Urban Northwest. Edited by Smith MW. New York, Columbia University Press, 1949, pp 37–76

Guthrie G, Szanton D: Folk diagnosis and treatment of schizophrenia: bargaining with the spirits in the Philippines, in Culture-Bound Syndromes, Ethnopsychiatry and Alternate Therapies. Edited by Lebra W. Honolulu, HI, University of Hawaii Press, 1976, pp 148–163

Hall R: Alcohol treatment in American Indian populations: an indigenous treatment modality compared with traditional approaches. Ann N Y Acad Sci 472:168–178, 1986

Harding TW: Traditional healing methods for mental disorders. World Health Organization Chronicle 31:436–440, 1975

Harner M: Hallucinogens and Shamanism. New York, Oxford University Press, 1973

Hartog J, Resner G: Malay folk treatment concepts and practices, with special reference to mental disorders. Ethnomedizin/Ethnomedicine (Hamburg) 1:353–372, 1972

Harvey YK: The Korean Mudang as a household therapist, in Culture-Bound Syndromes, Ethnopsychiatry and Alternate Therapies. Edited by Lebra W. Honolulu, HI, University Press of Hawaii, 1976, pp 189–198

Harwood A: Puerto Rican spiritism. Cult Med Psychiatry 1:69–95, 1977

Heath DB: Alcohol use among North American Indians: a cross-cultural survey of patterns and problems, in Research Advances in Alcohol and Drug Problems, Vol 7. Edited by Smart RG, Glaser FB, Israel Y, et al. New York, Plenum Press, 1983, pp 343–396

Heggenhougen HK: Traditional medicine and the treatment of drug addicts: three examples from Southeast Asia. Medical Anthropology Quarterly 16:3–7, 1984

Heggenhougen HK, Navaratnam V: A General Overview on the Practices Relating to the Traditional Treatment of Drug Dependence in Malaysia. Minden, Penang, National Drug Dependence Research Center, University of Science Malaysia, 1979

Heinze RI: Trance and Healing in Southeast Asia Today. Bangkok, Thailand, White Lotus, 1988

Hidayat MD: Traditional treatment in psychiatry in the Minahasa, in Traditional Healing Practices. Edited by Kusumanto S, Roan WM. Jakarta, Indonesia, Directorate of Mental Health, Ministry of Health, Republic of Indonesia, 1983, pp 433–437

Hofmann A: Die heiligen Pilze in der Heilbehandlung der Maria Sabina, in Ethnopsychiatry. Edited by Dittrich A, Scharfetter C. Stuttgart, Germany, Ferdinand Enke, 1987, pp 45–52

Holdsworth D: Medicinal Plants of Papua New Guinea. Technical paper no 175. Noumea, New Caledonia, South Pacific Commission, 1977

Hollweg MG: La 'locura' en los indigenas y mestizos Bolivianos. Revista de Humanidades, Ciencias Sociales y Relaciones Internacionales (Bolivia) 1:19–27, 1985

Hollweg MG: Locura, Cultura y Magia. Santa Cruz de la Sierra, Bolivia, Centro de Salud Mental, 1991

Holmstedt B, Lindgren JE: Chemical constituents and pharmacology of South American snuffs, in Ethnopharmacologic Search for Psychoactive Drugs. Edited by Efron D. Public Health Service publication no 1645. US Dept of Health, Education, and Welfare. Washington, DC, US Government Printing Office, 1967, pp 339–372

Hooper A: Tahitian healing, in Healing Practices in the South Pacific. Edited by Parsons C. Honolulu, HI, University of Hawaii Press, 1985, pp 158–189

Howard JH: The plains Gourd Dance as a revitalization movement. American Ethnologist 3:243–259, 1976

Janzen J: The Quest for Therapy in Lower Zaire. Berkeley, CA, University of California Press, 1978

Jaria A: Considerazioni sul problema della 'malattia mentale' e della medicina tradizionale in Somalia. Africa (Istituto Italo-Africano) 40:459–469, 1985

Jilek WG: Mental health and magic beliefs in changing Africa, in Contributions to Comparative Psychiatry, Part II. Edited by Petrilowitsch N. Basel, Switzerland, Karger, 1967a, pp 138–154

Jilek WG: The image of the African medicine-man, in Contributions to Comparative Psychiatry, Part II. Edited by Petrilowitsch N. Basel, Switzerland, Karger, 1967b, pp 165–178

Jilek WG: From crazy witchdoctor to auxiliary psychotherapist: the changing image of the medicine man. Psychiatria Clinica 4:200–220, 1971

Jilek WG: Salish Indian Mental Health and Culture Change. Toronto, ONT, Holt, Rinehart & Winston, 1974

Jilek WG: Native renaissance: the survival and revival of indigenous therapeutic ceremonials among North American Indians. Transcultural Psychiatric Research Review 15:117–147, 1978

Jilek WG: Anomic depression, alcoholism and a culture-congenial Indian response. J Stud Alcohol (suppl) 9:159–170, 1981

Jilek WG: Indian Healing: Shamanic Ceremonialism in the Pacific Northwest Today. Surrey, British Columbia, Hancock House, 1982

Jilek WG: Renaissance of folk healing and shamanism: a matter of worldwide interest. Curare (Heidelberg) 6:271–272, 1983

Jilek WG (ed): Traditional Medicine and Primary Health Care in Papua New Guinea. Port Moresby-Waigani, World Health Organization & University of Papua New Guinea Press, 1985

Jilek WG: Epidemics of "genital shrinking" koro: historical review and report of a recent outbreak in South China. Curare (Heidelberg) 9:269–282, 1986

Jilek WG: The impact of alcohol on small-scale societies in the circum-Pacific region. Curare (Heidelberg) 10:151–168, 1987

Jilek WG: Mental health, ethnopsychiatry and traditional medicine in the Kingdom of Tonga. Curare (Heidelberg) 11:161–176, 1988

Jilek WG: Therapeutic use of altered states of consciousness in contemporary North American Indian dance ceremonials, in Altered States of Consciousness and Mental Health. Edited by Ward C. Newbury Park, CA, Sage, 1989, pp 167–185

Jilek WG, Jilek-Aall L: Psychiatric concepts and conditions in the Wapogoro tribe of Tanganyika, in Contributions to Comparative Psychiatry, Part I. Edited by Petrilowitsch N. Basel, Switzerland, Karger, 1967, pp 205–228

Jilek WG, Jilek-Aall L: Transient psychoses in Africans. Psychiatria Clinica 3:337–364, 1970

Jilek WG, Jilek-Aall L: Die soziale Stellung des Epileptikers: eine trans-kulturell-historische Studie, in Psychopathologie im Kulturvergleich . Edited by Pfeiffer WM, Schoene W. Stuttgart, Ferdinand Enke, 1980, pp 184–202

Jilek WG, Jilek-Aall L: Shamanic symbolism in Salish Indian rituals, in The Logic of Culture. Edited by Rossi I. South Hadley, MA: JF Bergin, 1982, pp 127–136

Jilek WG, Jilek-Aall L: Veraenderungen traditioneller Heilkulte unter westlichem Einfluss: kulturgemaesse Behandlung von Neurotikern und Suchtkranken in Thailand und bei nordamerikanischen Indianern, in Ethnomedizin und Medizingeschichte. Edited by Sterly J. Berlin, Mensch und Leben, 1983, pp 311–323

Jilek WG, Jilek-Aall L: The mental health relevance of traditional medicine and shamanism in refugee camps of northern Thailand. Curare (Heidelberg) 13:217–224, 1990

Jilek WG, Knaub C: Patterns of traditional medicine practice in Papua New Guinea: three paradigms, in Traditional Medicine and Primary Health Care in Papua New Guinea. Edited by Jilek WG. Port Moresby-Waigani, Papua New Guinea, World Health Organization & University of Papua New Guinea Press, 1985, pp 122–128

Jilek WG, Todd N: Witchdoctors succeed where doctors fail: psychotherapy among Coast Salish Indians. Canadian Psychiatric Association Journal 19:351–356, 1974

Jilek-Aall L: Geisteskrankheiten und Epilepsie im tropischen Afrika. Fortschr Neurol Psychiatr 32:213–259, 1964

Jilek-Aall L: Alcohol and the Indian-White relationship. Confinia Psychiatrica 21:195–233, 1978

Jilek-Aall L: Acculturation, alcoholism and Indian-style Alcoholics Anony-mous. J Stud Alcohol (suppl) 9:143–158, 1981

Jilek-Aall L, Jilek WG: Therapeutischer Synkretismus in Latein-Amerikanischen Heilkulten, in Ethnomedizin und Medizingeschichte. Edited by Sterly J. Berlin, Mensch und Leben, 1983, pp 297–310

Jilek-Aall L, Jilek WG: Buddhist temple treatment of narcotic addiction and neurotic-psychosomatic disorders in Thailand, in Psychiatry: The State of the Art, Vol 8. Edited by Pichot P, Berner P, Wolf R, et al. New York, Plenum, 1985, pp 673–677

Johnson SH: Treatment of drug abusers in Malaysia: a comparison Int J Addict 18:951–958, 1983

Kaplan B, Johnson D: The social meaning of Navaho psychopathology and psy-chotherapy, in Magic, Faith and Healing. Edited by Kiev A. New York, Free Press, 1964, pp 203–229

Kappa P: The role of the traditional healer in Malawi and Zambia. Curare (Heidelberg) 3:205–208, 1980

Kennedy J: Nubian Zar ceremonies as psychotherapy. Human Organization 26:185–194, 1967

Ketter T: Cultural stylization and mental illness in Bali. Transcultural Psychiatric Research Review 20:87–106, 1983

Kiev A: The psychotherapeutic value of spirit possession in Haiti, in Trance and Possession States. Edited by Prince R. Montreal, Canada, RM Bucke Memorial Society, 1968, pp 143–155

Kiev A: Transcultural Psychiatry. New York, Free Press, 1972

Kinzie D, Teoh JI, Tan ES: Native healers in Malaysia in Culture-bound Syndromes, Ethnopsychiatry and Alternate Therapies. Edited by Lebra W. Honolulu, HI, University Press of Hawaii, 1976, pp 130–146

Kortmann F: Popular, traditional and professional mental health care in Ethiopia. Transcultural Psychiatric Research Review 24:255–274, 1987

Koss J: Expectations and outcomes for patients given mental health care or spiritist healing in Puerto Rico. Am J Psychiatry 144:56–61, 1987

Kramer B: Psychotherapeutic implications of a traditional healing ceremony: the Malaysian Main Puteri. Transcultural Psychiatric Research Review 7:149–151, 1970

Kusumanto Setyonegoro R, Salan R: Investigations into the psycho-sociocultural factors involved in traditional healing mechanisms in three geographical areas in Indonesia: Palembang, Semarang and Bali 1982. Curare (Heidelberg) special vol 5:299–310, 1986

Lambo TA: Neuropsychiatric observations in the western region of Nigeria. BMJ 2:1388–1394, 1956

Lapuz L: Psychosomatic illness and the herbolario, in Traditional Healing Practices. Edited by Kusumanto Setyonegoro R, Roan WM. Jakarta, Indonesia, Directorate of Mental Health, Ministry of Health, Republic of Indonesia, 1983, pp 110–114

Lebra TS: Taking the role of supernatural "other": spirit possession in a Japanese healing cult, in Culture-Bound Syndromes, Ethnopsychiatry and Alternate Therapies. Edited by Lebra W. Honolulu, HI, University Press of Hawaii, 1976, pp 88–100

Lebra W: Shaman-client interchange in Okinawa: performative stages in shamanic therapy, in Cultural Conceptions of Mental Health and Therapy. Edited by Marsella AJ, White GM. Dordrecht, Holland, D Reidel, 1982, pp 303–315

Lee RLM: Alternative systems in Malaysian drug rehabilitation: organization and control in comparative perspective. Soc Sci Med 21:1289–1296, 1985

Lemlij M: Primitive group treatment. Psychiatria Clinica 11:10–14, 1978

Levi-Strauss C: Structural Anthropology. New York, Basic Books, 1963

Levy R: Tahitian folk psychotherapy. International Mental Health Research Newsletter 9:12–15, 1967

Lombard J: Les cultes de possession en Afrique noire et le Bori Hausa. Psychopathologie Africaine 3:419–439, 1967

Ludwig A: Altered states of consciousness. Arch Gen Psychiatry 15:225–234, 1966

Mahania KM: La psychotherapie dans le systeme medical traditionel et le prophetisme chez les Kongo du Zaire. Psychopathologie Africaine 13:149–196, 1977

Makang Ma Mbog M: Essai de comprehension de la dynamique des psychotherapies africaines traditionelles. Psychopathologie Africaine 5:303–354, 1969

Makanjuola ROA: Yoruba traditional healers in psychiatry. Afr J Med Med Sci 16:53–59, 1987

Mala T: Alcoholism and mental health treatment in circumpolar areas: traditional and non-traditional approaches, in Circumpolar Health 84. Edited by R Fortuine. Seattle, WA, University of Washington Press, 1984, pp 332–334

Mala T: Alaska native "grass roots" movement: problem solving utilizing indigenous values. Arctic Med Res 40:84–91, 1985

Margetts E: Trepanation of the skull by the medicine-men of primitive cultures, with particular reference to present-day native East African practice, in Diseases in Antiquity. Edited by Brothwell D, Sandison AT. Springfield, IL, Charles C Thomas, 1967, pp 673–701

McGovern MP: Alcoholism in Southeast Asia: prevention and treatment. Int J Soc Psychiatry 28:36–44, 1982

McKenna D: On the comparative ethnopharmacology of malpighiaceous and myristacaceous hallucinogens. J Psychoactive Drugs 17:35–39, 1985

Messing S: Group therapy and social status in the Zar cult of Ethiopia, in Culture and Mental Health. Edited by Opler M. New York, Macmillan, 1959, pp 319–332

Meyer HJ: Pharmacology of Kava, in Ethnopharmacologic Search for Psychoactive Drugs. Edited by Efron D. Public Health Service publication no 1645. US Dept of Health, Education and Welfare. Washington, DC, US Government Printing Office, 1967, pp 133–140

Modarressi T: The Zar cult in South Iran, in Trance and Possession States. Edited by Prince R. Montreal, Canada, RM Bucke Memorial Society, 1968, pp 149–155

Monfouga-Broustra J: Phenomene de possession et plante hallucinogene. Psychopathologie Africaine 12:317–348, 1976

Muzaham F: The use of traditional healing practice, in Traditional Healing Practices. Edited by Kusumanto Setyonegoro R, Roan WM. Jakarta, Indonesia, Directorate of Mental Health, Ministry of Health, Republic of Indonesia, 1983, pp 406–417

Naka K: Yuta shamanism and community mental health on Okinawa. Int J Soc Psychiatry 31:267–274, 1985

Naranjo C: Psychotropic properties of the harmala alkaloids, in Ethnopharmacologic Search for Psychoactive Drugs. Edited by Efron D. Public Health Service publication no 1645. US Dept of Health, Education and Welfare. Washington, DC, US Government Printing Office, 1967, pp 385–391

Nebelkopf E: Herbal therapy in the treatment of drug use. Int J Addict 22:695–717, 1987

Nelson C: Self, spirit possession and world view: an illustration from Egypt. Int J Soc Psychiatry 17:194–209, 1971

Nicolas J: Culpabilite, somatisation et catharsis au sein d'un culte de possession: le Bori Hausa. Psychopathologie Africaine 6:147–180, 1970

Okasha A: A cultural psychiatric study of El-Zar cult in the United Arab Republic. Br J Psychiatry 112:1217–1221, 1966

Orley JH: Culture and Mental Illness. Nairobi, Kenya, East African Publishing House, 1970

Pascarosa P, Futterman S, Halsweig M: Observations of alcoholics in the peyote ritual: a pilot study, in Work in Progress on Alcoholism. Edited by Seixas F, Eggleston S. Ann N Y Acad Sci 273:518–524, 1976

Peltzer K: Some Contributions of Traditional Healing Practices Towards Psychosocial Health Care in Malawi. Frankfurt, Germany, Fachbuchhandlung fuer Psychologie, 1987

Peltzer K: The role of traditional and faith healers in primary mental health care: a southern African perspective. Curare (Heidelberg) 11:207–210, 1988

Peters L: Psychotherapy in Tamang shamanism. Ethos 6:63–91, 1978

Pfeiffer CC, Murphree HB, Goldstein L: Effect of Kava in normal subjects and patients, in Ethnopharmacologic Search for Psychoactive Drugs. Edited by Efron D. Public Health Service publication no 1645. US Dept of Health, Education and Welfare. Washington, DC, US Government Printing Office, 1967, pp 155–160

Pfeiffer W: Transkulturelle Psychiatrie. Stuttgart, Germany, Georg Thieme, 1971

Pineda DFL: Curanderismo y Brujeria en la Costa Peruana. Lima, Peru, Lytograf, 1986

Polack-Eltz A: Folk medicine in Venezuela. Curare (Heidelberg) special vol 5:75–80, 1986

Ponce OV: Hampicamayoc: Medicina Folklorica y su Substrato Aborigen en el Peru. Lima, Peru, Universidad Nacional Mayor de San Marcos, 1986

Ponglux D, Wongseripipatana S, Hadungcharoen T: Medicinal Plants. Bangkok, Thailand, First Princess Chulaborn Science Congress, Medicinal Plants Exhibition Committee, 1987

Poshyachinda V: Thailand: treatment at the Tam Kraborg temple, in Drug Problems in the Sociocultural Context: A Basis for Policies and Program Planning. Edited by Edwards G, Arif A. Public Health Papers no 73. Geneva, Switzerland, World Health Organization, 1980, pp 121–125

Poshyachinda V: Indigenous Drug Dependence Treatment in Thailand. Bangkok, Thailand, Drug Dependence Research Center, Institute of Health Research, Chulalongkorn University, 1982

Pressel EL: Heilungszeremonien in den Kulten von Umbanda Brasilien und Voodoo Haiti, in Ethnopsychotherapie. Edited by Dittrich A, Scharfetter C. Stuttgart, Germany, Ferdinand Enke, 1987, pp 102–113

Prince R: Some notes on Yoruba native doctors and their management of mental illness, in First Pan-African Psychiatric Conference, Abeokuta, Nigeria. Edited by Lambo TA. Ibadan, Nigeria, Government Printer, 1961, pp 279–288

Prince R: Indigenous Yoruba psychiatry, in Magic, Faith and Healing. Edited by Kiev A. New York, Free Press, 1964, pp 84–120

Prince R: Possession cults and social cybernetics, in Trance and Possession States. Edited by Prince R. Montreal, Canada, RM Bucke Memorial Society, 1968, pp 157–165

Prince R: The problem of spirit possession as a treatment for psychiatric disorder. Ethos 2:315–333, 1974

Prince R: Symbols and psychotherapy: the example of Yoruba sacrificial ritual. J Am Acad Psychoanal 3:321–338, 1975

Prins M: Tabernanthe iboga, die vielseitige Droge Aequatorial-Westafrikas: Divination, Initiation und Bessessenheit bei den Mitsogho in Gabun, in Ethnopsychotherapie. Edited by Dittrich A, Scharfetter C. Stuttgart, Ferdinand Enke, 1987, pp 53–69

Prinz A: Die traditionelle Heilkunde der Azande Nordost-Zaires. Mitteilungen der Oesterreichischen Gesellschaft fuer Tropenmedizin und Parasitologie 6:143–155, 1984

Rappaport H, Dent P: An analysis of contemporary East African folk psychotherapy. Br J Med Psychol 52:49–54, 1979

Reynolds B: Magic, Divination and Witchcraft Among the Barotse of Northern Rhodesia. London, Chatto Windus, 1963

Richeport M: Hypnose als Heilverfahren in aussereuropaeischen Gesellschaften Das Beispiel Brasilien, in Ethnopsychotherapie. Edited by Dittrich A, Scharfetter C. Stuttgart, Germany, Ferdinand Enke, 1987, pp 81–89

Roeder F, Opalic P: Der Einfluss des Hodschas magischer Heiler auf tuerkische psychiatrische Patienten in der Bundesrepublik. Psychiatr Prax 14:157–162, 1987

Roy C: Indian peyotists and alcohol. Am J Psychiatry 130:329–330, 1973

Ruiz P: Spiritism, mental health and the Puerto Ricans: an overview. Transcultural Psychiatric Research Review 16:8–43, 1979

Salan R, Maretzki T: Mental health services and traditional healing in Indonesia: are the roles compatible? Cult Med Psychiatry 7:377–412, 1983

Sanua V: Psychological intervention in the Arab world: a review of folk treatment. Transcultural Psychiatric Research Review 16:205–208, 1979

Sargant W: Witchdoctoring, Zar and Voodoo: their relation to modern psychiatric treatment. Proceedings of the Royal Society of Medicine 60:1055–1060, 1967

Sartorius N: Crosscultural psychiatry, in Psychiatrie der Gegenwart, Vol 1: Grundlagen und Methoden der Psychiatrie, Part I. Edited by Kisker KP. Berlin/Heidelberg, Springer, 1979, pp 711–737

Schultes RE: An overview of hallucinogens in the western hemisphere, in Flesh of the Gods: The Ritual Use of Hallucinogens. Edited by Furst P. New York, Praeger, 1972, pp 3–54

Seguin CA: Papel y funcion del curandero en la sociedad. Latino–Americana. Transcultural Psychiatric Research Review 8:81–83, 1971

Seguin CA: What folklore psychotherapy can teach us. Psychotherapy and Psychosomatics 24:293–302, 1974

Seguin CA (ed): Psiquiatria Folklorica. Lima, Peru, Ermar, 1979

Shakman R: Indigenous healing of mental illness in the Philippines. Int J Soc Psychiatry 15:279–287, 1969

Sharon D: The San Pedro cactus in Peruvian folk healing, in Flesh of the Gods: The Ritual Use of Hallucinogens. Edited by Furst P. New York, Praeger, 1972, pp 114–135

Sich D: Ein Beitrag zur Volksmedizin und zum Schamanismus in Korea. Curare (Heidelberg) 3:209–216, 1980

Singer M, Borrero M: Indigenous treatment of alcoholism: the case of Puerto Rican spiritism. Med Anthropol 8:246–273, 1984

Sofowora A: Medicinal Plants and Traditional Medicine in Africa. Chichester, England, John Wiley, 1982

Spencer CP, Heggenhougen HK, Navaratnam V: Traditional therapies and the treatment of drug dependence in Southeast Asia. Am J Chin Med 8:230–238, 1980

Stepan J: Patterns of legislation concerning traditional medicine, in Traditional Medicine and Health Care Coverage. Edited by Bannerman RH, Burton J, Wen-Chieh C. Geneva, Switzerland, World Health Organization, 1983, pp 290–313

Stubbe H: Zur Ethnopsychiatrie in Brasilien. Soc Psychiatry 14:187–195, 1979

Stumpfe KD: Die Heilmethoden der Medizinmaenner. Curare 6:25–31, 1983

Sundkler BGM: Bantu Prophets in South Africa. London, Oxford University Press, 1961

Suwaki H: Naikan and Danshukai for the treatment of Japanese alcoholic patients. Br J Addict 74:15–20, 1979

Suwaki H: Culturally based treatment of alcoholism, in Drug Problems in the Sociocultural Context: A Basis for Policies and Program Planning. Edited by Edwards G, Arif A. Public Health Papers no 73. Geneva, Switzerland, World Health Organization, 1980, pp 139–143

Suwanlert S: Phii Pob: spirit possession in rural Thailand, in Culture-Bound Syndromes, Ethnopsychiatry and Alternate Therapies. Edited by Lebra W. Honolulu, HI, University Press of Hawaii, 1976, pp 68–87

Suwanlert S, Visuthikosol Y: Phii Pha: folk group psychotherapy in northeast of Thailand, in Traditional Healing Practices. Edited by Kusumanto Setyonegoro R, Roan WM. Jakarta, Indonesia, Directorate of Mental Health, Ministry of Health, Republic of Indonesia, 1983, pp 142–146

Tan CT, Chee KT, Long FY: Psychiatric patients who seek traditional healers in Singapore. Singapore Med J 21:643–647, 1980

Tan Pariaman HHBS: Traditional healing in Indonesia, in Traditional Healing Practices. Edited by Kusumanto Setyonegoro R, Roan WM. Jakarta, Indonesia, Directorate of Mental Health, Ministry of Health, Republic of Indonesia, 1983, pp 147–155

Tart C (ed): Altered States of Consciousness. New York, John Wiley, 1969

Tella A: The practice of traditional medicine in Africa. Nigerian Medical Journal 9:607–612, 1979

Teo Hui Khian: Traditional healing: some observations of its use in drug addiction in West Malaysia, in Traditional Healing Practices. Edited by Kusumanto Setyonegoro R, Roan WM. Jakarta, Indonesia, Directorate of Mental Health, Ministry of Health, Republic of Indonesia, 1983, pp 105–114

Torrey EF: The Zar cult in Ethiopia. Int J Soc Psychiatry 13:216–223, 1967

Torrey EF: The Mind Game: Witchdoctors and Psychiatrists. New York: Emerson Hall, 1972

Trotter RT: Evidence of an ethnomedical form of aversion therapy on the United States-Mexico border. J Ethnopharmacol 1:279–284, 1979

Trotter RT, Chavira JA: Discovering new models for alcohol counseling in minority groups, in Modern Medicine and Medical Anthropology in the United States-Mexico Border Population. Edited by Velimirovic B. Scientific Publication no 359. Washington, DC, Pan American Health Organization/Regional Office of the World Health Organization, 1978, pp 164–171

Tseng WS: Folk psychiatry in Taiwan in, Culture-Bound Syndromes, Ethnopsychiatry and Alternate Therapies. Edited by Lebra W. Honolulu, HI, University Press of Hawaii, 1976, pp 164–177

Turner N: Traditional use of devil's club Oplopanax horridus; Araliaceae by native peoples in western North America. Journal of Ethnobiology 2:17–38, 1982

Walker S: Ceremonial Spirit Possession in Africa and Afro-America. Leiden, Netherlands, EJ Brill, 1972

Ward C: Therapeutic aspects of ritual trance: the Shango cult in Trinidad. Journal of Altered States of Consciousness 5:19–29, 1979

Ward C (ed): Altered States of Consciousness and Mental Health. Newbury Park, CA, Sage, 1989

Wassens SH: Anthropological survey of the use of South American snuffs, in Ethnopharmacologic Search for Psychoactive Plants. Edited by Efron D. Public Health Servive publication no 1645. US Dept of Health, Education and Welfare. Washington, DC, US Government Printing Office, 1967, pp 233–289

Wasson RG: Fly agaric and man, in Ethnopharmacologic Search for Psychoactive Plants. Edited by Efron D. Public Health Servive publication no 1645. US Dept of Health, Education and Welfare. Washington, DC, US Government Printing Office, 1967, pp 405–414

Wasson RG: What was the Soma of the Aryans? in Flesh of the Gods: The Ritual Use of Hallucinogens. Edited by Furst P. New York, Praeger, 1972, pp 201–213

Watt J: African plants potentially useful in mental health. Lloydia 30:1–22, 1967

Werner R: Die Behandlung von malaysischen Drogenabhaengigen mit den Methoden der traditionellen Medizin. Oeffentliches Gesundheitswesen 41:332–343, 1979

Werner R: Bomoh, Dukun, Poyang: The Wisdom of Traditional Medicine of West Malaysia. Kuala Lumpur, Malaysia, University of Malaya Press, 1984

Westermeyer J: Folk treatment for opium addiction in Laos. Br J Addict 68:345–349, 1973

Westermeyer J: Medical and nonmedical treatment for narcotic addicts: a comparative study from Asia. J Nerv Ment Dis 167:205–210, 1979

Westermeyer J: Treatment for narcotic addiction in a Buddhist monastery. Journal of Drug Issues 10:221–228, 1980

Westermeyer J: Poppies, Pipes, and People. Berkeley, CA, University of California Press, 1982

Wittkower E: Spirit possession in Haitian Vodun ceremonies. Acta Psychotherapeutica 12:72–80, 1964

Wyatt TA: Therapeutic uses of betel nut in Papua New Guinean traditional medicine, in Traditional Medicine and Primary Health Care in Papua New Guinea. Edited by Jilek WG. Port Moresby-Waigani, Papua New Guinea, World Health Organization & University of Papua New Guinea Press, 1985, pp 79–96

Yeoh OH: Malay psychiatric patients and traditional healers Bomohs. Med J Malaysia 34:349–357, 1980

Young A: Why Amhara get Kureynya: sickness and possession in an Ethiopian Zar cult. American Ethnologist 2:567–584, 1975

Young A: Internalizing and externalizing medical belief systems: an Ethiopian example. Soc Sci Med 10:147–156, 1976

Zarkasi M: A preliminary exploratory study on three traditional healing practices in Jakarta, in Traditional Healing Practices. Edited by Kusumanto Setyonegoro R, Roan WM. Jakarta, Indonesia, Directorate of Mental Health, Ministry of Health, Republic of Indonesia, 1983, pp 270–289

Zempleni A: La dimension therapeutique du cult des Rab. Psychopathologie Africaine 2:295–439, 1966

Zolla E: Lo sciamanesimo Coreano. Conoscenza Religiosa Florence 76(3/4):392–407, 1982

Phytotherapeutica

1. Sedatives / Tranquilizers

Plants with scientifically established effective sedative/tranquilizing properties. These plants are used in traditional medicine. Their side effects are dose dependent and controllable by experienced practitioners. *Rauwolfia. Rauwolfia spp.* contain many bioactive alkaloids, including reserpine. *Rauwolfia serpentina* is used in Ayurvedic medicine and in Thai (Ponglux et al. 1987) and Japanese traditional treatment of agitation, anxiety, and restlessness. *Rauwolfia vomitoria* root powders or decoctions are well-known tranquilizing remedies in the indigenous treatment of psychotics in West and Central Africa (e.g., Yoruba, Togolese, Azande) (Ahyi 1978; Sofowora 1982; Watt 1967). *Boophone disticha* (bulbs containing hyoscine-like alkaloids) are hypnotic and are used in Cape Bantu medicine. *Conopharyngia pachysiphon,* root bark medicines, control maniform behavior (used in Nigeria, Ghana). *Dioscorea spp.* (containing dioscorine, diosgenine), is used in many parts of Africa. *Fagara xanthoxyloides*, a soporific, is used in Nigeria, Guinea (Watt 1967). *Limosella major*, a soporific used in Hehe medicine, is used in Tanzania (Edgerton 1971). *Morinda citrifolia fruit* (containing anthraquinones with sedative action), is used in Tongan folk medicine management of hysterical and psychotic states (Jilek 1988). *Moringa pterygosperma* root is administered as a sedative in Central Africa and India (Watt 1967). *Solanum nigrum* ("Black Night Shade") contains solanine and other bioactive alkaloids. It is found in infusions known as soporifics in West African, Papua New Guinean, and New Caledonian medicine (Holdsworth 1977; Watt 1967). *Whithania somnifera* (containing somniferine) is a hypnotic and is used in East Africa and southern Africa (Watt 1967).

Plants with reported sedative/tranquilizing action.   Scientific confirmation of the action of these plants by laboratory investigation pending. *Apocynaceae, Asclepiadaceae,* and *Euphorbiaceae spp.* are the basis of sedative traditional remedies in West Africa (Ahyi 1978). *Casuarina equisetifolia* bark extracts are used to calm aggressive mental patients in Papua New Guinea and Malaysia (Holdsworth 1977). *Pongamia pinnata* leaf sap and Samanea saman leaf decocts are applied internally to tranquilize agitated infants in Papua New Guinea (Holdsworth 1977).

Canavalia maritima, Vigna marina, Evodia hortensis leaf sap, decoctions, and macerations are used in Polynesian traditional medicine (Tonga) to treat hysterical and psychotic patients, as is the bark of *Erythrina variegata* (Jilek 1988).

Sedative medicines prepared from the following plants are used by Amerindian herbalists of the Northwest Pacific coast tribes: *Arctostaphylos uva-ursi (bear-berry leaves), which containing psychoactive glycosides); Chamaecyparis nootkatensis* (yellow cedar branch tips); *Glaux maritima* (sea milkwort roots); *Ledum palustre* (Labrador tea) (Marles 1977; Nebelkopf 1987).

2. Anxiolytics / Muscle Relaxants

Piper methysticum (kava, yanggona) contains alpha-pyrones with anxiolytic, muscle relaxant, and anti-epileptic properties (Meyer 1967; C. C. Pfeiffer et al. 1967). Beverages prepared from the powdered rhizome of the kava shrub dissolved in water are used for medicinal and ceremonial purposes throughout Polynesia and parts of Melanesia and Micronesia. Today kava has a role as a substitute for alcohol in recreation and in the rehabilitation of alcohol abusers (Jilek 1987).

3. Central Nervous System Stimulants / Euphorants

Areca catechu L. (betel nut) is chewed with *Piper betle* and slaked lime. The betel nut contains arecoline and arecaidine, which have euphorizing and relaxing effects (assumed memory enhancement was not verified in tests made by this author). It has medicinal, ceremonial, and recreational uses in South and Southeast Asia and Papua New Guinea, including being used in the traditional treatment of mental disorders. It is reported to be effective as a mood elevator (Burton-Bradley 1979; Wyatt 1985). *Tabernanthe iboga*, a root containing ibogaine, tabernantheine, and iboluteine, has central nervous stimulant effects; high doses may produce a cataleptic state in clear sensorium. It is taken by participants in curative possession ceremonials (Bwiti, Mbiri) among the Fang and Mithsogo of West Central Africa; its main effectiveness is reported in dysphoric and psychosomatic symptom formation among women (Dobkin de Rios 1984; Fernandez 1972; Prins 1987; Watt 1967). *Alchornea floribunda* and *Elaeophorbia drupifera* are also taken in similar ceremonials with reported similar effects; no biochemical evaluation has been done (Fernandez 1972).

Schumanniophyton klaineanum is known as a tonic stimulant in Gabonese traditional medicine. *Hartogia capensis* is known as a stimulating and alerting medicine among Bantu populations in South Africa (Watt 1967).

Strychnos spp., containing strychnine and other alkaloids and having central nervous system stimulant and emetic properties, are used in traditional medicine, such as in Thailand (Ponglux et al. 1987). It is also used in Tanzania among the Wapogoro by specialized healers for the termination of psychotic states, together with *Stereospermum kunthianum* and *Pteleopsis myrtifolia* (Jilek and Jilek-Aall 1967).

4. Hallucinogens

The following plants with proven hallucinogenic properties have been shown to be of therapeutic value when used in group therapeutic context under the guidance of experienced ritual leaders in well-structured ceremonials. Their therapeutic effectiveness is documented in the area of prevention, treatment, and rehabilitation of neurotic and psychophysiological symptom formation found with depression and anxiety, especially if this is associated with alcohol abuse. These conditions are today often generated by sociocultural alienation. The function of hallucinogenic plants is the induction of altered states of consciousness that permit catharsis under group support, depatterning of faulty traits and habits, and opening for therapeutic suggestions conducive to positive personality reconstruction. It should be emphasized here that Western-type individualistic-hedonistic motivation of hallucinogen use, which leads to autistic and antisocial behavior, is foreign to the tradition-directed cultures in which these hallucinogenic plants are used.

4.1. Hallucinogenic plants with analyzed psychoactive agents.   The top part of *Lophophora williamsii* (peyote cactus) contains several psychoactive alkaloids, including mescaline, that induced multisensory hallucinations and feelings of tranquility. It has a traditional use in Amerindian populations of Mexico and the southwestern United States among the Huichol, Cora, Tarahumara, Navaho tribes for shamanic ceremonies, divination, and healing (Aberle 1966; Benzi 1972; Dobkin de Rios 1984; Schultes 1972). Other hallucinogenic cacti such as *Ariocarpus fissuratus*, *Epithelanta micromeris*, and *Pachycereus pecten* are also used for ceremonial and medicinal purposes among Amerindians in Mexico (Schultes 1972). *Trichocereus pachanoi* (San Pedro cactus), which contains mescaline and other psychoactive substances, is used by traditional healers in Peru (north coastal area) (Dobkin de Rios 1984; Lemlij 1978; Sharon 1972).

Psilocybe spp., *Conocybe spp.*, *Panaeolus sphinctrinus*, and *Stropharia cubensis* contain tryptophan derivatives and psilocybin, which have hallucinogenic and muscle relaxant properties. These substances are found in mushrooms ingested in curing ceremonials of Mexican Indian tribes, especially the Oaxaca tribe (Dobkin de Rios 1984; Hofmann 1987; Schultes 1972). *Amanita muscaria* (fly agaric mushroom), which contains muscarine, muscimol, bufotenine, and so on), is used in paleo-Siberian shamanic divination and curing rites (Dobkin de Rios 1984; Wasson 1967, 1972).

Sophora secundiflora seed ("mescal bean"), which contains the hallucinogenic alkaloid cytisine), induces altered states of consciousness with ceremonial and curative aims in "medicine societies" of North American Indian tribes (e.g., Apache, Comanche) (Dobkin de Rios 1984; Schultes 1972).

The hallucinogenic action of *Banisteriopsis spp. (B. caapi, B. amazonica, B. inebrians, B. rusbyana)* and *Psychotria viridis* is due to dimethyltryptamines, which are activated by monoamine oxidase inhibiting betacarbolines also present in these plants, is an example of monoamine oxidase inhibitors in phytotherapy (McKenna 1985). Liquid medicines prepared from the bark of *Banisteriopsis spp.* (ayahuasca,

yaje, caapi drinks) are imbibed in curing ceremonies conducted by shamans of Amerindian tribes in the Amazon region, especially in Peru.
Today they also feature prominently in the syncretistic group therapy
practiced by traditional healers among Peruvian urban populations, with
documented effectiveness in the treatment of psychosomatic, depressive,
and anxiety symptoms (Baer 1987; Chiappe 1979; Dobkin de Rios 1984;
Jilek-Aall and Jilek 1983; Lemlij 1978; Naranjo 1967; Schultes 1972).

Anadenanthera/Piptadenia peregrina is ground into a ceremonial
and medicinal snuff in the West Indies (cohoba) and in the Orinoco basin
(yopo). *Anadenanthera colubrina* is used in the same way by Amerindians in western and central South America (vilca snuff), as is *Virola
spp.* by the Waika tribes of the Rio Negro basin (parica and epena
snuffs)(Wassen 1967). These plants contain various hallucinogenic substances (methyltryptamines, apparently also harmine and derivatives,
and bufotenine) (Dobkin de Rios 1984; Holmstedt and Lindgren 1967;
Schultes 1972).

Datura spp. contains tropane alkaloids like hyoscyamine and scopolamine. *Datura stramonium* (jimson weed) was used by North American
Indian tribes for personality depatterning in initiation rites (Dobkin de
Rios 1984; Schultes 1972). Today it is still medicinally applied in the
traditional treatment of psychiatric patients, including psychotics, in
West Africa and among South African Bantu tribes (Shagana, Tsonga)
(Ahyi 1978; Watt 1967). *Datura metel* root preparations are ingested by
participants in the Bori cult of Niger, a curative possession ceremonial
run by female ritualists reportedly with considerable success for women
with psychophysiologic complaints or having psychosocial problems
(Monfouga-Broustra 1976). Medicinal beverages made from *Datura
spp.* help induce altered states of consciousness for diagnosis and curing
by traditional healers among Amerindian populations, (e.g. *Datura in-
oxia* in Mexico, *Datura candida, Datura speciosa* [toë], *Datura arborea*
[misha] in Colombia, Ecuador, and Peru [Baer 1987; Schultes 1972]).

Methysticodendron amesianum, containing scopolamine and hyoscyamine, also plays a role in divination and healing among Amerindians
of southern Colombia (Schultes 1972). Seeds of morning glory plants
(*Ipomoea sidaefolia/Rivea corymbosa* and *Ipomoea violacea*), which
contain lysergic acid derivatives, were widely used by Mexican Amerindians in pre-Columbian times for divinatory and ceremonial purposes

(ololiuqui) and continue to be in use in Oaxaca (Dobkin de Rios 1984; Schultes 1972). Likewise utilized as a "divination leaf" in Mexico are *Salvia divinorum*, of the mint family (essential oils containing hallucinogenic substances), and *Heimia salicifolia* (sinicuichi) with quinolidizine alkaloids that induce euphoria and auditory hallucinations (Schultes 1972).

4.2. Hallucinogenic plants whose psychoactive properties have not been analyzed. The stem, root, and inner bark of *Monesis uniflora* (wild snowdrops leaves) and *Oplopanax horridus* (devil's club—ginseng family) were taken orally and are still applied externally in shamanic ceremonials of Northwest Pacific Amerindian tribes (Marles 1977; Turner 1982). *Monadenium lugardae* root is ground to medicine by Bantu diviners and healers in Transvaal (Watt 1967).

CHAPTER 12

Cultural Aspects of Treatment: Conceptual, Methodological, and Clinical Issues and Directions

Anthony J. Marsella, Ph.D.
Joseph Westermeyer, M.D., M.P.H., Ph.D.

Introduction

Cultural factors play a major role in all aspects of the treatment process, including assessment, diagnosis, and therapy content and process. They influence the patient's conceptualization, experience, and expression of his or her problem, and they influence the doctor's diagnostic processes and therapeutic decisions. Indeed, it can be safely said that there is no aspect of the doctor-patient relationship that escapes cultural influence and determination. This is because both the patient and the doctor are members of ethnocultural traditions that encode and socialize various assumptions and premises regarding health and illness, and because the doctor belongs to a medical subculture that also has encoded and socialized various assumptions and premises about health and disease.

Statement of Purpose

The purpose of this chapter is to provide an overview of the theory and research on the relationship between culture and therapy. The chapter is divided into eight main sections: 1) definition of important terms, 2) cultural aspects of treatment, 3) cultural factors in the conceptualization of illness and health, 4) cultural factors in diagnosis and classification, 5) cultural factors in assessment and the problem of equivalency, 6) culture and treatment, 7) cultural factors affecting course and outcome of disorder, and 8) the importance of preserving ethnic diversity.

Definition of Terms

Ethnocentrism

One of the major reasons that cultural factors in treatment are often ignored is the frequent ethnocentrism of our medical knowledge and medical care systems. There may be failures in recognizing that culture influences these systems, and that they are not necessarily universal in their applicability. How can this be? How can something as obvious as ethnocultural tradition and experience be disregarded or dismissed as inconsequential in treatment? The answer is ethnocentrism. *Ethnocentrism* can be defined as

> A habitual, and often unconscious, tendency or disposition to evaluate foreign people or cultures by the standards and practices of one's own ethnocultural group. An inclination to view one's own way of life as the only proper or moral way with a resulting sense of personal and cultural superiority. (*Webster's Third New International Dictionary* 1981, p. 420)

Everyone is to a greater or lesser degree ethnocentric. Yet it is precisely our unwillingness as human beings, constrained as we are by the limits of our experience, to move beyond that which is obvious to us that is the major source of the problem. Ethnocentrism limits our capacity to accept the fact that culture directly shapes and fashions the realities that we live by. And to the extent that cultures differ, so will our realities.

To ask people from a scientifically, technically oriented culture to accept the obvious fact that people from a nonscientifically, nontechnically oriented culture are different may not seem like a major problem.

But to ask people from the former group who are medical and mental health professionals to accept the fact that as a result of these differences, concepts and practices regarding medical and mental disorders may be different in their distribution, expression, course, and outcome has proven to be a difficult, but not impossible task. It requires an extraordinary effort to acknowledge that one's world view is not an actual representation of the reality, but simply a perspective that is a function of cultural experience. This is true for both the patient and the doctor. Enhancing our awareness of ethnocentrism is a major challenge for the health and medical professions because it is unlikely that our patients will be less willing to change their fundamental views.

Culture

Although the term *culture* is frequently used by both the general public and by academics, there is considerable confusion about its meaning. Years ago, Kroeber and Kluckhohn (1962) published a book that summarized and compared 150 definitions of culture used in the past century. They noted that culture had a wide array of denotative and connotative meanings. However, a sizable number of the definitions acknowledged that culture has behavior implications.

Building on a definition first used by the famous anthropologist, Ralph Linton, Marsella (1987) proposed that *culture* could be defined as

> Shared learned behavior which is transmitted from one generation to another for purposes of individual and group adaptation, adjustment, and growth and development. Culture has both internal and external referents. External referents include artifacts, role patterns, and institutions. Internal referents include values, attitudes, beliefs, cognitive styles, epistemologies, and patterns of consciousness. (pp. 8–9)

This definition is valuable for understanding the relationship between culture and treatment because it articulates the simple but essential fact that culture is not only something external to the person, but is also something that is part of each person's experience of reality. If one accepts this definition and its implications, then it is clear that cultural factors cannot be separated from treatment. The cultural experience shapes the entire perception and experience of illness. We cannot acknowledge cultural differences among people and then apply unmodified theories and therapies.

In our opinion, all medical and mental health professionals should be trained to consider the meaning and definition of culture in the treatment process. Indeed, Pedersen and Marsella (1982) raised serious questions about the ethics of rendering mental health services to patients if the professional or health worker was unfamiliar with the patients' cultural background and experience.

Ethnocultural Identity

Ethnocultural identity is different from culture. Ethnocultural identity can be defined as "the extent to which an individual or group is committed to both endorsing and practicing a set of values, beliefs, and behaviors which are associated with a particular ethnocultural tradition" (Marsella 1990, p. 14).

In contrast to culture, ethnocultural identity is the term that refers to actual involvement in a cultural life-style or way of life. Much research and commentary simply compares ethnic groups or races but does not consider ethnic identity. Thus comparisons are made among different ethnic groups (e.g., Japanese, Chinese, Black, and Hispanic). The use of ethnocultural identity provides a much more detailed and specific variable for grouping individuals. Because of this, ethnocultural identity offers researchers the capacity to recognize and distinguish the contributions of ethnocultural variables to health and disease. Marsella (1990) cited a number of strategies for assessing ethnocultural identity.

Among ethnocultural minorities, variations in behavior within a given ethnocultural group are dramatic and profound, and any effort to group people together for research on the basis of the largest possible ethnocultural dimension (e.g., Asian, Black, and Hispanic) is contributing excessive error variance to the design. Even within these larger categories, the shared culture may be minimal because of geographical, genetic, and psychocultural variation. For example, those peoples considered Hispanic—Cubans, Puerto Ricans, Mexicans, and Central Americans—differ from one another in spite of certain common historical traditions such as language, religion, food, and so forth. Indeed, even the fact that Spanish is the common language does not acknowledge the numerous variations in the denotative and connotative linguistic meanings specific to the different groups. In brief, we must emphasize the variations and patterns within an ethnocultural tradition and heritage, and not simply use the general category when conducting research or considering treatment strategies.

Kitano (1982) proposed a framework that offers insight into these distinctions (Figure 12–1). According to Kitano, one can separate people along two dimensions on a high-versus-low basis: degree of Westernization and degree of traditional culture. This yields four categories of possible life-styles: bicultural, traditional, Westernized, and alienated.

Within this framework, one can see that there are at least four possibilities of ethnocultural identity that a patient may assume. Each of these have different implications for treatment. For example, in the United States, when one is treating a Middle Eastern refugee, the extent of the refugee's Westernization must be considered. If refugees are living a traditional life-style, their assumptions about the nature of their problem

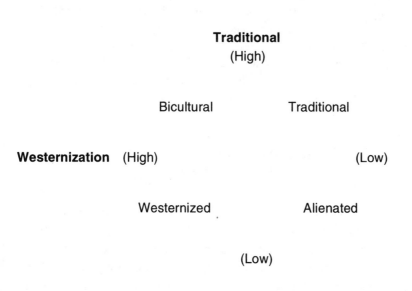

Figure 12–1. Ethnic identity alternatives.
Source. Adapted from Kitano 1982.

and their expectations for treatment may differ profoundly from those of the doctor, and this can effect the treatment process. The doctor must not be misled by the patient's language or appearance. Patients may speak fluent English and dress in Western styles but they may still adhere to traditional cultural notions regarding health and disease.

The Concept of Healing

An effective treatment process involves more than assessment, diagnosis, classification, and therapy; it also involves healing. Healing is a qualitative dimension of treatment and, in many cases, it is absent even though treatment has been rendered. Healing requires respect for and incorporation of the cultural aspects of the treatment process. It is an approach that considers the patient's total life circumstances and not simply the disease. As Kleinman and Sung (1976) wrote

> Healing is not so much a result of the healer's efforts (as it is) a condition of experiencing illness and care within the cultural context of the health care system. Healing is a necessary activity that occurs to the patient, and his family and social nexus, regardless of whether the patient's disorder is affected or not. The health care system provides psychosocial and cultural treatment . . . for the illness by naming and ordering the experience of illness, providing meaning for that experience, and treating the personal, family, and social problems which comprise the illness, and thus it heals, even if it is unable to effectively treat the disease. (pp. 55–56)

Cultural Aspects of Treatment: An Overview

Patient and doctor are both sources of cultural input into the treatment process. To the extent that there are similarities in their cultural construction of health, illness, and the treatment process, there is an increased likelihood of patient understanding, cooperation, and compliance. There is also a reduced risk of misdiagnosis and erroneous treatment. However, when cultural factors in the treatment process are ignored or denied, there is an increased probability that positive treatment effects will be minimized or eliminated. A key to effective treatment is understanding the cultural bases of communication (see Furnham 1989).

Cultural Dimensions of Patient-Doctor Interaction

Some important cultural dimensions of the patient-doctor/healer interaction include the following:

Patient

1. Holds implicit and explicit assumptions and premises about the nature, causes, and control of health and illness
2. Holds expectations about the role of the doctor/healer
3. Holds preferences for treatments and services
4. Expresses symptoms in modes and dimensions that are culturally determined (e.g., somatic mode, interpersonal mode, existential mode)
5. Communicates his or her personal (cultural) construction of the disorder to the doctor/healer in channels deemed to be appropriate and effective (e.g., verbal, nonverbal, and paraverbal)
6. Accepts and/or rejects treatment proposed and offered; complies with therapeutic regimens and/or rejects them
7. Appraises mental and physical conditions against culturally constructed concepts of health and disorder to index health status.

Doctor/Healer

1. Holds implicit and explicit assumptions and premises about the nature, cause, and control of health and illness; is skilled in various treatment and prevention technologies that reflect these assumptions and premises
2. Holds expectations and preferences about the patient's role
3. Holds preferences for treatments and services
4. Examines and tests for certain signs and symptoms that are associated with their constructs of health and illness
5. Communicates professional (cultural) diagnostic and therapeutic decisions and conclusions to the patient via different channels of communication (e.g., verbal, nonverbal, and paraverbal)

6. Implements treatment and preventive strategies and technologies. May or may not be aware of all the above, and may or may not be culturally sensitive

Patient-Doctor Expectations Regarding Treatment

Of all the sources of possible cultural variations in the treatment process, patient-doctor expectations regarding treatment may well play the most important role in patient cooperation and compliance. It is clear that both the patient and the doctor come to the treatment encounter with expectations; however, age, gender, class, ethnic, and professional differences can produce sizable variations in these expectations. These differences can result in increased tensions between the two parties. For patients, the doctor's failure to conform to their idea of what is supposed to occur can lead to a sense of uncertainty, distrust, fear, and anger. They may lose confidence in the doctor because the doctor is not acting in ways that they consider appropriate. Even though their expectations may be simply constructed and formed, they nevertheless constitute the reality on which their feelings toward treatment are based. As Kleinman (1980) pointed out, patients are not passive vessels in the treatment process. Like doctors, they have explanatory models about the nature of their illness and its treatment. While they may initially yield to professional opinions, recommendations, and suggestions, especially if therapeutic success is rapid, less immediate success may result in noncompliance and termination of the relationship.

Case Example 1

A 30-year-old Samoan immigrant to the United States comes to a state mental health clinic because he is sad. He has no job, no housing, no car, and few family resources to rely on. He has started to drink and get in fights. He does not want to seek help from the local chief or church. After the initial intake interview by the social worker, the psychiatrist prescribes antidepressant medication and begins a psychodynamically oriented course of psychotherapy. The psychotherapy focuses on the patient's self-concept and his relationship to his family members, especially his mother and father. The patient comes for two sessions and then stops.

A posttreatment evaluation of the case reveals that the patient wanted help with his immediate problems and was not interested in medication and discussion of his family dynamics and personality. He felt a job and housing were all he needed to feel happy. The patient was upset by the side effects of the medication. The psychiatrist wanted to help by using a Western psychiatric model that considered the patient's problems to be a function of personal responsibility and neurochemical imbalances.

Although there may be considerable cultural variations in any or all of these patient and doctor/healer dimensions, it is also important to note that there are certain pan-human aspects to the patient–doctor/healer relationship. These aspects include the following:

1. Doctors/healers are sought when the problem exceeds the patient's and/or family's capacity to deal with the it.
2. Doctors/healers need to access certain information regarding the patient to begin the treatment process. This access process may take a variety of forms (e.g., tests, divination).
3. Doctors/healers reach a diagnosis and assign the disorder to a classification system. The principles and categories of the classification vary across cultures.
4. Doctors/healers render treatment and receive compensation.

Non-Western Medical and Therapeutic Systems

The widespread use of Western (i.e., scientific, technical, reductionistic, North American/European) traditions, medicine's *modus operandi*, even in the face of national and cultural differences, means that people all around the world have had exposure to the process of history taking, mental and physical examination, tests, diagnosis, and treatment. But it is important to recognize that there are numerous non-Western alternatives to Western medicine that have broad appeal and support. These systems include, but are not limited to, the following: 1) American Indian medicine, 2) Ayurvedic medicine (India), 3) Chinese medicine (Sino cultures), 4) Hawaiian medicine, 5) Tibetan medicine, 6) Unani (Arabic Medicine).[1]

All medical systems, Western and non-Western, reflect the themes and epistemologies of the cultures in which they were derived and developed. Thus, the application of any medical system imposes upon the patient, either implicitly or explicitly, a particular cultural world view and set of assumptions. In this respect, the indiscriminate application of Western medicine can have pernicious consequences because it actually promotes cultural change with all of its attendant cultural conflicts. Fortunately, however, one of the characteristics of Western medicine is a growing sensitivity and explicit awareness of ethnocultural issues in care and service delivery.

Lock (1976) described the concept of sickness within the context of some non-Western medical and therapeutic systems:

> Sickness ... is not seen so much in terms of an intruding agent, although this aspect of disease causation is acknowledged, but rather due to a pattern of causes leading to disharmony. These causes can be environmental, social, psychological, or physiological. . . . The function of diagnosis is not to categorize a patient as having a specific disease, but to record the total body state and its relationship to the macrocosm of both society and nature as fully as possible. . . . The model allows for explanations for the benefit of the patient to be broad psycho/social and environmental terms which are readily understandable and cognitively acceptable. These explanations can be used by the patient to account for the occurrence of suffering in the context of his or her own life history at that moment. . . . Therapy is designed to act on the whole body—removal of the main symptoms is not considered adequate as all

---

[1] The Society for the Study of Traditional Asian Medicine is a well-known professional and scholarly group that is devoted to understanding traditional Asian medicines. There are also many scientific and scholarly journals that are devoted to the study of traditional and non-Western medical and health care systems and theories, including *Medical Anthropology Quarterly, Culture Medicine and Psychiatry*, and *Transcultural Psychiatric Research Review*. Leslie's (1976) classic book, *Asian Medical Systems*, remains one of the best resources for understanding these systems. It is also important to note that there are scores of alternative healing systems even within the Western culture (see LaPatra [1978]) for a summary of more than 60 alternative systems, including chiropractic, homeopathy, naturopathy, and osteopathy).

parts of the body are thought to be interdependent—in this sense the model is holistic. . . . It is believed that the functioning of man's mind and body is inseparable. (pp. 15–17)

Higginbotham and Marsella (1988) raised serious questions about the homogenization of mental health services around the world under pressures from both national and international agencies. This homogenization, designed along the lines of Western assumptions about the nature of mental health and the delivery of mental health services, has created treatment contexts that are often incongruent with existing financial, religious, familial, legal, and medical care institutions and values. Traditional models of health and sickness may no longer be viable within the Western care systems. One result is that patients may not receive care previously available through folk and indigenous health care systems. Furthermore, the new systems are often inaccessible and unacceptable to patients.

Higginbotham (1984) offered a scale for assessing the cultural accommodation of mental health services to the indigenous culture. It should be noted, however, that Higginbotham's book identifies that changes are occurring. Scientific medicine is beginning to address the problems of bias and ethnocentricity, within the tradition of the scientific impulse and method.

Cultural Factors in the Conceptualization of Illness and Health

Disease

The patient and the doctor both have assumptions about the nature, cause, and control of illness. In a classic study, Murdock (1980), using the Human Relations Area Files (HRAF), reviewed the models of disease held by different cultural groups around the world. The HRAF is a detailed research data pool that contains the formal and informal observations and findings from the field work of thousands of anthropologists who have studied hundreds of cultures throughout the world. It is like a cultural atlas. These research findings are available to researchers who may wish to conduct similar studies, or who may wish to compare different cultures on a similar variable (e.g., toilet training, child-rearing patterns, healing practices).

On the basis of his research, Murdock divided these models into a number of different categories based on the primary assumptions of causality. He first separated illness into theories of natural causation and theories of supernatural causation. He then further subdivided the latter category into theories of mystical causation, animistic causation, and magical causation. Each of these theory categories was further subdivided into types of disorder. (Because of space limitations, in this chapter only an outline of Murdock's efforts is presented. The interested reader is referred to Murdock [1980].) Murdock's final ordering is presented in Table 12–1.

Table 12–1.   Theories of illness

I. Theories of natural causation: any theory, scientific or popular, that accounts for the impairment of health as a physiological consequence of some experience of the patient in a manner that would appear reasonable to modern science.
  A. Infection
  B. Stress
  C. Organic deterioration
  D. Accident
  E. Overt human aggression

II. Theories of supernatural causation: any theory that accounts for the impairment of health as a consequence of some intangible force
  A. Theories of mystical causation (impersonal force)
    1. Fate
    2. Ominous sensations
    3. Contagion
    4. Mystical retribution
  B. Theories of animistic causation (personalized entity)
    1. Soul loss
    2. Spirit aggression
  C. Theories of magical causation (actions of evil force)
    1. Sorcery
    2. Witchcraft

Source.   Adapted from Murdock 1980.

It is noteworthy that Kleinman and Sung (1976) made a distinction between the concepts of illness and disease. They stated,

> Let us call disease any primary malfunctioning in biological and psychological processes. And let us call illness the secondary psychosocial and cultural responses to disease (e.g., how the patient, his family, and social network respond to his disease). . . . At present, modern professional health care tends to treat disease but not illness; whereas, in general, indigenous systems of healing tend to treat illness, but not disease. (p. 4)

Health and Well-Being

Cultural concepts of health have not been studied to the same extent that concepts of disease and illness have been. Nevertheless, it is clear that cultures vary with respect to the former as much as they differ about the latter, and that these variations impact on treatment in significant ways. The World Health Organization (WHO) definition of health included in WHO's constitution offers a good starting point for a brief discussion about this concept: "a state of complete physical, mental, and social well-being and not merely the absence of disease."

As is well known, the WHO goal of "Health for All by the Year 2000" requires "the attainment by all peoples of the highest possible level of health" (World Health Organization 1981). It is hoped that as a minimum, all people in all countries should have at least such a level of health that they are capable of working productively and of participating actively in the social life of the community in which they live. However, this statement acknowledges that there may be considerable national and cultural variations.

Walsh and Shapiro (1983) edited an exceptional volume of essays on concepts of health in Western and non-Western cultures. One of the themes to emerge from their book was that Western scientific concepts of health often tend to separate mind, body, and spirit whereas Eastern concepts of health often tend to emphasize holistic integration; mind-body interaction; harmony among people, family, ancestral sectors; and life-styles that emphasize congruence between religion, daily life, and health. In many non-Western cultures, the spiritual dimension of being is an integral part of human health, and many health-related activities are closely linked to spiritual practices (e.g., yoga [Indian culture], *santeria* [Caribbean and Hispanic cultures], and meditation [Buddhist cultures]). Doctors may need to familiarize themselves with alternative health care systems if their practice includes many non-Western populations because, for these populations, concepts of health may require greater attention to holism and integration. The possibility of incorporating indigenous healers into the care cycle needs to be considered. The healers can function as consultants, gatekeepers, and therapists (see Marsella and Higginbotham 1984).

A good example of a non-Western conception of health is discussed by Setynegoro (1979). He described the Japanese concept of *kebathinan*, which seeks to establish harmony between spiritual, psychological, and physical functioning:

> *Kebathinan* therefore, is a metaphysical search for harmony within one's inner self, harmony between one's fellow man and nature, and harmony with the universe, the almighty God. . . . One should be aware of the mystical power of communicating with the supernatural [through] which one [will] be able to sense, realize, and understand [one's] relation to environment, the society, and the universe. . . . To be Japanese means to understand and demonstrate appropriate manners [*pantas dan patut*], to understand and maintain an ordered existence in which persons, matters and things in their "place," "time," and "space" [*tempat, waktu, dan kedudukannya*, respectively], as if everybody and everything and every matter has a predictable "orbit." Disorder and disharmony—ill health, illness, and disease—are hence derangement and confusion of concept and matter. (Setynegoro 1979, pp 1–2)

Setynegoro's last statement regarding disorder and disharmony highlights the important role that many non-Western culture's place on the relationships between psychological and physical functioning. While Western culture has long separated mind and body, non-Western cultures have sought to develop integrated notions in which the *psyche* and *soma* are indivisible. It may well be that the psychosomatic and holistic medicine movements in the West will alter future Western thinking. However, for the time being, concepts of health and disease continue to vary considerably across cultures.

Cultural Factors in Diagnosis and Classification

The Diagnostic Process

Diagnosis is the process by which the doctor arrives at a conception of the nature and causes of a disorder by an analysis of the symptoms and signs with which the patient presents and an analysis of various psychological and physical examinations and tests. By describing and naming the disorder, the doctor is able to classify it. The classification of the disorder should offer insights into treatment and prevention.

In Western medicine and psychiatry, the diagnosis and classification of physical and mental disorders reflects the cultural and historical influences of Western culture. The *Diagnostic and Statistical Manual of Mental Disorders* (DSM) of the American Psychiatric Association and the *International Classification of Diseases* (ICD) of WHO reflect Western assumptions and theories about disease. However, every society has its own set of assumptions about health and disease, and these may vary considerably from DSM and ICD in the expressive symptomatology and categorical premises. One can imagine trying to diagnosis paranoid schizophrenia among a sub-Saharan tribal society in which there are considerable beliefs regarding evil spirits, astronomical deities, animism, and similar non-Western thought contents and processes. The validity of assigning a diagnosis of paranoid schizophrenia, even among Western people, is low. When the burden of separating cultural contents and processes from pathology is added, the task becomes formidable. Yet the task is not impossible. Sound research, which is sensitive to cultural variables, can help us understand alternative world views and their contributions to the shaping of psychopathology.

One approach to this problem is to ignore the classification category and focus on specific behaviors in question. By using culturally informed consultants and by mapping the behaviors for their frequency, severity, duration, situational appropriateness, and other overt behavior indexes, the risk of making interpretive errors—assigning diagnostic labels—is reduced. In working with ethnic minorities and non-Western people, diagnostic labels may not be as important as understanding observable symptoms and syndrome patterns within the context of cultural norms.

Culture and Symptoms

Clement (1982) noted that Samoan Society has five major categories of mental disorder. In contrast, DSM-III-R (American Psychiatric Association 1987) has over 200 categories of mental disorders. The reasons for this variation can be traced to the cultural differences of the two societies in their social construction of *disorder* and *health*. Marsella (1985) remarked that a culture's construction of a disorder is closely related to its conception of self-hood or personhood. In the Japanese culture, many of the disorders surround interpersonal behavior because the Japanese concept of self is sociocentric. In contrast, American society's construction of mental disorders surround individual existential functioning because of the emphasis on personal autonomy, choice, and purpose.

An early study by Marsella et al. (1973) found that somatic symptoms were a central theme of depressive disorders among Chinese Americans, interpersonal symptoms were a central theme of Japanese Americans, and existential symptoms were a central theme of European-Americans. Many subsequent reports have supported these views of culture and symptom variation (e.g., Kleinman and Good 1986). In recent years, there has been an emphasis on studying *idioms of distress* (Kirmeyer 1989; Nichter 1981; Parsons and Wakely 1991) and *folk disorders* (e.g., Westermeyer and Wintrob 1979) to increase cross-cultural sensitivity in medical and psychiatric care.

Cultural variations in psychopathology are also demonstrated via the numerous culture-specific disorders that have been identified (Simons and Hughes 1985). While some researchers believe these culture-specific disorders can be accommodated within Western diagnostic systems such as DSM-III-R, others point out that they are distinct and that all mental disorders are actually culture-specific because no mental disorders can escape cultural experience in their patterning, expression, and phenomenological experience (see Marsella 1982).

Case Example 2

A 55-year-old Japanese-American female is a hospitalized in state hospital for trying to hang herself from a closet bar in her home. The family reports that she has been upset for a number of months because of internal family problems. When she is interviewed at the state hospital, the Caucasian psychiatric resident reports that the patient shows few signs of depression. He notes that she smiled pleasantly throughout the interview and was very cooperative. He further notes that she denied family problems and provided no explanation for her suicidal attempt. The psychiatric resident wonders whether the patient is faking depression for the sake of attention. Several days later, the patient tries to commit suicide in the state hospital. At issue here is the psychiatric resident's lack of knowledge about Japanese culture and behavior. The lady smiled through much of her interview because she wished to be polite to the doctor. She did not wish to be a burden. She denied problems because, within Japanese culture, problems are to be accepted and shouldered. This is part of the Buddhist tradition. She was in fact sad and ashamed. However, the psychiatric resident did not pick up her communication of symptoms, including a desire to be by herself and not be a bother to her family, as indications of depression. He was unfamiliar with Japanese symptom pattern variations.

Thus effective treatment requires an understanding of the role that cultural factors play in the symptom phenomenology. Research suggests that there is cultural variation in the onset, expression, course, and outcome of mental disorders. The careful researcher and professional will give special attention to the role of culture in his or her diagnostic and clinical processes because they recognize the risks of misdiagnosis and classification, and ultimately erroneous treatment.

Cultural Factors in Assessment: The Problem of Equivalency

The term *equivalency* has become a popular part of the cross-cultural research lexicon in the past two decades. Equivalency refers to the extent to which a word, concept, scale, or norm of a measuring instrument can be considered similar or equivalent across cultures. Obviously, to the extent that cultures are similar, equivalency is not a problem and cultural bias is reduced. However, to the extent that cultures differ, there is a risk of bias in assessment. Marsella and Kameoka (1989) discussed the risks of ethnocultural bias in the assessment of psychopathology. In brief, they noted that researchers and practitioners must consider the problem of equivalency across all aspects of the assessment process. They cited three important areas of concern:

- *Linguistic equivalency*: Is the assessment instrument in a valid translation of the language? In order to achieve this end, back-translation procedures are recommended. Effective translation requires an understanding of both denotative and connotative meanings.
- *Conceptual equivalency:* Is the concept being assessed relevant to the cultural background of the patient? For example, in American culture, dependency is considered a negative character attribute. It suggests immaturity and helplessness. American culture has always prized independence, autonomy, and self-reliance. When American researchers go to Japan to study dependence, they encounter a strange phenomenon. The Japanese have a concept called *amae*, which translates as dependency; in Japan this concept has a positive connotation. The Japanese think it is good to be dependent and to rely on others. They do not like behavior that reflects individual autonomy and self-reliance.
- *Scale equivalency:* Is the scale appropriate for the cultural background of the patient? While Western people are accustomed to rating scales (e.g., Likert scales, true-false scales, semantic differential scales), many non-Western patients are not. As a result, the information derived from the scales may be erroneous. It should be remembered that the entire concept of being able to scale or quantify an inner experience or opinion is very much a function of cultural world views.

Culture and Therapy

Psychotherapy and Counseling

Every society has some form of counseling and psychotherapeutic healing activity (e.g., Kiev 1964; Lebra 1976; Marsella and White 1982; Prince 1968). However, these forms differ across cultures in their emphasis on theories of illness, roles for patient and therapist, and the use of specific principles of behavior change. Some of the more well-known non-Western healing systems include the following: acupuncture (Chinese), Ayurveda (India), Morita therapy and Naikan therapy (Japan), Ho'oponopono (Hawaii), possession states (Bali, Caribbean, Africa), spirit guides (American Indian), yoga (India), Zen therapy (Japan).

It is important to understand that each of these systems represents a viable and effective means of treatment when appropriately applied to members of that culture. The principles of behavior change may vary across cultures but effectiveness is still a function of the problem, therapist, patient, and dynamics. Some of the important principles of behavior change that are used include catharsis, cognitive attribution, fear reduction, hope, persuasion, reduction of uncertainty, and suggestion (see Marsella 1982).

Case Example 3

A 17-year-old Hawaiian male has become a severe behavior problem. He has dropped out of school and has had several encounters with police regarding fights, suspected robbery, substance abuse, and vandalism. He presents as a tough and hardened rowdy. Repeated efforts by mental health professionals to help him have failed, and it is likely that he will end up in jail as a chronic criminal offender. The family decides to conduct *ho'oponopono*, an indigenous form of group therapy and calls upon a *kupuna*, a revered elder in the community for assistance. The young man, all the family members, and the kupuna gather at a house. The session opens with a *pule* (prayer) to bring peace and harmony to the group. After the pule, each member of the family is offered the chance to speak their feelings regarding the young man's behavior and its impact upon them. Some of the members express anger, some sadness, some guilt and shame, some fear. All present speak their piece. The young man also shares his feelings, including his sadness and anger. The kupuna expertly guides the group, permitting negative emotions to be expressed, but always assisting in their resolution and always moving toward a forgiveness of the young man for his errant ways. By the end of the meeting, all present are crying and expressing love for one another. They promise to pull together, to help one another, to be sensitive to one another's feelings, and to try to prevent problems before they develop. The hardened young man is crying like a young child. He is once again accepted by his family.

Ho'oponopono means "to smooth over" or "to make right." Using ancient Hawaiian beliefs about personal and family harmony, the kupuna has deftly restored family harmony and given the young man another chance to be a part of his culture and community. He is no longer alienated. He belongs to a group. A number of months later, all is still well.

Within the last decade, there has been a proliferation of clinical and research literature on cross-cultural counseling and psychotherapy (e.g., Leong 1986; Pedersen and Marsella 1982; Pedersen et al. 1989; Sue and Sue 1990). These publications call attention to the importance of understanding cultural variations in the therapeutic process. While it is not easy to conduct cross-cultural counseling and psychotherapy, it is possible if the doctor is willing to learn how culture influences psychopathology and psychotherapy.

Ethnopsychopharmacology

Cultural and ethnic factors also play an important role in the use of psychoactive medications. Interest in this topic is relatively new; however, within the span of just a decade, there has been a proliferation of research on the topic. Much of this research points to ethnic and cultural variations in responses to psychopharmacological medications. K. M. Lin, a Taiwanese psychiatrist who immigrated to the United States, has been a leader in this area. While doing his residency in the United States, Lin was surprised to find that his Caucasian schizophrenic patients were being given 10 times the dosage of haloperidol (Haldol) that schizophrenic patients in Taiwan received. Differences such as this prompted him to begin a major research project on ethnopharmacology. He now directs a National Institute of Mental Health–funded research center for the study of the psychobiology of ethnicity at University of California in Los Angeles (see "Drug Responses Differ" 1992, p. 5).

Dr. Lin found differences between Western and Asian populations in such areas as metabolic rates for medication, hormonal responses to medications, dosage level requirements, and side effects. For example, he reported that Blacks have more lithium in their cells than Caucasians after taking lithium carbonate for bipolar disease. Trevisan et al. (1984) reported similar ethnic differences.

Studies done on tricyclic antidepressants, benzodiazepines, neuroleptics, and other medications also report racial and ethnocultural variations in dosage level requirements and side effects (e.g., Allen et al. 1977; Branch et al. 1978; Escobar and Tuason 1980; Ghoneim et al. 1981; Kalow et al. 1986; Lin and Finder 1983; Pi et al. 1986; Yang 1985). In general, Caucasians tend to show lower blood levels of a psychoactive medication at a given dose, need higher doses to attain specific blood levels, and have differences in side effects and complications than non-Caucasian groups.

It is important to note that diet and climate must also be considered in prescribing medications. For example, monoamine oxidase inhibitors may be troublesome to administer in a culture that eats pickled fish, aged cheese, or mammalian organs (e.g., kidneys, liver, heart). Lithium given to individuals who do heavy work in tropical climates can lead to lithium toxicity because of excessive perspiration without replacement of salt and fluids. Extreme heat can also disrupt anticholinergic medication, causing hyperthermia or hypotension. Issues such as temperature, humidity, activity levels, and consumption of alcohol, caffeine, salt, and sugar may need to be considered (e.g., Itil 1975; Lin and Finder 1983).

Cultural Factors Affecting
Treatment Course and Outcome

Once the patient enters treatment, there are a number of cultural factors that may affect the course and outcome of the disorder. This is especially true of psychiatric disorders where the patient's personal and social resources may become potent mediators of the course the disorder may follow, as well as its final resolution. For example, two major WHO international studies (i.e., the International Pilot Study of Schizophrenia [WHO 1979] and the study on the Determinants of Outcome of Severe Mental Disorders [Sartorius et al. 1986]) have shown that outcome for schizophrenic disorders was significantly better in developing countries than in developed countries. Based on research in Sri Lanka, Waxler (1979) reported findings that agreed with this conclusion, citing the important role of social supports and indigenous conceptions of illness. A more recent publication by Cohen (1992) questioned the accuracy of these reports. However, the debate has raised important questions regarding cultural factors that may mediate course and outcome.

Marsella (1992) noted a number of cultural factors that may impact on the course and outcome of mental disorders: conceptions of illness that limit personal responsibility and causation, lower social rejection of the ill member, continuous family care and involvement of the ill member (i.e., low personal burden), greater emphasis on role performance, reduced stress, lower competency requirements, greater social and religious involvement, lower emphasis on institutionalization and custodial care, reduced substance abuse and alcoholism, and sensitivity to class and ethnic differences between patient and professional. In brief, in some non-Western cultures, the course and outcome of the patient's disorder may be improved because there are many cultural factors that mediate the disorder.

Culturally Appropriate Medical and Mental Health Services

In assessing mental health needs of ethnocultural minorities and non-Western people, it is essential that a broad spectrum of variables (listed in Table 12–2) be examined that are sensitive to ethnocultural influence, ranging from the location and physical setting of the health service to the possible integration of indigenous healers and caretakers into the system. A systematic assessment of these variables would do much to accommodate to ethnocultural factors in service delivery (see Higginbotham 1984; Kleinman 1980; Marsella 1987; Marsella and Higginbotham 1984; Pedersen et al. 1989). While the variables listed in Table 12–2 are neither comprehensive nor exclusive to ethnocultural minorities and/or non-Western populations, they represent a reasonable sampling of the variables that must be considered in developing culturally sensitive mental health services.

Special Populations

Yet another perspective on culture and therapy comes from the growing research on treatment of special populations such as refugees, torture

Table 12–2. Variables to be considered in developing culturally sensitive mental health services

A. Population parameters
1. Population demographic characteristics (e.g., age, gender, socioeconomic status, educational level, ethnocultural background, languages, and religious distributions)
2. Population conceptions of health and disorder
3. Population conceptions of personhood and self
4. Population expectations and preferences for health services

B. Service provider characteristics
1. Service provider characteristics, conceptions of health and disorder, and expectations and preferences for health services
2. Service provider talents, skills, attitudes, and values, and also service provider training and experiences with culturally different patients

C. Health and disorder parameters
1. The distribution of disorders in the population (i.e., epidemiology such as incidence, point prevalence, and period prevalence rates) according to both Western and indigenous conceptions of disorder
2. The distribution of clinical parameters of disorders in the population including onset, diagnosis, symptomatology, course, outcome, correlates, and treatment responsivity
3. Outcome criteria regarding normality and abnormality
4. Outcome criteria regarding discomfort, distress, and disease, and also coping, competence, and actualization

D. Assessment and therapeutic parameters
1. The availability and acceptability of indigenous healers
2. The use of assessment methods and techniques that have linguistic, conceptual, and measurement equivalence
3. The range of services needed: emergency; crisis; inpatient; outpatient; partial hospitalization; transitional care; special services for diagnosis, assessment, and prevention activities; and special services for children, alcoholic people, and elderly people
4. Reliability and validity of existing data regarding the population to be served, especially with reference to the source of data bases
5. Therapeutic options available in service system (e.g., biochemical therapies, psychotherapies, behavioral therapies, and indigenous therapies [e.g., ho'oponopono, naikan therapy, and shamanism])
6. Opportunities for family involvement and participation
7. Design, furnishing, and ambience of physical settings

victims, sojourners, and migrants. There is a rapidly growing body of clinical and research literature on treating these populations, all pointing to the importance of considering ethnocultural factors in the treatment process. Professionals involved in serving these populations are encouraged to read this literature to avoid diagnostic errors, assessment problems, iatrogenic effects, and noncompliance problems (see Marsella et al., in press; Westermeyer et al. 1992; Williams and Westermeyer 1986).

The Importance of Preserving Ethnic Diversity

In the rush to offer mental health services to ethnocultural minorities and non-Western people, little attention has been given to the pernicious consequences that these services may have for the patient's nonclinical life. All health care services carry both direct and indirect cultural meanings and communications. All forms of Western medical therapy and psychotherapy are carriers of Western cultural traditions and practices. In this regard, when ethnocultural minority or non-Western patients receive these services, they are being socialized into the Western culture. Is this good? Is this right? These are difficult questions to answer and each case must be considered separately. However, a central issue that must not be ignored is the danger associated with cultural homogeneity.

Ethnic diversity offers the world a series of choices and these choices must be preserved. Diversity and variation are the basis of life. They must be preserved and defended, not dismissed as inconsequential by short-sighted thinkers. The Mexican poet, Octavio Paz, argued these points much more eloquently. He stated,

> What sets worlds in motion is the interplay of differences, their attractions and repulsions. Life is plurality, death is uniformity. By suppressing differences and peculiarities, by eliminating different civilizations and cultures, progress weakens life and favors death. The ideal of a single civilization for everyone implicit in the cult of progress and technique, impoverishes and mutilates us. Every view of the world that becomes extinct, every culture that disappears, diminishes a possibility of life.

In providing treatment, the emphasis should be placed on developing and offering services that accommodate and are sensitive to cultural traditions and life-styles. This is important not only because such services will be more effective and obtain more compliance, but also because they will help preserve rather than destroy cultural alternatives. By so doing, life is enhanced rather than constrained.

References

Allen J, Rack P, Vaddadi K: Differences in the effects of clomipramine on English and Asian volunteers. Postgrad Med J 53:79–86, 1977

American Psychiatric Association: Diagnostic and Statistical Manual of Mental Disorders, 3rd Edition, Revised (DSM-III-R). Washington, DC, American Psychiatric Association, 1987

Branch R, Sahih S, Momeida A: Racial differences in drug metabolizing ability: a study with antipyrines in the Indian. Clin Pharmacol Ther 24:283–286, 1978

Clement D: Samoan folk knowledge of mental disorders, in Cultural Conceptions of Mental Health and Therapy. Edited by Marsella AJ, White G. Boston, MA, G. Reidel, 1992, pp. 193–214

Cohen A: Prognosis for schizophrenia in the third world: a re-evaluation of cross-cultural research. Cult Med Psychiatry 16:53–76, 1992

Drug responses differ among ethnic groups. ADAMHA News. Rockville, MD, Alcohol, Drug Abuse, and Mental Health Administration, 1992

Escobar J, Tuason V: Antidepressant agents: a cross-cultural study. Psychopharmacol Bull 16:49–52, 1980

Furnham A: Communicating across cultures: a social skills perspective. Counselling Psychology Quarterly 2:205–222, 1989

Ghoneim M, Korttila K, Chiang C, et al: Diazepam effects and kinetics in Caucasians and Orientals. Clinical Pharmacology and Therapy 19:749–756, 1981

Higginbotham H: Third World Challenge to Psychiatry: Cultural Accommodation and Mental Health Care. Honolulu, HI, University Press of Hawaii, 1984

Higginbotham H, Marsella AJ: International mental health consultation and the homogenization of third world psychiatry. Soc Sci Med 27:553–561, 1988

Itil T: Transcultural Neuro-Psychopharmacology. Istanbul, Bozak Publishing, 1975

Kalow W, Goedde H, Agarwal D: Ethnic Differences in Reactions to Drugs and Xenobiotics. New York, Alan R Liss, 1986

Kiev A: Magic, Faith, and Healing. Glencoe, IL, Free Press, 1964

Kirmeyer L: Cultural variations in the response to psychiatric disorders and emotional distress. Soc Sci Med 29:327–339, 1989

Kitano H: Counseling and psychotherapy with Japanese-Americans, in Cross-Cultural Counseling and Psychotherapy. Edited by Marsella AJ, Pedersen P. New York, Pergamon, 1982

Kleinman A: Patients and Healers in the Context of Culture. Berkeley, CA, University of California Press, 1980

Kleinman A, Good B: Culture and Depression. Berkeley, CA, University of California Press, 1986

Kleinman A, Sung B: Why do indigenous practitioners successfully heal? Paper presented at the Conference on the Healing Process. Michigan State University, East Lansing, Michigan, April 8–10, 1976

Kroeber A, Kluckhohn C: Culture: A Critical Review of Concepts and Definitions. New York, Random House, 1962

LaPatra J: Healing: The Coming Revolution in Holistic Medicine. New York, McGraw-Hill, 1978

Lebra W (ed): Culture Bound Syndromes, Ethnopsychiatry, and Alternative Therapies. Honolulu, HI, University Press of Hawaii, 1976

Leong F: Counseling and psychotherapy with Asian-Americans: review of the literature. Journal of Counseling Psychology 33:196–206, 1986

Leslie C (ed): Asian Medical Systems. Berkeley, CA: University of California Press, 1976

Lin KM, Finder E: Neuroleptic dosage in Asians. Am J Psychiatry 140:490–491, 1983

Lock M: Oriental medicine in urban Japan. Unpublished doctoral dissertation, University of California, Berkeley, CA, 1976

Marsella AJ: Culture and mental disorder: an overview, in Cultural Conceptions of Mental Health and Disorder. Edited by Marsella AJ, White G. Boston, MA, G Reidel, 1982

Marsella AJ: Culture, self, and mental disorders, in Culture and Self: Asian and Western Perspectives. Edited by Marsella AJ, Devos G, Hsu F. New York, Tavistock Press, 1985

Marsella AJ: Health, public policy, and culture: the issue of ethnocentricity, in Yale University Symposium on Healthy Public Policy. Edited by Draper R, Leaf P Levin L. New Haven, CT, Yale University Press, 1987

Marsella AJ: Ethnic identity: the "new" independent variable in cross-cultural psychology. Focus: Newsletter of the Ethnic Minority Division of the American Psychological Association 4:14–15, 1990

Marsella AJ: Toward the development of culturally relevant treatments for the seriously mentally disordered. Keynote presentation to the Workshop on Chronicity and Culture, Hawaii State Hospital, Kaneohe, HI, April 28, 1992

Marsella AJ, Higginbotham H: Traditional Asian medicine: applications to psychiatric services in developing nations, in Mental Health Services: The Cross-Cultural Context. Edited by Pedersen P, Sartorius N, Marsella AJ. Beverly Hills, CA, Sage, 1984

Marsella AJ, Kameoka V: Ethnocultural issues in the assessment of psychopathology, in Measuring Mental Illness: Psychometric Assessment for Clinicians. Edited by Wetzler S. Washington, DC, American Psychiatric Association, 1989

Marsella AJ, White G (eds): Cultural Conceptions of Mental Health and Therapy. Boston, MA, G Reidel, 1982

Marsella AJ, Kinzie D, Gordon P: Ethnocultural variations in the expression of depression. Journal of Cross-Cultural Psychology 4:435–458, 1973

Marsella AJ, Borneman T, Ekblad S, et al (eds): Amidst Peril and Pain: The Mental Health and Well-Being of the World's Refugees. Washington, DC, American Psychiatric Association, (in press)

Murdock G: Theories of Illness: A World Survey. Pittsburgh, PA, University of Pittsburgh Press, 1980

Nichter M: Idioms of distress: alternatives in the expression of psychological distress: a case study from South India. Cult Med Psychiatry 5:379–408, 1981

Parsons C, Wakeley P: Idioms of distress: Somatic responses to distress in everyday life. Cult Med Psychiatry 15:111–132, 1991

Pedersen P, Marsella AJ: The ethical crisis in cross-cultural counseling and psychotherapy. Professional Psychology 13:492–500, 1982

Pedersen P, Draguns J, Lonner W, et al: Counseling Across Cultures. Honolulu, HI, University Press of Hawaii, 1989

Pi E, Simpson G, Cooper T: Pharmacokinetics of desipramine in Caucasian and Asian volunteers. Am J Psychiatry 143:1174–1176, 1986

Prince R: Trance and Possession States. Montreal, Canada, R. Burke Society, 1968

Sartorius N, et al: Early manifestations and first contact incidence of schizophrenia in different cultures: a preliminary report of the evaluation phase of the WHO Collaborative Study of the Determinants of Outcome of Severe Mental Disorders. Psychol Med 16:909–928, 1986

Setynegoro K: Some Indonesian concepts of mental health. Paper presented at the First International Conference on Traditional Asian Medicine, Canberra, Australia, August 1979

Simons R, Hughes R: The Culture-Bound Syndromes. Boston, MA, G Reidel, 1985

Sue DW, Sue D: Counseling the Culturally Different: Theory and Practice. New York, John Wiley, 1990

Trevisan M, Ostrow D, Cooper R, et al: Sex and race differences in sodium-lithium countertransport and red cell sodium concentration. Am J Epidemiol 120:537–541, 1984

Walsh R, Shapiro D: Beyond Health and Normality: Explorations of Exceptional Psychological Well-Being. New York, Van Nostrand Reinhold, 1983

Waxler N: Is outcome for schizophrenia better in non-industrial societies? J Nerv Ment Dis 167:144–158, 1979

Webster's Third International Dictionary. New York, Merriam-Webster, 1981

Westermeyer J, Wintrob R: "Folk" explanations of mental illness in rural Laos. Am J Psychiatry 136:901–905, 1979

Westermeyer J, Williams C, Nguyen N (eds): Refugee Mental Health and Social Adjustment: A Guide to Clinical and Preventive Services. Washington, DC, US Dept. of Health and Human Services, 1992

Williams C, Westermeyer J (eds): Refugee Mental Health in Resettlement Countries. Washington, DC, Hemisphere Publishing, 1986

World Health Organization: The International Pilot Study of Schizophrenia. Chichester, England, Wiley, 1979

World Health Organization: Global Strategy for Health for All by the Year 2000. Health for All Series, No 3. Geneva, Switzerland, World Health Organization, 1981

Yang Y: Prophylactic efficacy of lithium and its effective plasma levels in Chinese bipolar patients. Acta Psychiatr Scand 71:171–175, 1985

Section VI

Quality of Care and Care of Quality

Introduction to Section VI

This final section deals with variations in treatment models and practices according to the level of care and with the assessment of the quality of care.

There is great inequity in the distribution of treatment resources; while a minority of the world's population has easy access to many forms of treatment, the vast majority lacks access to minimum proven treatments. Resources must be used more justly. In recent years, the World Health Organization has worked out a strategy based on *graded* treatment possibilities; better description of each profession's task at different levels of care; and supervision and referral chains for quality control. Information regarding the main components of this strategy is provided and discussed by Wig in the first chapter of this section.

In the second chapter, Bertolote deals with the assessment of the quality of care. The detection of unexpectedly large variations in many aspects of care, together with the growing costs of medical care and the dissatisfaction of some consumers, has been one of the main reasons for the growth of quality assurance programs in mental health. A quality assurance program has therefore become an essential component of any mental health program that aims at a balanced, rational utilization of scarce resources.

CHAPTER 13

Rational Treatment in Psychiatry: Perspectives on Psychiatric Treatment by Level of Care

Narendra N. Wig, M.D., D.P.M., F.R.C.Psych., F.A.M.S.

Introduction

Rational treatment in any branch of medicine is generally accepted as a specific intervention that removes the cause of disease wherever possible and restores a previous state of health. In psychiatry, where the cause of most disorders is still uncertain, such an ideal situation for treatment is often not possible. Most of the time psychiatrists deal with conditions where the cause of symptoms is unknown or only partly understood. Available treatment is often empirical, or just symptomatic, and restoration to the premorbid state of health is not always attainable. Further, the multifactorial nature of most psychiatric disorders limits the applicability of a specific intervention as a complete solution to the problem.

In spite of these inherent limitations, psychiatric treatment has done relatively well during the last 50 years. Since the early 1950s, a whole new range of psychotropic drugs has become available. The scope of psychological treatments has greatly increased with the introduction of various forms of behavior therapy and cognitive therapy. Social and community models of treatment and rehabilitation have provided new frameworks for psychiatric care. Stricter criteria for psychiatric diagnosis and classification, and better means for neuroradiological assessment, now offer hope of better treatment of psychiatric illness. However, despite these dramatic developments, the current situation remains far from satisfactory and the following conclusions seem justified.

1. Many currently proposed methods of treatment, be they psychological, physical, or pharmacological, have not been adequately assessed in a rigorous scientific way and in different sets of populations over sufficient length of time, to accept claims that one is the most appropriate and rational treatment for a particular condition.
2. There is an enormous wastage of resources in supporting inadequately proven treatments (e.g., in the training of therapists in special forms of psychotherapy or in the flooding of the market with a large number of nonessential drugs).
3. There is scarcity among plenty. While a small proportion of the world population has access to many varieties of psychiatric treatment, elsewhere a large number of psychiatrically ill people live without even the most basic minimum of proven treatment. Available treatment resources need to be distributed better.
4. The majority of individuals who have psychiatric disorders, both in developing and developed countries, are never seen by psychiatrists. Nonpsychiatric health workers—such as general physicians, health staff, persons working in primary care, and, in many countries, practitioners of traditional systems of medicine—carry the load of providing treatment to the bulk of psychiatrically ill individuals. Any plan of rational psychiatric treatment for those who need it most must take this reality into account.

The concept of rational psychiatric treatment, therefore, is much more than the notion of providing a specific treatment for (if they exist) single pathologies; it has much more to do with the deployment of therapeutic approaches that are of established efficacy, are economically possible, and are appropriate to both the individual being treated and the wider community. The concept of psychiatric treatment, in the strict sense, is a relatively limited one, failing to embrace notions of prevention and rehabilitation and the processes needed to promote mentally healthy living. Such a wider concept is implied in the term *mental health care.*

Within this expanded context, as in the treatment situation, it is vital that rational (as defined above) care systems be set up. Such is the objective that has motivated the World Health Organization (WHO) perspectives on mental health care.

A World Health Organization Perspective on the Development of Psychiatric Services

Existing systems for the delivery of health care, including mental health care, have largely failed to meet the needs of most of the world's population. Many of these systems are centralized, hospital based, and disease oriented, with care delivered by medical personnel in a one-to-one doctor/patient relationship. Such care is often inconsistent with the principles of social equity, particularly in developing countries (World Health Organization 1990a).

The member states of WHO have agreed that the key to achieving the goal of health for all by the year 2000 is primary health care. This is care based on the needs of populations rather than on the needs of health systems and centralized specialist facilities; this care is decentralized, requires the active participation of the community and family, and is undertaken by nonspecialized general health workers collaborating with personnel in other governmental and nongovernmental sectors. The health sector should be structured to support these decentralized activities. The key components are thus decentralization, delegation of certain medical tasks to general health care workers and to people themselves, and a permeation of health knowledge and techniques into other sectors, using those who are not health care personnel to promote health (World Health Organization 1990a).

Since its inception, WHO has been greatly involved in helping member countries, especially developing countries, to organize mental health services in keeping with the needs and resources of their population. A significant WHO event was the publication of the 16th report of the Expert Committee on Mental Health, which was titled "Organization of Mental Health Services in the Developing Countries" (World Health Organization 1975).

During the 1970s, a number of experiments were started in different parts of the world to bring mental health services to previously unserved populations. One of the best known of such studies was the WHO Collaborative study on "Strategies for Extending Mental Health Care in the Community" (Climent et al. 1980; Harding et al. 1980; Sartorius and Harding 1983). This study was carried out simultaneously in Colombia, India, Senegal, and the Sudan, and later in Brazil, Egypt, and the Philippines. Subsequently, similar work was carried out in a number of other countries (e.g., Tanzania [Schulsinger and Jablensky 1991], Guinea Bissau [De Jong 1987], and Pakistan [Mubbashar et al. 1986]).

In many cases these studies have stimulated the development of national programs of mental health in which mental health services are being organized along the lines of principles that have evolved from the studies: 1) the integration of mental health into general health services and 2) the delivery of mental health services at the primary care level. Through such national programs, mental health services have now become available as an integral part of primary health care services in many rural areas of the world (e.g., India, Tanzania, Iran, and the Yemen) (Wig 1989; World Health Organization/Eastern Mediterranean Regional Office 1991a).

Although these projects differ considerably in the details of implementation, they highlight a common set of principles relevant to introducing mental health care into primary health care (Sartorius 1988; Wig et al. 1981; World Health Organization 1990a; World Health Organization/Eastern Mediterranean Regional Office 1989).

These principles can be summed up as follows:

1. Mental health care should be an integral part of a comprehensive health system and, where relevant, should also include sectors other than health.
2. An awareness of the importance of mental health should permeate all aspects of health care.
3. Activities designed to promote mental health and to prevent and treat mental and neurological disorders should be decentralized, with patients being cared for within or as close as possible to their own communities.
4. For the decentralization of services, it is important to integrate men-

tal health care with general health care, with mental health care being delivered through existing infrastructures of health care services.

5. Mental health care can best be organized through appropriate task-oriented training, with graded responsibility from the primary through the secondary and tertiary levels (e.g., from a health worker to a general physician to a specialist).

6. Mental health services must begin in the community and be for the maximum benefit of the population, and they must use existing resources such as those of family, social networks, religious and cultural institutions, and traditional healers for the promotion of mental health and for the prevention, treatment, and rehabilitation of mental disorders.

The Concept of Graded Responsibility in Mental Health Care

In the implementation of these emerging mental health services, one of the crucial question is, Who should do what at various levels of mental health care? What should be the role (if any) of a village health volunteer, a supervisory health worker (a nurse or medical assistant), a general physician, a psychiatric specialist, or of those many others in the chain of delivery of mental health care? If agreement can be reached on the mental health tasks at various levels of health care, it will become easier to organize such subsequent steps as appropriate training for each category, the selection of appropriate neuropsychiatric drugs, the establishment of a sensible referral chain, and the development of an appropriate data base and recording system.

In a recent publication, *The Introduction of a Mental Health Component into Primary Health Care* (World Health Organization 1990a), this issue has been examined in detail. The following passages have been largely adopted from that publication.

Mental Health Tasks at the Primary Level

Individual communities constitute the primary level at which health care operates. In many countries, the first health personnel are locally selected village or community health workers or volunteers. They are unlikely to be educated beyond the primary or middle school level or to have had more than a few months' training in basic health care principles. They may work only part time, having a number of other family or community commitments. It would be unrealistic to expect such people to have an approach to health problems more sophisticated than one of common sense, but they do have the particular advantage of having an intimate knowledge of the community.

The mental health activities that can be entrusted to village health workers include monitoring the psychological development of children, identifying patients who have major mental and neurological disorders and referring them to the next level of care, understanding the principles of long-term treatment regimens and ensuring that patients receive and take their medication, and undertaking limited education about mental health issues. Their cooperation with, and supervision by, better qualified primary health care workers is essential if they are to make their fullest contribution to community health care.

Primary health care workers who are sufficiently well qualified to be given supervisory responsibilities are likely to have had secondary or high school education and 2 or more years' professional health training, perhaps as a nurse or medical assistant. The clinics or dispensaries from which they work may have one or two overnight beds but are principally concerned with the care of ambulatory patients.

Health workers in this category may assist, educate, and supervise several village or community health workers. In addition, they will have regular contact with visiting staff from secondary-level facilities and should be capable of informed discussion with them about individual patients and about the mental health needs of the community as a whole. The mental health care tasks of these supervisory health workers include the following:

- Providing basic health service to both patients with mental disorders and those with physical complaints
- Identifying patients with mental disorders designated as priority conditions, such as epilepsy, a chronic psychotic disorder, severe depression, dependence on drugs or alcohol, and emotional and psychological crises

- Identifying patients who should be seen by visiting secondary-level personnel or referred to a higher level health facility
- Keeping a register of patients referred back to the community from higher level health facilities and maintained on long-term medication, thereby ensuring continuity of treatment
- Providing education on the maintenance of good mental health, and providing liaison in this area with other concerned and influential members of the community
- Initiating programs for personal development (training in relaxation techniques, promotion of recreational activities and exercise, and counseling on involvement in community activities)
- Using communication skills to mobilize and motivate mutual-support and self-help groups and to involve voluntary agencies in community development activities
- Identifying individuals whose mental health may be under threat for any number of reasons, such as family stress, poverty, physical hardship, adverse working conditions, and so forth

Mental Health Tasks at the Secondary Level

The secondary level of health care is generally represented by district hospitals or by large health centers serving between 50,000 and 500,000 people. In some systems, smaller health centers occupy an intermediate position between these and community clinics. Depending on their size, district hospitals will have at least one general clinician and probably a number of specialists. These centers should have a qualified psychiatrist, a psychiatric assistant, or a senior nurse with specialized psychiatric training. Currently, however, in many countries such district centers are lacking in psychiatric resources.

In existing health systems there may be no formal administrative or functional link between district and first-referral levels (i.e., between district hospitals and primary health care facilities). It is important to promote close cooperation between the two, for example by requiring district hospital staff to spend a substantial proportion of their working time visiting primary health clinics and dispensaries.

The principal functions of mental health personnel (a mental health–trained physician or a psychiatrist) at this level include the following:

- Diagnosis, treatment, and follow-up of patients, including those referred from primary-level clinics. Both in- and outpatients will be seen. Mental health personnel should also act in a consultative capacity to other hospital departments where patients may have disorders that are essentially psychological, rather than physical, in origin.

- Continued education, support, and supervision of primary health care workers and personnel from other sectors concerned with mental health. To fulfill this role, mental health personnel will require training in social and behavioral sciences, community planning, and organization and evaluation of services.

- Liaison with other relevant sectors in the district to promote mental health, raise awareness of mental health issues both within and outside the hospital, and foster mental health skills in all hospital departments.

- Application of treatments for mental disorders, including drugs, electroconvulsive therapy, and psychotherapeutic counseling.

- Efficient and comprehensive record-keeping, particularly for the follow-up and continued treatment of long-term patients who return to their communities to be cared for by primary health care workers.

Mental Health Tasks at the Tertiary Level

In mental health care, the tertiary or second-referral level is represented by qualified psychiatric personnel working in specialized mental health facilities, which may be independent or part of large general hospitals. Such specialized facilities may also be teaching institutions. At this level, mental health specialists will deal with complex problems of diagnosis and treatment referred from secondary and primary levels; will organize training in mental health for all levels of the health service; will have supervisory responsibilities for secondary-level facilities; will undertake research and evaluation work for the entire health system; and will act in an advisory capacity to governments and health administrators.

In integrating mental health care into primary health care, it is important to clarify the role of the psychiatric specialist working at the tertiary—and sometimes secondary—level. Where ignorance of mental health problems, particularly of acute and chronic psychotic disorders, is common at the primary level, specialist facilities may be inundated by referred (or self-referred) patients thought to need the type of care that can only be provided at this level. Paradoxically, many of these patients have disorders that could be diagnosed and adequately managed within their own communities, and therefore represent a significant and unnecessary drain on scarce specialist resources.

Although it is becoming increasingly evident that nonspecialist health care workers are capable of diagnosing and treating a wide range of mental and neurological disorders, qualified psychiatric specialists are sometimes reluctant to risk what they perceive as a loss in their own status by delegating the treatment of mental illness to general health personnel. It needs to be realized that the role of such specialists is increasingly one of education, consultation, supervision, and research and evaluation. Specialists' importance in the diagnosis and management of the more complex and intractable mental health problems will remain undiminished, but this change in emphasis demands new skills from mental health specialists, and this must be reflected in their training.

The administrative and conceptual changes involved in this new approach to mental health care may have to be the subject of government intervention. Formal mechanisms may have to be established to control referral patterns and to modify the role played by senior mental health professionals. Above all, there must be cooperation between the various levels of health care and sufficient flexibility in the system to ensure that health care is delivered effectively and with appropriate regard for people's differing cultural and political values.

The Role of Neuropsychiatric Drugs in Primary Health Care

Treatment with drugs forms only one part of the effective management of mental and neurological disorders. There is, however, convincing evidence that appropriate drug therapy provides one of the most powerful means available for the treatment and control of a number of neuropsychiatric disorders of public health importance. Over the last 30 years, a large number of new drugs for psychiatric and neurological disorders have been introduced into medical practice, and these have transformed treatment possibilities.

Harding and Chrusciel (1975), in their classic paper "The Use of Psychotropic Drugs in Developing Countries," outlined the following five essential steps for facilitating the rational use of psychotropic drugs. The steps listed imply a series of interdependent actions, designed to increase the rational and effective use of psychotropic drugs. It is not intended that such steps be carried out in any particular numerical order.

Focus on a limited number of conditions. Effective training will not be possible if the target conditions are poorly defined or too numerous. Health workers at most levels should not be expected to master the complicated psychiatric classifications used by psychiatrists, nor can they be expected (in view of the limited time available) to cope with the whole range of mental disorders, even if they are clearly defined. In the preliminary phase, therefore, it is necessary to focus on a very limited range of conditions that are known to be prevalent, that have marked harmful consequences, and for which drug therapy is of clear benefit. The selection of priority conditions must be carried out in each country and should reflect prevalence, the expressed needs of the people, and the general level of socioeconomic development. These conditions will have to be defined clearly with an agreed terminology that is precise and easily understood. This requires close collaboration between those responsible for training and those concerned with providing services.

Make available a limited range of drugs for defined situations. The definition of a limited range of psychotropic drugs for use in a particular country facilitates bulk purchase or local manufacture and helps to ensure a relatively cheap and constant supply. It also allows a more rational and efficient approach to training, because trainers can ensure that information is relevant to subsequent practice. Unnecessary duplication, different dosage regimens, and confusing nomenclature should be avoided. Psychiatrists and physicians may resist "restriction of freedom to prescribe." In countries with a large private health sector, there will be problems of implementation. There will inevitably be disagreements about which drugs should be included in the limited range, and this could lead to a situation in which drug suppliers might use pressures of various kinds to influence decisions. Nevertheless, the potential advantages of a defined, limited range of drugs are such that it is essential to overcome these problems.

Simplify the division of tasks in the use of drugs. The division of tasks in the use of drugs is usually rather rigid. A physician makes a decision concerning the choice of drug and its dose, route of administration, and duration. This decision is translated into a written prescription, often supplemented by direct verbal information and explanation to the patient. The prescription is interpreted by a pharmacist or a nurse who supplies the drug to the patient. Further decisions concerning change of dose, cessation of treatment, use of other drugs, and so forth are made by the physician on the basis of clinical observation and information given by the patient. In some cases this may be supplemented by information from nurses or the patient's family. The limiting factor in such a system is the physician, as he or she must be available for all decision making.

In view of the great shortage of physicians, particularly those with adequate training in the use of psychotropic drugs, the effective use of these drugs is severely limited. A more flexible system is required in which those observations and assessments on which decisions are based are collected and recorded by all health workers concerned, and decision making is delegated to the most appropriate worker in each case. In such a system there needs to be clearly defined criteria and standards for the performance of such tasks to ensure that task sharing does not lead to low standards of care and inadequate precautions.

Coordinated training programs. The successful introduction of the approach described would depend primarily on the provision of appropriate and effective training (and retraining) of all health workers involved. This would require an integrated approach so that training of each category of health worker matched the subsequent work requirements. Sensible training programs must also take into account problems posed by side effects, by abuse potential, by failure to take drugs as prescribed, by the risks of overdose, and by the fact that for some psychiatric conditions effective drug treatments are not yet available.

There is often too little continuity between the training of health workers and their subsequent work. Physicians and nurses are usually trained in hospitals where teaching on psychotropic drugs may be based on selected populations and may reflect the particular views and practices of one or more hospital-based psychiatrists. In actual practice the physician or nurse may have to deal with a different range of conditions in a different environment. Drugs used in the training hospital may not be available or may have a different name. In addition, there is a need for close coordination between those responsible for ordering and distributing drugs, the training institutions, and health service administrators. Lack of coordination may lead to drugs being supplied for which health personnel have not received training.

The setting up of a central policy body. None of the above steps can be instituted without the full agreement and cooperation of practicing psychiatrists, nurses, and those responsible for training, administration, and health planning. There may be problems of legal responsibility and professional rivalry. There need to be safeguards and regulations to limit the abuse of drugs. This could be achieved by a central planning body for mental health within the health ministry with access to the various professional groups, training schools, and institutions involved.

Selection of Essential Neuropsychiatric Drugs

Not all countries can afford to have all patients treated by a medical doctor. In many of the developing countries, over 80% of outpatient consultations are done by medical assistants, clinical officers, nurses, and village health workers operating from district hospitals, health centers, dispensaries, and dressing stations right down to the village level. In many other countries, all consultations are done by doctors, and the health center or hospital outpatient clinic may be the first level of care, rather than a referral level.

Whatever the health care system, the lowest level health care worker is usually not adequately trained in neuropsychiatry. The selection of essential neuropsychiatric drugs for that level should, therefore, be considered carefully.

At a recent WHO consultation on appropriate neuropsychiatric drugs for primary health care (World Health Organization/Eastern Mediterranean Regional Office 1991b), the question of selection of drugs at various levels of care was considered in detail. The recommendations of the consultation in this regard are shown in Table 13–1. As a general model, four levels of professional training are assumed, using the level rather than the type of institution as a criterion for the selection of drugs. These are the psychiatrist specialist, the general physician, the medical assistant, and the village health worker.

In preparing a model list of drugs for each training level, a task-oriented approach was chosen. For each of the levels, a list of diseases was drawn up that should be diagnosed and treated. This model list is shown in Table 13–1. Such a list may not only be used for the selection of drugs, but can also be used as the basis for a training program for prescribers, and for a specific record system for neuropsychiatric pathology at various levels of care.

For each of the diseases listed in Table 13–1, first line drugs are chosen. The criteria for selection are efficacy, optimal benefit/risk ratio, large therapeutic margin, and low cost. No combination preparations have been selected as they usually do not offer any benefit over and above the components given separately. Most drugs are widely available as generic drugs.

For several diseases that require long-term treatment, continued treatment can be given and its effect monitored at a lower level than that at which the diagnosis was made and treatment initiated. Such *down-referral* has been indicated by drugs shown in brackets.

For other diseases, drugs constitute only one part of the total treatment; making the drug available may, however, lead to overemphasis on drug treatment alone or may lead to irrational prescribing. The use of tranquilizers to treat anxiety or insomnia is a case in point. In Table 13–1, such drugs are marked with a "?"; emphasis should be placed on adequate training in their proper use.

Drugs designated for use by specialist psychiatrists are, in general, all those neuropsychiatric drugs included in the most recent WHO model list of essential drugs (World Health Organization 1987). The only two additions recommended here are trifluoperazine and imipramine. Trifluoperazine is a long-acting phenothiazine with actions and uses similar to those of chlorpromazine, which can be given once daily and is therefore a good alternative to one tablet of chlorpromazine every 8 hours and monthly injections of fluphenazine used to treat chronic psychosis. It is

Table 13–1. Essential neuropsychiatric drugs for primary health care

Levels of health workers / Conditions	Drugs that could be presented by			
	Psychiatrist specialist	> 6 years training (e.g., general physician)	Health workers — 2–3 years training (e.g., medical assistant)	< 1 year training (e.g., village health worker)
Neurotic Disorders				
Anxiety	Diazepam (DZP)	DZP?[a]		
Depression	Imipramine[b] (IMI)	IMI	(IMI)	
	Amitriptyline			
Psychotic disorders				
Schizophrenia	Chlorpromazine (CPZ)	CPZ	CPZ	(CPZ)[c]
	Fluphenazine injection (inj)	FPZ	(FPZ)	
	Biperiden (BP)	BP	(BP)	
	Trifluoperazine[d] (TPZ)	TPZ		
Other	Lithium carbonate			
	Haloperidol			
	Haloperidol injection			
Epilepsy				
Grand mal	Phenobarbital	PB	PB	(PB)[c]
	Phenytoin	PHT		
Other	Carbamazepine			
	Ethosuximide			
	Valproic acid			

Emergencies			
Acute psychosis	Chlorpromazine	CPZ	CPZ
Acute alcohol withdrawal	Chlorpromazine / Diazepam inj	CPZ inj / DZP inj	CPZ inj
Status epilepticus	Diazepam inj	DZP inj	
Other disorders			
Drug/alcohol withdrawal	Chlorpromazine	CPZ	
Insomnia	Diazepam	DZP?[a]	

[a] Diazepam is often overprescribed, and careful training in its rational use is mandatory.

[b] Imipramine and amitriptyline are nearly equivalent. Although the latter is included in the World Health Organization (WHO) Model List of Essential Drugs (1987), imipramine is recommended because of its lower cost and more general availability.

[c] In several country programs, village health workers have been trained to follow up on treatment with chlorpromazine and phenobarbitone initiated at a higher level.

[d] It is recommended that trifluoperazine, although not on the WHO List of Essential Drugs, should also be available.

also the second cheapest phenothiazine after chlorpromazine. Imipramine is nearly equivalent to amitriptyline, which is on the WHO model list; it is preferred as it is more widely available in developing countries.

The Role of Training

One of the key elements for the introduction of good mental health care into primary health care is the provision of proper training for all categories of health staff. It is clear that general health personnel—be they doctors, nurses, or other health care workers, particularly in developing countries—receive very little training in mental health and behavioral sciences during their medical or other education. If mental health services are to be decentralized, then this situation must be remedied. Because changing medical curricula in universities and health institutes is a major undertaking requiring considerable effort, many countries, as an immediate measure, are organizing short, task-oriented training programs for in-service health personnel. The principles for such training (e.g., the necessary content of teaching and methods of evaluation) have been well documented in reports from various parts of the world (Srinivasa Murthy and Wig 1983; World Health Organization/Eastern Mediterranean Regional Office 1988). These training programs are essentially task oriented. They stress the preparation of the primary care physician or worker for mental health care in his or her daily work. The following principles sum up the scope of such training (World Health Organization/Eastern Mediterranean Regional Office 1988):

1. Training should be relevant to the daily work of primary care personnel. Emphasis should be on the acquisition of skills rather than on just acquiring knowledge.
2. The course should affect the attitude of the trainee. As a result, there ought to be an increased awareness of the importance of psychosocial factors in health and disease.
3. Training should increase knowledge of and enhance correct management of mental illness, while avoiding unnecessary complexity or the use of technical jargon that bears no meaningful relationship to the everyday work of the primary care physician or worker.

4. Training should have an impact on existing services by decreasing the number of unnecessary secondary referrals, laboratory tests, and hospitalizations.

For such training programs to be successful, it is important that mental health tasks be presented in as simple and clear a manner as possible, especially for nonphysician health personnel. A number of trainers have developed and used flow charts and algorithms (e.g., Essex and Gosling 1983). There has also been an extensive growth of relevant training manuals and "how to" books. The World Health Organization has recently prepared an annotated directory of such manuals (World Health Organization 1990b), listing 60 mental health training manuals written in thirteen different languages. Their number is still growing.

Summary and Conclusions

During the last half century, there have been many advances in psychiatric treatment. Many treatments in use, however, still remain inadequately assessed. Furthermore, there is great inequity in the distribution of treatment resources; while a minority of the world's population has easy access to many forms of treatment, the vast majority lack access to minimum proven treatments. Resources must be used more justly.

In recent years, WHO has worked out a strategy based on graded treatment possibilities, better description of each profession's task at different levels of care, and supervision and referral chains for quality control. Introduction of this strategy for mental health care in primary health care is proving successful in many countries and offers hope of a more rational approach to treatment in psychiatry.

References

Climent CE, Diop BSM, Harding TW, et al: Mental health in primary health care. World Health Organization Chronicle 34(6):231–236, 1980

De Jong JTVM: A Descent into African Psychiatry. Amsterdam, Royal Tropical Institute of The Netherlands, 1987

Essex B, Gosling H: An algorithmic method for management of mental health problems in developing countries Br J Psychiatry 143:451–459, 1983

Harding TW, Chrusciel TL: The use of psychotropic drugs in developing countries. Bulletin of the World Health Organization 52:357–367, 1975

Harding TW, De Arango MV, Baltazar J, et al: Mental disorders in primary health care: a study of their frequency and diagnosis in four developing countries. Psychol Med 10:231–241, 1980

Mubbashar MH, Malik SJ, Zar JR, et al: Community-based rural mental health care program. World Health Organization/Eastern Mediterranean Region Health Services Journal 1:14–20, 1986

Sartorius N: Mental health in primary health care. Int J Ment Health 17(3):5–12, 1988

Sartorius N, Harding TW: The WHO collaborative study on strategies for extending mental health care. I: the genesis of the study Am J of Psychiatry 140:1470–1473, 1983

Schulsinger F, Jablensky A (eds): The national mental health program in the United Republic of Tanzania: a report from WHO and DANIDA. Acta Psychiatr Scand Suppl 83:364, 1991

Srinivasa Murthy R, Wig NN: The WHO collaborative study on strategies for extending mental health care. IV: a training approach to enhancing the availability of mental health manpower in a developing country. Am J Psychiatry 140:1486–1490, 1983

Wig NN, Srinivasa Murthy R, Harding TW: A model for rural psychiatric services—Raipur Rani experience. Indian J Psychiat 23(4):275–290, 1981

Wig NN: The future of psychiatry in developing countries—the need for national programs of mental health. National Institute of Mental Health and Neurosciences Journal 7(1):1–11, 1989

World Health Organization: Organization of Mental Health Services in Developing Countries. Technical Report Series No 564. Geneva, Switzerland, World Health Organization, 1975

World Health Organization: The Use of Essential Drugs. Technical Report Series, No 770. Geneva, Switzerland, World Health Organization, 1987

World Health Organization: The Introduction of a Mental Health Component into Primary Health Care. Geneva, Switzerland, World Health Organization, 1990a

World Health Organization: Annotated Directory of Mental Health Training Manuals. WHO/MNH/MND/906. Geneva, Switzerland, World Health Organization, Division of Mental Health, 1990b

World Health Organization/Eastern Mediterranean Regional Office: Intercountry Workshop on Training on Mental Health in Primary Health Care, Islamabad, Pakistan. WHO-EM/MENT/114-E. Alexandria, Egypt, World Health Organization, 1988

World Health Organization/Eastern Mediterranean Regional Office: Intercountry Meeting on the Progress of National Programs of Mental Health, Isfahan, Islamic Republic of Iran. WHO-EM/MENT/115-E. Alexandria, Egypt, World Health Organization, 1989

World Health Organization/Eastern Mediterranean Regional Office: The Second Intercountry Meeting on Progress Achieved in National Mental Health Programs, Nicosia, Cyprus. WHO-EM/MENT/116-E. Alexandria, Egypt, World Health Organization, 1991a

World Health Organization/Eastern Mediterranean Regional Office: Report on Regional Consultation on Appropriate Neuropsychiatric Drugs for Primary Health Care, Alexandria, Egypt. WHO-EM/MENT/117-E. Alexandria, Egypt, World Health Organization, 1991b

CHAPTER 14

Quality Assurance in Mental Health Care

José M. Bertolote, M.D., M.Sc., Ph.D.

Introduction

Gone are the times when medical practice aimed at the divine, times when doctors consoled themselves with maxims such as *Sedare dolorem opus divinum est* and *Primum non nocere*. While not abandoning these maxims, the ultimate goal of medical practice these days goes well beyond such aphorisms and aims at contributing to

- The attenuation of symptomatology
- The improvement of quality of life
- Good social adaptation
- The enhancement of patient satisfaction
- The alleviation of family burden
- The enhancement of caregiver satisfaction

In order to guarantee the attainment of each of these ambitious objectives, and also to keep a balance among them all, some sort of system of internal control must be established. Such systems have been called *quality assurance* (QA).

In this paper, I briefly review the following:

- The basic concepts in the literature relating to QA
- Issues relating to the introduction of QA in health care, and more particularly in mental health care
- Approaches geared to QA in public mental health

443

- Those guidelines and criteria necessary for the development and implementation of this approach
- Mechanisms for ensuring quality

Basic Concepts

In the specialized literature on QA are to be found recurrent terms and concepts inconsistently used. Key concepts in this area are those of *guidelines, criteria, standards,* and *indicators.* In addition, terms such as *quality control* and *quality assurance* are also used in an inconsistent manner. In order to avoid misunderstandings it is important to provide working definitions of these terms. Corresponding related concepts will also be discussed.

Guidelines are texts providing help in making risk management decisions, based on epidemiological findings and other scientific evidence. They concern public health protection and disease control. They are derived from ideal, desired health situations, irrespective of reality constraints. Guidelines, as instructions on how to do things, need to be distinguished from the use of the term *guideline* to refer to an approximate standard.

Criterion is the phenomenon one counts or measures in order to assess the quality of care (Donabedian 1981); it is a gauge allowing for the precise delimitation of a topic (e.g., bacterial contamination, infant mortality) within an otherwise too broad or complex domain (e.g., water quality, human development). It is also a sign, a notion, or a set of elements selected to make comparisons and discriminations. It has been mostly used to indicate things we want to measure (as in the examples above). Recently, however, the use of *criteria* as a checklist to determine limits has been widespread, such as in expressions like *diagnostic criteria* to precisely indicate signs and symptoms of a specific disease, or *admission criteria* to select those subjects who are allowed to enter a hospital or a group in a research project.

Standards define "the boundary between acceptable and unacceptable care" (World Health Organization 1988, p. 14), and therefore place some aspects of guidelines in specific context. They may be legal impositions enacted by means of laws, regulations, or accepted technical norms. These are usually established by authorities (national or otherwise) through a process of adapting guidelines to national priorities. This process takes into account local technical, economical, social, cultural, and political conditions (Hespanhol and Prost 1991). A standard represents a certain point in a scale defining a criterion.

Indicators are variables that help to measure change. This measurement may be direct or indirect, and should identify the extent to which the objectives and targets of a program are being attained (World Health Organization 1984). In the literature related to QA, it is now usual to classify indicators in the areas of structure, process, and outcome (Donabedian 1988; Vuori 1989). In some instances this division may be too limiting. For example, some programs for staff in-service training, some legal procedure provisions, or some funding for rehabilitation programs may, properly, be considered as both *structure* and *process*. The above terms and concepts are shown in Table 14–1 for different domains.

Donabedian (1981) has elaborated on different types of standards, describing two varieties: *categorical* or *monotonic* standards (all or nothing), used for elements "of which the more we have the better or the less we have the better" (p. 411) (e.g., survival on the one hand or death on the other); and *inflected* standards, referring to those "phenomena which have their most desirable value at some maximum or minimum point, on either side of which the valuation placed upon them is less" (p. 412). The definition of categorical standards usually poses less problems than that of inflected standards because the latter require the definition of two thresholds. Some standards may move from one variety to the other (or from one pole to the opposite one in the same category) or may be subject to historical or ideological variation, such as has been the case with mental hospitals, boarding schools, breast-feeding, or psychoanalysis.

In the health sector QA has been defined as a "planned and systematic approach to monitoring and assessing the care provided, and the services being delivered, in the expectation that this will provide opportunities for improvement, and a mechanism for taking action to make and maintain improvement" (Rosen et al. 1989, p. 381). It is a system that ensures the effectiveness of the quality control. Indeed, QA requires the application of both quality control and evaluation (or assessment), here defined as a set of measures aimed at "ascertaining whether the objectives of a program or activity have been achieved," and "does not neces-

Table 14–1. Elements for the establishment of some selected health standards

Domain	Criterion	Indicator	WHO guidelines	Local standards
Air quality	SO$_2$ content	$\mu g/m^3$	40–60	United Kingdom <35
Water quality	Bacterial contamination	Coliforms/100 ml	0	Canada 0 United States 1 Sudan 3
Human development	Infant mortality	Number of deaths per 1,000 live births within the first year after birth	Targets variable according to region	Japan <5 Cuba <11 Tunisia <45
Access to general health care	Availability of highly qualified medical experts	Doctors/population	—	Sweden 1/400 Kenya 1/10,000
Access to mental health care	Availability of inpatient treatment facilities	Beds/population	—	Japan 1/280 Brazil 1/2,000
	Availability of highly qualified psychiatric experts	Psychiatrists/population	—	Sweden 1/10,000 The Netherlands 1/43,000

sarily comprise any attempts to fill the gaps between the objectives and the actual situation" (World Health Organization 1988, p. 6). Evaluations and control of quality are the technical components feeding the larger administrative and decisional level represented by QA.

Quality control, on the other hand, can be understood as a system of activities aimed at the production of a good quality product. According to Dávalos and Quevedo (1991), the purpose of quality control is to provide a satisfactory level of quality of a product, including safety, reliability, and affordability in the process of producing it. Specific objectives of quality control include

- To keep the product and the process within acceptable levels
- To identify mistakes, keeping them at a minimum
- To verify the appropriateness, correctness, and precision of procedures, allowing for their immediate correction in case of any deviance

Figure 14–1 allows for visualization of the QA process. The main steps in the establishment of QA programs are the following:

- *Step 1*: Identification of goals and objectives
- *Step 2*: Selection of interventions
- *Step 3*: Definition of criteria and standards
- *Step 4*: Provision of care
- *Step 5*: Evaluation of care
- *Step 6*: Comparison between practice and standards
- *Step 7*: Implementation of remedial recommendations

The model basically revolves around an interaction between observed practices and established standards. According to some authors (e.g., Vuori 1989), Steps 1 and 2 would correspond to technology assessment and would not be an intrinsic part of QA; the selection of these technologies, however, is an essential component of QA programs. Although not mentioned in the model, there are also the crucial issues of who sets the standards, who observes practice, and who implements changes. These aspects will be dealt with in the section "Guaranteeing Quality," below.

Quality Assurance in Health Care

Following the introduction of measures to control and ensure the quality of products in industry, similar ideas were adopted, and adapted, by the health sector for the control of the quality of health services "products." When initiated in the medical area, there was an initial period during which QA programs were closely associated with expenditure control, with all the limitations involved in such an association. Currently the approach is more balanced.

Among numerous existing examples of QA in health care one should mention the Finnish Model Health Care Program Project, the Finnish

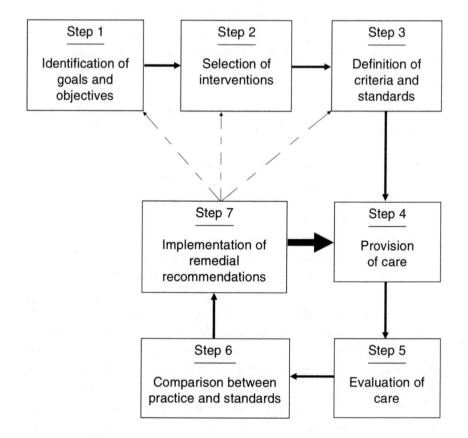

Figure 14–1. Components of quality assurance.
Sources. Chambers 1985; Dávalos and Quevedo 1991; Fowkes 1982.

Model Health Care Program for Stroke (World Health Organization 1989a), and the World Health Organization Care Programs for Care (World Health Organization 1989b).

The Quality Assurance Project (1982), funded by the Australian Department of Health under the aegis of the Royal Australian and New Zealand College of Psychiatrists, represents a completed example of QA in the field of psychiatry. It produced 10 treatment outlines for schizophrenia, depression, anxiety, somatoform disorders, and personality disorders. Each treatment outline presented a review of the literature, based on a meta-analysis of published studies; a survey of current practice carried out among a representative sample of Australian psychiatrists; and advice from selected experts in a particular topic.

Quality Assurance in Mental Health: Guidelines and Criteria

Most of the examples of QA in health care correspond to a *vertical* approach, in the sense of a program that can be set up in isolation without organic, structural links with the remaining organization of the health services. Mental health activities, on the other hand, might be best dealt with using an approach based on full integration into the primary health care system (World Health Organization 1990a). During a consultation held in Geneva in September 1990 (World Health Organization 1990b), such an approach was discussed. One of the recommendations of that meeting was that instruments for QA should be developed that take into account a country's national mental health policy, structure, and program. To this end, one can envisage a three-level system of QA.

The *first level* looks at the nature of the local (national or regional) mental health policy and its organization. Topic areas for the application of QA in a mental health policy include

- Decentralization
- Intersectoral action
- Comprehensiveness
- Equity
- Continuity

- Community participation
- Periodic reviews

whereas topic areas for the application of QA to mental health programs include

- Range of actions
- Components of plan of work
- Monitoring and evaluation
- Community participation

At the *second level* are specific mental health care programs and settings. These include primary health care facilities delivering mental health care, outpatient psychiatric facilities (e.g., mental health centers, emergency care rooms, crisis intervention centers), inpatient facilities (e.g., mental hospitals and psychiatric wards in general hospitals), and residential facilities (e.g., nursing homes, forensic psychiatric facilities).

Finally, at the *third level*, QA is relevant to specific interventions (e.g., for psychopharmacotherapy and psychotherapy) or for the management of specific disorders such as schizophrenia, affective disorders, and agoraphobia.

The public mental health approach calls for an integration of all three of these levels. Examples and models, however, are available mainly for the third level (e.g., the above-mentioned Australian QA Project) or for undertakings that are part of hospital or mental health center accreditation programs (e.g., see Canadian Council on Hospital Accreditation 1986; Joint Commission on Accreditation of Hospitals 1986). To develop QA for all levels within an integrated public mental health approach, it is necessary to define guidelines and criteria on which to base indicators and standards, these being the elements with which programs can be evaluated. The most relevant areas for the development of criteria, indicators, guidelines, and standards are those related to the following areas.

Service Structure and Organization

Service structure and organization are highly dependent on local sociocultural and economic characteristics. Diversity is such that so far it has prevented the emergence of useful categorizations. Most of the current descriptions are organized around dichotomies: hospital-based/community-based facilities on the one hand, and state-funded/privately funded facilities on the other. What is found in practice is often more complex than these simple dichotomies, and hybrid models are the rule rather than the exception.

Physical Characteristics of Facilities

It is not difficult to describe characteristics and indicators in this area (Baker et al. 1959); however, selecting criteria and indicators and standardizing them is more of a problem. Physical (architectural) characteristics of facilities are to a great extent dictated by the ideology governing service structures and organization, although awareness of this is surprisingly low. The same objective indicator can be valued as being of good quality in one ideological system and as being undesirable in another. For instance, close observation units or wards can be variously seen as conferring clinical or security advantages, or as an intrusion into patients' privacy.

The number of psychiatric beds has probably been the most frequently used indicator of mental health services (e.g., see Royal College of Psychiatrists 1988). This indicator is usually expressed as a ratio (e.g., per 1,000 or 10,000 population). According to available information this can vary between less than 0.05 per 1,000 (as in Angola and Ethiopia) to more than 4.0 per 1,000 (as in Finland and Ireland). To some the lower figure is better, because it is an indirect indicator of a noninstitutionalization policy. To others the higher figures are an indication of a more careful and caring mental health policy. In fact, there are indications pointing to a certain relationship between the availability of psychiatric beds and the degree of national wealth (as measured by gross national product); within certain limits richer countries or regions tend to have more psychiatric beds—and other resources as well—than poorer countries or regions, with some exceptions (J. M. Bertolote and G. de Girolamo, manuscript in preparation). Nonetheless, no consensus has been reached concerning a good or acceptable standard for the number of psychiatric beds per population, and maybe this is an example of an inflected standard, according to Donabedian's terminology (Donabedian 1981).

Staffing

The definition of professional roles in mental health is still an issue open for debate. Basic topics such as 1) statutory definitions and regulations governing different professions and specialties, 2) who should be involved in mental health activities, 3) who does what, and 4) which hierarchical model should be used, present very different pictures when examined in different countries or among people with different professional backgrounds (World Health Organization 1991b).

Once, in a given culture, agreement is reached in relation to the above, a more difficult question reveals itself: how to define the optimum level of staffing for a given region or facility. Here is the same problem as discussed previously in relation to the physical characteristics of units and facilities. The range is so wide as to produce meaningless guidelines (see Table 14–1). Some professions have, however, their own internal standards of operation, which guarantees a certain degree of quality.

Sacks (1992) has already noted that staffing levels is an important issue that cannot be avoided, and unless mental health professionals firmly contribute to its definition, "staff-patients ratios will be determined by forces outside our control such as availability of funds, public attitudes toward psychiatric hospitalization, and, increasingly as a last resort, judicial intervention" (Sacks 1992, p. 309).

In practice, as far as staffing is concerned, the most urgently needed consensus on standards relates to the types of professions to be involved in specific mental health activities; less urgent is the number of professionals per population unit.

Nomenclature and Classification

Several national classifications of mental disorders are now available, as well as the World Health Organization's *International Classification of Diseases, 10th Edition* (ICD; World Health Organization 1992). The most recent classifications have put more emphasis on reliability than on validity; what could be seen as an epistemological problem turns out to be an asset for QA programs. One of the greatest advantages of using internationally acceptable classifications lies in the standardization of language and of concepts they provide. An additional benefit—to both people and psychiatry—is that they make less probable the use of psychiatric diagnoses for nonmedical reasons (e.g., the unwarranted use of otherwise precise psychiatric diagnostic labels for controlling undesirable social behavior and political dissension).

The ICD is currently used by most countries in their official external correspondence (e.g., to send periodical statistical reports to WHO). National classifications have also been developed, usually by psychiatric associations, in several countries; in some cases psychiatrists in other countries have also used these in practice (e.g., the *Diagnostic and Statistical Manual of Mental Disorders*, prepared by the American Psychiatric Association). The current DSM (DSM-III-R; American Psychiatric Association 1987) is however translatable into ICD-9 (World Health Organization 1977), and the next revision of the DSM—DSM-IV—as well as other important national classifications are compatible with and translatable into ICD-10. Standardization is, therefore, reasonably developed in this area of classification.

Procedures for Clinical Examination (Structured Interviews)

Classifications alone cannot make certain uniform diagnoses—hence the importance of standardized screening instruments and techniques for conducting clinical interviews. Currently there are several well-tested instruments available for screening purposes (e.g., the General Health Questionnaire [Goldberg 1972], the Self-Report Questionnaire [Harding et al. 1980]), for diagnostic confirmation (e.g., Present State Examination [Wing et al. 1974], Schedules for Clinical Assessment in Neuropsychiatry [Wing et al. 1990]), for specific populations (e.g., for elderly people, the Geriatric Mental State Schedule [Copeland et al. 1976] and the Cambridge Examination for Mental Disorders of the Elderly [Roth et al. 1988]), for specific diagnostic categories (e.g., Standardized Assessment of Depressive Disorders [Sartorius et al. 1980] for depression), for the use of non-medical interviewers (e.g., the Composite International Diagnostic Interview [Robins et al. 1988]), and so on. Some of these instruments have been designed and developed for research purposes but many of them have conquered the field of clinical practice and become routine tools. On the other hand, fewer satisfactory instruments have been created for the assessment of other domains highly relevant to QA (mental health) such as quality of life, burden on caregivers, and degree of client satisfaction.

Treatment Characteristics: Modalities, Indications, and Processes

What exactly constitutes a treatment of high quality—an issue beyond the scope of the present chapter—is a problem not just in the mental health field, but in that particular field practitioners are not even close to having a consensus. Regarding of health care in general—and this could be applied to treatment as well—the Council on Medical Service of the American Medical Association identified the following elements characterizing high quality of care:

- Emphasize health promotion, disease and disability prevention, and early detection and treatment
- Provide care in a timely manner, without inappropriate delay, interruption, premature termination, or prolongation of treatment
- Pursue patient's cooperation and participation in the decisions and process of his or her treatment
- Base foundations on accepted principles of medical science, and the skillful and appropriate use of other health professionals and technology
- Provide care with sensitivity to the stress and anxiety that illness can cause with concern for the patient's and family's overall welfare
- Use technology and other resources efficiently to achieve the treatment goal
- Sufficiently document the patient's medical record to allow continuity of care and peer evaluation. (American Medical Association 1988)

Until very recently some of the most widespread treatment modalities in psychiatry rested on their prestige alone, without well-documented demonstration of efficacy and with a clear disrespect for several of the elements indicated above. Currently the utilization of some of these highly prestigious techniques is being questioned and scrutinized, and some counterindications and/or caveats in relation to their use have been proposed (see Chapter 8, "The Benefits of Psychotherapy"). WHO's "Evaluation of Methods for the Treatment of Mental Disorders" (World Health Organization 1991a) sets out guidelines for the evaluation of treatment methods. These guidelines will, however, have to be adapted to treatment provided in different countries and for distinct ethnic, cultural, age, and gender groups.

An examination of Figure 14–1 shows that evidence for efficacious and efficient health care intervention is a prerequisite for any QA program in the health care field. The Quality Assurance Project (1982) constituted a remarkable attempt to define standard treatment practices for certain diagnostic classes. It represented a model that could be adapted and checked in different cultural and ethnic settings.

Outcome Measures

Most of the work related to quality indicators in mental health have dealt with what has been called *structure and process indicators* (Donabedian 1988). Outcome measures in psychiatry have mostly been developed to measure changes in psychopathology and to examine the side effects of therapeutic interventions, but they have not been developed in other areas.

As noted in the Introduction, above, other outcome indicators—such as patient and caregiver satisfaction, family burdens, social integration, and, most of all, quality of life—have acquired so great a social importance that a mental health program that does not take them into account must be regarded as not being fully warranted.

On the other hand, care-process indicators in use in mental health services have been borrowed from other areas in which the industrial origins of QA programs are more visible. Assembly line measurements are readily adapted to areas such as those of hospital infections, surgical procedures, and food control. In many mental health activities relevant indicators must examine what has been called *soft variables* (for example, quality of relationships, overall climate in the ward, subjective well-being) that evade simple classification as structure, process, or outcome variables.

Nevertheless, outcome measures have acquired a great relevance and represent a major area of interest for many health authorities. From a public health perspective, justification for most of the infrastructure, inputs, activities, personnel, and expenditures should be based on the outcome they produce. In the words of the Council of Medical Service of the American Medical Association,

> Patient outcome reflects the degree of effectiveness with which health professionals combine their own skill and compassion with the use of technology for the patient's benefit. Implicit in the definition is the need to develop more precise and meaningful criteria of "favorable" outcomes. (American Medical Association 1986, p. 1032)

Notwithstanding the present importance appropriately attached to outcome indicators, a grain of caution should be introduced, particularly in relation to evaluations based mainly on outcome measures. In the words of Mirin and Namerow,

> Although there is general agreement that measuring outcome of care is desirable, there are substantial impediments to accomplishing this task. Mental health care affects the entire person—from the ability to perform basic activities of daily living to the complex cognitive and affective processes that go into making relationships. Moreover, changes in patients' symptoms, or in their functional abilities, are matters of degree along a continuum rather than absolutes. Nor is treatment outcome unidimensional in time; rather it is an evolving process that affects many aspects of a patient's life over many years. Finally, whether or not a psychiatric patient experiences clinical symptoms, performs well at school or work, or functions appropriately within a family unit is determined not only by the treatment he or she may have received, but also by a multitude of cultural, socioeconomic, and interrelational factors. (Mirin and Namerow 1991, pp. 2–3)

In summary, outcome indicators probably represent the most needed components for the establishment of good QA programs. Therefore, efforts should be directed toward their development. Their inclusion in QA programs will not only make mental health programs more comprehensive but will also give them more social relevance and legitimacy.

Legislation

Work initiated by WHO in 1975 resulted in the publication in 1978 of *The Law and Mental Health* (Curran and Harding 1978). This book established guidelines as to how legislation could be used to harmonize mental health goals with other social goals and with the rights of patients. In many countries it has been the basis for the passing of new legislation in these areas.

In 1991, the United Nations General Assembly approved the "Principles for the Protection of Persons With Mental Illness and the Improvement of Mental Health Care." This set of principles deals mainly with the rights of the mentally ill, particularly in situations related to, or similar to, those of involuntary admissions to mental hospitals.

Currently, WHO is conducting a study in which legislation related to mental health and social support systems in 45 countries is being reviewed. The final goal of this project is to establish guidelines for better access to mental health services as well as to ensure its integration with wider social support systems, using legislation as the instrument for improvement.

This, therefore, is one area in which principles exist. The main need now is for their transformation into local standards.

Guaranteeing Quality: Assessment and Implementation

People are crucial in QA. The interests, professional orientation, and personal biases and prejudices of the staff can be highly influential in relation to the direction a QA program takes. In already established QA programs, planning and implementation has been mostly a task for professionals, and *peer review* has been the basic model for monitoring (Mattson 1992).

However, Article 4 of the Declaration of Alma-Ata affirmed that "people have the right and duty to participate individually and collectively in the planning and implementation of their health care" (World Health Organization 1978, p. 3). According to the QA model being proposed here, planning, implementation, and evaluation are interconnected aspects of the same endeavor. Community involvement, therefore, should be sought at every stage of the QA process. More comprehensive community involvement could be obtained from

1. Service users (those who may be current patients in mental health care facilities, or may have been patients in the past; these are also designated as primary consumers)
2. Family groups
3. Community groups (such as women's groups, groups representing ethnic minorities or others who are disadvantaged, and churches and other religious groups)
4. Representatives of local government and health care organizations
5. Representatives of trade unions or other professional groups within the health and social care delivery system
6. Special community agencies
7. Self- and citizen-advocacy groups specifically set up to assist consumers of mental health services (World Health Organization 1989c)

In mental health—and particularly in community mental health activities—primary consumers are an important segment that should be taken into consideration. This is especially relevant in the evaluation of services. Insofar as specific methodologies for monitoring QA programs are concerned, more and more importance has been given to qualitative ethnographic approaches in which consumers' opinions can more easily be obtained and incorporated into the final evaluation (Richards and Barham, in press).

Conclusions

One practical remark concerns the introduction of QA programs. There is always the risk of dissipating efforts through being too ambitious. It is preferable to install a QA program that focuses on one or two areas, gradually adding others when appropriate, until more complete coverage is achieved. The selection of the initial areas is a delicate task; the more broadly based it is, the lesser the dangers of failure and future discontentments are.

QA programs, like any other component or activity in the health field, should always be evaluated and appropriate corrective measures introduced when needed. As stated by the Canadian Psychiatric Association in its position paper on Quality Assurance in Psychiatry (Cahn and Richman 1985),

> The efficacy of the quality assurance program itself can and should be evaluated. For the quality assurance program to be effective, we must be assured that the problems have been or are being solved, that there are no major omissions, and where there has been exceptional performance it has been appropriately verified. (p. 151)

References

American Medical Association, Council on Medical Service: Quality of Care. JAMA 256:1032–1034, 1986

American Psychiatric Association: Diagnostic and Statistical Manual of Mental Disorders, 3rd Edition, Revised (DSM-III-R). Washington, DC, American Psychiatric Association, 1987

Baker A, Davies RL, Sivadon P: Psychiatric Services and Architecture. PHP 1. Geneva, World Health Organization, 1959.

Cahn C, Richman A: Quality assurance in psychiatry: the position paper of the Canadian Psychiatric Association. Can J Psychiatry 30:148–151, 1985

Canadian Council on Hospitals Accreditation: Guide to Accreditation of Canadian Mental Health (Psychiatric) Centers. Ottawa, ONT, Canadian Council on Hospitals Accreditation, 1986

Chambers LW: Quality Assurance in Long-Term Care: Policy, Research and Measurement. Copenhagen, Denmark, World Health Organization, 1985

Copeland JMR, Kelleher MJ, Kellet JM, et al: A semi-structured clinical interview for the assessment of diagnosis and mental state in the elderly. the Geriatric Mental State Schedule. I. development and reliability. Psychol Med 6:439–449, 1976

Curran W, Harding T: The Law and Mental Health: Harmonizing Objectives. Geneva, World Health Organization, 1978

Dávalos YO, Quevedo F: Garantía de la Calidad de los Laboratórios de Microbiología Alimentaria. Washington, DC, Organizacion Panamerican de la Salud/Organizacion Mundial de la Salud, 1991

Donabedian A: Criteria, norms and standards of quality: what do they mean? Am J Public Health 71:409–412, 1981

Donabedian A: The quality of care: how can it be assessed. JAMA 260(12):1743–1748, 1988

Fowkes FGR: Medical audit cycle: a review of methods and research in clinical practice. Med Educ 16:228–238, 1982

Goldberg D: The Detection of Psychiatric Illness by Questionnaire. Maudsley Monographs. London, Oxford University Press, 1972

Harding TW, De Arango MV, Baltazar J, et al: Mental disorders in primary health care: a study of their frequency and diagnosis in four developing countries. Psychol Med 10:231–241, 1980

Hespanhol I, Prost A: The role of guidelines and standards for public health protection and the World Health Organization guidelines for the use of wastewater for irrigation. WHO/CWS/91.8. Geneva, World Health Organization, 1991

Joint Commission on Accreditation of Hospitals: Consolidated Standards Manual/87. Chicago, IL, Joint Commission on Accreditation of Hospitals, 1986

Mattson MR (ed): Manual of Quality Assurance. A Report of the American Psychiatric Association Committee on Quality Assurance. Washington, DC, American Psychiatric Association, 1992

Mirin SM, Namerow MJ: Why study treatment outcome? in Psychiatric Treatment: Advances in Outcome Research. Edited by Mirin SM, Gossett JT, Grob MC. Washington, DC, American Psychiatric Press, 1991, pp 1–14

The Quality Assurance Project: A methodology for preparing "ideal" treatment outlines in psychiatry. Aust N Z J Psychiatry 16:153–158, 1982

Richards H, Barham P: The Consumer Contribution to Qualitative Evaluation in Mental Health Care. Geneva, World Health Organization, in press

Robins LN, Wing J, Wittchen HU, et al: The Composite International Diagnostic Interview. Arch Gen Psychiatry 45:1069–1077, 1988

Rosen A, Miller V, Parker G: Standards of care for area mental health services. Aust N Z J Psychiatry 23:379–395, 1989.

Roth M, Huppert FA, Tym E, et al: CAMDEX: The Cambridge Examination for Mental Disorders of the Elderly. Cambridge, England, Cambridge University Press, 1988

Royal College of Psychiatrists: Psychiatric Beds and Resources: Factors Influencing Bed Use and Service Planning. London, Gaskell/RCP, 1988

Sacks MH: Considerations in Determining Staff-Patient Ratios (editorial). Hosp Community Psychiatry 43:309, 1992

Sartorius N, Jablensky, A, Gulbinat W, et al: World Health Organization collaborative study: assessment of depressive disorders. Psychol Med 10:743–749, 1980

United Nations: The Protection of Persons With Mental Illness and the Improvement of Mental Health Care. A/46/119. New York, United Nations, 1991

Vuori H: Research needs in quality assurance. Qual Assur Health Care 1:147–159, 1989

Wing JK, Cooper JE, Sartorius N: Measurement and Classification of Psychiatric Symptoms: An Instruction Manual for the PSE and Catego Program. London, Cambridge University Press, 1974

Wing JK, Babor T, Brugha T, et al: SCAN: Schedules for clinical assessment in neuropsychiatry. Arch Gen Psychiatry 47:589–593, 1990

World Health Organization: Glossary of Terms Used in the "Health for All" Series Nos 1–8. Geneva, World Health Organization, 1984

World Health Organization: International Classification of Diseases, 1975 revision. Geneva, World Health Organization, 1977

World Health Organization: Primary Health Care. Report of the International Conference on Primary Health Care, Alma-Ata, USSR, September 6–12, 1978. Geneva, World Health Organization, 1978

World Health Organization: Quality Assurance of Health Services: Research Implications. ACHR29/88.14. Geneva, World Health Organization, 1988

World Health Organization, Working Group: Principles of development of model health care programs. Qual Assur Health Care 1:161–178, 1989a

World Health Organization, Care Program Committee: Development of care programs for cancer. Qual Assur Health Care 1:179–192, 1989b

World Health Organization: Consumer Involvement in Mental Health and Rehabilitation Services. WHO/MNH/MEP/89.7. Geneva, World Health Organization, 1989c

World Health Organization: The Introduction of a Mental Health Component Into Primary Health Care. Geneva, World Health Organization, 1990a

World Health Organization: Quality Assurance in Mental Health. WHO/MNH/MND/90.11. Geneva, World Health Organization, 1990b

World Health Organization: Evaluation of Methods for the Treatment of Mental Disorders. Report of a World Health Organization Scientific Group. TRS 812. Geneva, World Health Organization, 1991a

World Health Organization: The Contribution of Different Professional Roles to Mental Health. Report on an Informal Consultation. MNH/MND/91.18. Geneva, World Health Organization, 1991b

World Health Organization: The ICD-10 Classification of Mental and Behavioral Disorders. Clinical Descriptions and Diagnostic Guidelines. Geneva, World Health Organization, 1992

CHAPTER 15

Conclusions:
Cure, Relief, and Comfort

Gavin Andrews, M.D., F.R.A.N.Z.C.P., F.R.C.Psych.
G. Allen German, M.B.Ch.B.(Aber.Hons.),
F.R.C.P.(Edin.), F.R.C.Psych., F.R.A.N.Z.C.P.
Leon Eisenberg, M.D.
Giovanni de Girolamo, M.D.
Norman Sartorius, M.D., M.A., D.P.M., Ph.D., F.R.C.Psych.

Introduction

The treatment of individuals with mental disorders remains one of the most challenging tasks in medicine, posing problems commensurate with the complexity of human mental function. Given the difficulty of the task, it is essential to focus on answerable questions. Empiricism and pragmatism must take precedence over ideology and polemic. The objectives of treatment must include the relief of symptoms, an increase in the quality of life, a reduction in handicap, and a minimization of the stigma associated with mental illness. As is outlined in the present volume, considerable progress has been made in terms of treatment over the past two decades in the prevention of some disorders and in the amelioration of the symptoms of other disorders. It is now possible to minimize impairment due to illness and maximize functional capacity, so that some persons who were once doomed to live lives of misery and degradation can now experience fulfilling lives with higher self-esteem.

Specific and Nonspecific Treatments

It is not enough to know which treatment is likely to benefit which disorder. Once specific treatments become available, the real task begins. That task is to ensure that treatment is acceptable in different cultures and to disseminate relevant information about treatment to people of different levels of sophistication. Health professionals, at both primary care and specialist levels, need to be retrained so that they are able to discard less effective approaches and incorporate new treatments into their practice. At present, the application of knowledge to everyday clinical practice is lagging behind the knowledge produced by therapeutic trials, even though attempts have been made to encourage the adoption of this knowledge. The World Health Organization (WHO) Technical Report on the treatment of mental disorders (World Health Organization 1991), which led to this book, is one such example; the National Institute of Mental Health (NIMH) consensus conferences in the United States and the Australian Quality Assurance Project are two others.

Still, too many "treatments" that are costly and of no established value are promoted by practitioners who insist that they are justified simply because the last patient they treated in this way appeared to improve. The problem is also cultural, for many health professionals prefer to use, and indeed insist on using, treatments that fit their world view, and also their view of the nature of the disorder. The time has come when it is no longer acceptable to use a particular treatment for reasons of philosophy and tradition alone.

While the researcher may have the luxury of deferring judgment on a particular treatment pending further evidence, the clinician has an obligation to respond promptly to the patient's requests for help by using the most effective therapy available. When adequate information is not yet at hand, clinical practice must be guided by the clinical wisdom of senior practitioners as well as by the clinician's own experience. But when the necessary evidence does become available, it is then unethical for the clinician to ignore it.

Evaluation of treatment in medicine, generally, is bedeviled by the fact that most patients recover from most illness episodes without any specific treatment at all (Beeson 1980). Many illness episodes are self-limiting, and patients will naturally improve over time, even if they receive no specific treatment for their malady. Another reason for improvement is that the very act of consulting a physician brings relief (regardless of the type of treatment recommended), and this can be one manifestation of the so-called placebo effect. A third reason is that patients with chronic disorders tend to visit their doctor when their symptoms are particularly bad and leave treatment when their symptoms are particularly good. This is known as *regression to the mean* in symptom severity. Historically, patient and physician alike have assigned credit for the improvement, or "cure," to whatever specific agent was in use when the remission occurred. While such things as natural improvement, regression to the mean, and the placebo response are a bonus for the clinician, they are a bane to the researcher.

The problem of evaluating treatment efficiency in the face of these confounding variables applies to all medical disorders. Evaluation that controls for these natural phenomena became possible when the randomized controlled trial, developed for agriculture by Fisher (1926), was introduced to medicine by Bradford Hill (1962). The randomized controlled trial was introduced into psychiatry shortly after the discovery of the first neuroleptic drug, chlorpromazine, and is now a prerequisite for regulatory authorities to approve new drugs. What has lagged has been the application of this "gold standard" methodology to the evaluation of psychological treatments. Only recently have data about some of the psychological treatments begun to meet Bradford Hill's criteria for identifying a specific treatment. These criteria include a strong treatment effect, a dose-response relationship, a lack of temporal ambiguity in response, and a response that is coherent with the perceived nature of the disorder.

Evaluation of treatment efficiency should also involve recognition of the negative aspects of treatment. Many treatment methods, although beneficial, may produce side effects and severe complications. There is a clear ethical duty to weigh these risks carefully against the advantages produced by the treatment. The Hippocratic idea *primum non nocere* reminds us that the first, inescapable goal for the therapist has to be the avoidance of harm to the patient. Harm, not outweighed by significant benefit, has been too frequent in the history of psychiatry, and recent progress has stemmed as much from the elimination of these dangers as from the discovery of new treatment methods. The study of persons who do not respond to treatment is a crucial step in this direction, allowing recognition of the limits that are inherent in many treatments. The awareness of these limits can enhance the wisdom of uncertainty and prevent the creation of therapeutic myths.

New Treatments or Old

New drugs and new psychological treatments continue to appear. In most countries the introduction of new drugs is subject to regulations that require that their safety and usefulness be demonstrated before a license for their use is issued. There is, however, no requirement that the drug be shown to be more useful or less expensive than any other existing drugs. Despite the steady stream of new drugs introduced over the past 30 years, many researchers consider that no significant breakthrough has occurred since the introduction of the prototypical drugs—chlorpromazine, imipramine, lithium, and diazepam. Since it was first published in 1977, the WHO List of Essential Drugs has consistently listed only six drugs, a tribute to the power of the randomized controlled trial to identify that the new treatments are not, in broad terms, more effective than the original six are.

The situation with respect to the introduction of new psychological treatments is worse, and no regulatory agencies seem to be concerned with the safety or utility of these treatments. The difficulties involved in making clinicians accept the need for rigorous evaluation have led to the uncontrolled growth of diverse psychological techniques. In 1986 Karasu reported that more than 400 presumably different types of psychotherapy had been identified and the NIMH report on research on child and adolescent mental disorders noted that "more than 230 psychotherapeutic techniques . . . are in use" (National Institute of Mental Health 1990). These very high numbers clearly signal that the authors could not decide which treatments were appropriate or inappropriate for each disorder. The present book makes it clear that evidence on the efficacy of psychological treatments is now available. If a list of essential psychological remedies was to be published, then possibly as few as three psychotherapies would rank alongside the list of six essential drugs: the cognitive behavioral techniques for anxiety and depression; interpersonal psychotherapy for depression; and psychoeducational family interventions for schizophrenia. Identifying three proven treatments is very different to listing 450 possible therapies.

With respect to the introduction of both new drugs and new psychological treatments, we would do well to recall Cochrane's injunctions (1972) concerning the improvement of Britain's National Health Service: "To prevent the introduction of new drugs and therapeutic procedures unless they are more effective (or equally effective and cheaper) than existing therapies. To evaluate all existing therapies, slowly excluding those shown to be ineffective or too dangerous. . . ."

This volume provides a description of treatments of established efficacy; it also summarizes other treatments in common use that take their warrant from clinical practice even though the controlled trials remain to be done. From this material and that published elsewhere the relative costs and benefits of different approaches can be estimated, and the balance between likely gains from therapy and losses from unwanted side effects can be gauged with some certainty. It is thus possible to base decisions about treatment on a foundation of data that were not available 20 years ago. These data should be considered in light of each patient's individual needs and wishes. One patient may be adverse to drugs and insist on psychological treatment, even when told that such treatment is usually less effective than drugs. Another may reject psychological treatment out of hand and prefer medication, despite the risk of severe side effects. This is similar to the choice that patients with coronary artery disease must make between bypass surgery and medical treatment. It is the patient that must make the decision because, when two treatments have been shown to be equally effective, the choice between risk and benefit is inevitably a personal one.

In this book, the authors have largely emphasized evaluation of specific or individual treatments simply because that was the way in which the book was organized. Evaluation of quality of care is equally important but the ultimate validator of quality of care is the effectiveness of treatment in producing health and satisfaction. Treatment is not just the application of proven and acceptable remedies; it also depends on the skills and attitudes of the therapist and their congruence with the sociocultural context in which the treatment is applied. The conduct of the interpersonal process between therapist and patient must meet individual and societal expectations about privacy, confidentiality, and informed choice, as well as expectations about concern, empathy, honesty, and sensitivity.

Good Clinical Care

About half the improvement observed in most disorders is due to the nonspecific benefits of good clinical care (Shepherd and Sartorius 1989). That is, benefits accrue from such things as diagnosis, counseling of patient and relatives, realistic goal setting in terms of the cultural milieu, and encouragement and support from the sanctioned health care worker. Although good treatment is always better than the sum of the parts, bad treatment detracts from whatever specific benefits might have been available to a good clinician.

Ambroise Pare (1510–1590) defined the tasks of medicine as "cure sometimes, relieve often and comfort always." Although the last two decades have seen a rapid expansion in our ability to cure and relieve, good and bad physicians can still be distinguished by their ability to comfort and support, to encourage optimal functioning, and to minimize damage in persons for whom specific treatments are either not yet available or not sufficiently effective. Good clinical care involves the physician or health care worker in a number of steps. These steps can be summarized as follows:

Step 1: Focus on presenting problems.   Take a detailed history of the presenting problems: how long they have been present, how the symptoms have developed since then, how they have interfered with the patient's life and activities, what seems to make them worse or better, and what the patient sees as likely to have contributed to the onset and development of symptoms. This step is essential to validate the patient and the symptoms he or she brought to therapy.

Step 2: Establish the diagnosis.   The symptoms elicited from the history of the presenting complaint form the basis of a provisional clinical diagnosis when mapped onto the ICD-10 (World Health Organization 1992) diagnostic criteria. The diagnosis can be confirmed by using an appropriate structured diagnostic interview, such as the Composite International Diagnostic Interview (Robins et al. 1988), the Schedule for Clinical Assessment in Neuropsychiatry (Wing et al. 1990), or the International Personality Disorder Examination (Loranger et al. 1991). Further support for the diagnosis can be derived by measurement of known risk factors associated with the probable diagnosis, items such as a positive family history for schizophrenia or depression or a vulnerable personality in the neuroses. When all data concur, confidence in the validity of the diagnosis rises. Once the diagnosis is established the physician should concentrate on therapy, reviewing the diagnosis if therapy is not successful, but not repeatedly reviewing the diagnosis as a defense against having to provide therapy.

Step 3: Match treatment to diagnosis.   A successful therapist is not bound to use one particular type of therapy for all disorders, but accepts that different specific treatments have been shown to be most effective with particular disorders. Where there is more than one specific and effective treatment for a disorder, then the choice of which to use should depend not only on the therapist's bias or convenience but on careful consideration as to which of the proven treatments is likely to be most effective with this particular patient. Good therapists also realize that nonspecific approaches, with their potential to enhance the effects of specific treatment, are fundamental, for after one has matched treatment to diagnosis there is the problem of compliance, the option of adjuvant psychological remedies that may also be of benefit, and the necessity of ensuring that either the patient lives in circumstances consistent with recovery or that patients learn appropriate skills to ensure that they can make the necessary arrangements and changes themselves.

Step 4: Expect improvement.   Thirty years ago hospitalization for a psychosis meant hospitalization for an average of 18 months. Now hospitalization in some countries averages 2 weeks and some intensive care units take an average of 5 days to diagnose, institute treatment, and resolve concurrent crises, discharging patients to be cared for in the community. Many patients are, of course, now managed in the community without recourse to hospitalization at all. Thirty years ago treatment for a neurosis could mean long-term psychotherapy with no certainty of relief. Treatment with the cognitive behavioral therapies now averages 20–30 hours, the improvement being permanent and extending to symptoms, behavior, and amelioration of the underlying personality risk factors. Long-term treatment in or out of the hospital can be associated with harm, at best resulting in a fixing of roles between the "caring doctor" and the "helpless patient," at worst resulting in exploitation of the patient by the therapist or institution. Even in chronic disorders one should now expect to see improvement in particular facets of the disorder within a short period of time. If this does not occur, one should review the diagnosis and treatment plan and, if nothing seems awry, call for a second opinion. Treatment failures are too often associated with the doctor's ignorance or indolence, not with patient incurability.

Step 5: Define criteria for ending treatment. During the initial diagnostic interviews, one should determine the patient's definition of being well. Goals should be made explicit (e.g., the symptoms will abate or the patient will be able to sleep, enjoy, socialize, travel, work, and so on) and progress measured. Therapy should end when the changes defined at the beginning of therapy have been attained; otherwise, both patient and therapist will escalate the degree of change they both seek. Many good clinicians become despondent about their therapeutic competence simply because the majority of their clinical time is spent with slow-to-improve patients, with the quick-to-respond patients swiftly ceasing clinical contact and, being well, getting on with their lives. Doing a follow-up study of a cohort of patients is therefore a salutary experience, for one then sees the full range of improvement. Even though the majority of clinic time may have been spent with patients who needed the greatest help and who perhaps made the smallest gains, the other patients may be found to have benefited considerably and remained robustly well.

Mental Health for All

In an ideal world, one in which all diagnoses were valid and treatments specific to each diagnosis were identified and proven, there would still be important therapy issues to take into account. One such issue relates to the observation that treatment in primary care centers is different, but not necessarily inferior, to treatment in research centers, where the majority of very expert health professionals are. Another issue concerns the way treatment delivery is altered by the social and cultural milieu in which the treatment is carried out.

A third issue relates to the lack of uniformity in service delivery, both within and among countries. Regrettably, not everyone has equal access to optimal health care. Within most countries skilled health care staff tend to congregate in the larger cities and services are disproportionately used by the educated and wealthy. The poor and rural populations in general commonly find difficulty in accessing skilled help. In developing countries this problem is acute, but even in wealthy developed countries like the United States social class will determine who will be treated and who will not. In other countries, where universal health insurance has removed economic barriers, rural populations are still deprived by a lack of facilities. Treatment frequently does not reach the people most in need. From the Epidemiological Catchment Area Study, Robins and Regier (1991) reported only one-fifth of the identified cases of active mental disorder received any specialized mental health care at all.

Unequal access to optimal health care is accompanied by significant variations in patterns of care both within and among countries. Significant variations have been reported in length of hospital stay, in referral and hospitalization rates, in the use of drugs, in lengths of psychotherapy, and in pathways to care. Differences in patient mix, demography, and severity of disease may explain a proportion of this variation but one is left with the very uncomfortable realization that many of the variations are so gross as to indicate a serious variation in quality of care. When such variations (e.g., a fivefold variation in length of stay, a tenfold variation in length of psychotherapy) occur among countries that are socioeconomically comparable, one is left to conclude that it is not clinical need that determines the service delivery pattern, but structural factors in the way hospitals are funded or therapy is paid for.

What we do not know still far exceeds what we do know, but there have been very considerable advances in our understanding of the psychobiology of mental disorders and of the ways of treating those disorders. The new treatments in psychiatry have powerful effects in reducing symptoms and in restoring personal effectiveness—not for all patients, but for many; not always, but often; not forever, but for substantial periods of time. What is of concern is the fact that these treatments are not being delivered to many of the patients who could benefit from them. All over the world the largest gap is in primary health care.

Psychiatric disorders are the cause of extensive suffering and functional impairment in a substantial number of patients seen in primary care. All too often the source of the patient's complaint is not recognized by the primary health care provider as being psychiatric. When it is, and when treatment is recommended, such care as the patient is likely to receive is delivered by that provider. Yet despite the fact that depression and anxiety are the most common problems physicians will encounter in the primary care setting, most physicians are poorly trained to diagnose and treat these disorders. Furthermore, the way doctors are reimbursed may penalize the conscientious practitioner who does take the time needed for appropriate clinical management. The result is predictable: underrecognition and ineffective care persist despite rigorous research that shows that depression and anxiety can be effectively treated by drugs and cognitive behavior therapy.

If the majority of persons with mental disorders are either untreated or treated by nonspecialist health professionals, then it becomes vital to increase, within the community in general and in the health professionals in particular, the ability to recognize the characteristics and to know the treatments of the common mental disorders. There is a considerable need, in both developed and developing countries, to prepare workbooks and teaching programs to ensure that the common disorders are recognized and treated. Under the auspices of WHO, some distinguished programs to make mental health care widely available have been established (World Health Organization 1990) but there is a need in most countries to ensure that community mental health workers and family physicians receive additional training so that they can recognize and treat people with mental disorders appropriately.

What is to be done in order to improve the care patients receive? The answer does not always lie in referral to mental health specialists. Any realistic hope of change must rest on improving the quality of care in the general medical sector. For this, no single solution will suffice. We will need to increase the general medical practitioner's knowledge of, and change the public's attitude toward, psychiatric disorders. Specifically, we will need to help generalists improve their interviewing skills; develop a range of practical therapeutic options that they can use; and reshape the way primary health care workers are educated, the way they are credentialed, and the way they are paid, if we are to make the next quantum of progress.

References

Beeson PB: Changes in medical therapy during the past half century. Medicine 59:79–9, 1980

Cochrane AL: Effectiveness and Efficiency: Random Reflections on Health Services. London, Nuffield Hospitals Trust, 1972

Fisher RA: The arrangement of field experiments. Journal of the Ministry of Agriculture 33:503–513, 1926

Hill AB: Statistical Methods in Clinical and Preventive Research. Oxford, England, Oxford University Press, 1962

Karasu TB: The specificity versus nonspecificity dilemma: towards identifying therapeutic change agents. Am J Psychiatry 143:687–695, 1986

Loranger AW, Hirschfeld RMA, Sartorius N, et al: The WHO/ADAMHA International Pilot Study of Personality Disorders. Journal of Personality Disorders 5:296–306, 1991

National Institute of Mental Health: National Plan for Research on Child and Adolescent Mental Disorders. DHHS Publication No (ADM)90-1683, Washington, DC, 1990

Robins LN, Regier DR (eds): Psychiatric Disorders in America. New York, Free Press, 1990

Robins LN, Wing J, Wittchen HU, et al: The Composite International Diagnostic Interview. Arch Gen Psychiatry 45:1069–1077, 1988

Shepherd M, Sartorius N (eds): Non-Specific Aspects of Treatment. Bern, Switzerland, Hans Huber, 1989

Wing JK, Babor T, Brugha T, et al: SCAN: Schedules for clinical assessment in neuropsychiatry. Arch Gen Psychiatry 47:589–593, 1990

World Health Organization: The Introduction of a Mental Health Component Into Primary Health Care. Geneva, World Health Organization, 1990

World Health Organization: Evaluation of Methods for the Treatment of Mental Disorders. Report of a WHO Scientific Group. Technical Report Series, No 812. Geneva, World Health Organization, 1991

World Health Organization: The ICD-10 Classification of Mental and Behavioral Disorders. Clinical Descriptions and Diagnostic Guidelines. Geneva, World Health Organization, 1992

Index

*Page numbers printed in **boldface** type refer to tables or figures.*

DATE DUE

		JUN 2 5 2014
NOV 2 8 2005		
DEC - 9 2008		
DEC 1 8 2009		

Demco, Inc. 38-293